FIRST INTERNATIONAL SYMPOSIUM
CURRENT ISSUES OF DRUG ABUSE TESTING

Editors
Jordi Segura
Rafael de la Torre

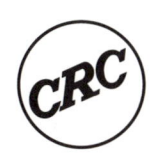

CRC Press
Boca Raton Ann Arbor London

Library of Congress Cataloging-in-Publication Data

International Symposium on Current Drug Abuse Testing (1st : 1990 : Lloret de Mar, Spain)
    First International Symposium on Current Issues of Drug Abuse Testing / editors, Jordi Segura and Rafael de la Torre.
        p.   cm.
    Includes bibliographical references.
    Includes index.
    ISBN 0-8493-4283-X
    1. Drug testing —Europe—Congresses.   I. Segura, Jordi.
II. Torre, Rafael de la Torre.   III. Title.
    [DNLM: 1. Drug and Narcotic control—methods—congresses.
2. Substance Abuse Detection—congresses.   WM 270 I638f 1990]
HV5823.5.E81581990
616.86—dc20
DNLM/DLC   91–11005
for Library of Congress   CIP

    This book represents information obtained from authentic and highly regarded sources. Reprinted material is quoted with permission, and sources are indicated. A wide variety of references are listed. Every reasonable effort has been made to give reliable data and information, but the author and the publisher cannot assume responsibility for the validity of all materials or for the consequences of their use.

    All rights reserved. This book, or any parts thereof, may not be reproduced in any form without written consent from the publisher.

    Direct all inquiries to CRC Press, Inc., 2000 Corporate Blvd., N.W., Boca Raton, Florida, 33431.

© 1992 by CRC Press, Inc.

International Standard Book Number 0-8493-4283-X

Library of Congress Card Number 91–11005
Printed in the United States 0 1 2 3 4 5 6 7 8 9

PREFACE

This book is based upon papers and discussions from the International Symposium on Current Issues on Drugs of Abuse Testing held on March 28–30, 1990 in Lloret de Mar, Spain. The activity was organized by the Department of Pharmacology and Toxicology of the Institut Municipal d'Investigació Mèdica of Barcelona City Council jointly with the Commission of the European Economic Community, the Spanish Administration (Plan Nacional sobre Drogas), and the Autonomous Government of Catalunya (Organ Tècnic sobre Drogodependències).

THE EDITORS

Jordi Segura, Ph.D., is the Chief of the Department of Pharmacology and Toxicology at the Municipal Institute for Medical Research, IMIM (Institut Municipal d'Investigació Mèdica) of the Barcelona City Council, Spain. Main research interests in this department are analytical toxicology of drugs of abuse and doping control, drug metabolism, drug-drug interactions, and clinical trials of new drugs.

The Analytical Laboratory directed by Dr. Segura is the coordinating center for the Spanish National Proficiency Testing Program on Drugs of Abuse and also holds the accreditation as Official Antidoping Laboratory for the International Olympic Committee. In this regard, Dr. Segura will be the Technical Director of the antidoping testing in the 1992 Olympic Games.

Previous activities of Dr. Segura were mainly in the development and direction of pharmaceutical research. At present, he is involved as a consultant in some multinational organizations (United Nations, European Economic Community, and Association of South East Asian Nations) for aspects related to drug analysis. He is Associate Professor of Pharmacology at the Autonomous University of Barcelona, Spain, and has published over 70 research papers in different fields.

Rafael de la Torre, Ph.D., is the Deputy Head of the Department of Pharmacology and Toxicology at the Municipal Institute for Medical Research, IMIM (Institut Municipal d'Investigació Mèdica) of the Barcelona City Council, Spain. Main research interests in this department are analytical toxicology of drugs of abuse and doping control, drug metabolism, drug-drug interactions, and clinical trials of new drugs.

Previous activities of Dr. de la Torre were mainly in the Hospital del Mar of Barcelona as being responsible for the Laboratory of Drug Analysis in the Department of Clinical Pharmacology and Toxicology. At present, he is involved as a consultant in some aspects related to drugs of abuse analysis. He is Associate Professor of Pharmacology at the Autonomous University of Barcelona, Spain, and has published over 30 research papers in different fields.

CONTRIBUTORS

C. Barceló
Hewlett Packard
División Química Analítica
Avd. Diagonal 605
08028 Barcelona, Spain

G. Barnett
Biometrics Research Institute
1401 Wilson Blvd., Suite 400
Arlington, Virginia 22209

R. C. Baselt
Chemical Toxicology Institute
1167 Chess Drive, Suite E
P.O. Box 8209
Foster City, California 94404

A. Berlin
Santé Publique
Direction Santé et Sécurité
Commission des Communautés Européennes
Bâtiment Jean Monnet
L-2920, Luxembourg, Luxembourg

R. V. Blanke
Consultant Toxicologist
4222 Croatan Road
Richmond, Virginia 23235

A. L. Calvo
Roche Diagnostica
Ctra. Carabanchel a Andalucia s/n
28025 Madrid, Spain

J. Camí
Director
Institut Municipal d'Investigació Mèdica
Passeig Marítim, 25-29
08003 Barcelona, Spain

A. S. Christophersen
National Institute of Forensic Toxicology
Sognsvannsvein 28
0372 Oslo 3, Norway

C. E. Cook
Research Triangle Institute
Chemistry and Life Sciences Unit
P.O. Box 12194
Research Triangle Park, North Carolina 27709

M. Donike
Deutsche Sporthoschule
Institute für Biochemie
Carl-Diem-Weg 6 Köln
Germany

B. S. Finkle
Center of Human Toxicology
University of Utah
417 Wakara Way, Room 290
Salt Lake City, Utah 84108

D. Fraisse
Service Centrale d'Analyse
C.N.R.S.
Echangeur de Solaize B.P.22
69390 Vernaison, France

A. C. Gabiola
Servicio Vasco de Salud
Dirección de Salud de Vizcaya
c/Maria Diaz de Haro 60
48010 Bilbao, Spain

E. Gelpí
Consejo Superior de
Investigaciones Científicas
c/Jorge Girona Salgado, s/n
08034 Barcelona, Spain

B. Griepink
Commission des Communautés Européennes
Bureau Communautaire de Réference
Rue de la Loi 200
B-1049 Brusselles, Belgique

F. Hervás
Laboratorio Central
Hospital Gomez Ulla
c/Glorieta del Ejercito s/n
28047 Madrid, Spain

K. Kelly
Syva Company
900 Arastradero Road
Palo Alto, California 94303

P. Lafargue
I.R.C.G. 1
Boulevard Théophile-Suer
93111 Rosny sous Bois Cedex
France

D. Lehane
E. I. Du Pont de Nemours & Company, Inc.
Glasgow Site
Wilmington, Delaware 19898

M. R. Moeller
Department of Forensic Medicine
University of Saarland
6650 Homburg/Saar
Germany

R. A. Moore
Managing Director
EURO/DPC Ltd.
31 Station Lane
Witney, Oxon, OX8 6AN
United Kingdom

E. Myers
Commission des Communautés Européennes
Bureau Communautaire de Réference
Rue de la Loi 200
B-1049 Brusselles, Belgique

M. Repetto
Director
Department Territorial de Sevilla
Instituto Nacional de Toxicología
Cra. San Jerónimo Km. 0.4, Apdo. 863
41080 Sevilla, Spain

M. Rodamilans
Department de Medicina Legal, Laboral
 y Toxicología
Hospital Clínico y Provincial
c/Villarroel 170
08036 Barcelona, Spain

L. San
Secció de Toxicomanies
Hospital del Mar
Passeig Maritim 25-29
Barcelona 08003, Spain

J. Segura
Department of Pharmacology
 and Toxicology
Institut Municipal d'Investigació Mèdica
Passeig Maritim 25-29
08003 Barcelona, Spain

S. Stewart
Abbott Laboratories
One Abbott Park Road
Abbott Park, Illinois 60064

I. Sunshine
4173 Hubbartt Drive
Palo Alto, California 94306

C. Sutheimer
Cuyahoga County Coroner Office
2121 Adelbert Road
Cleveland, Ohio 44106

K. Szendrei
Applied Scientific Research and
 Technical Information Division
Narcotic Drugs Division
Vienna International Center
P.O. Box 500
A-1400 Vienna, Austria

R. de la Torre
Department of Pharmacology
 and Toxicology
Institut Municipal d'Investigació Mèdica
Passeig Marítim, 25-29
08003 Barcelona, Spain

S. de Torres
Plan Nacional sobre Drogas
Ministerio de Sanidad y Consumo
Paseo del Prado, 28
28014 Madrid, Spain

TABLE OF CONTENTS

Chapter 1
Introduction 1
Jordi Segura and Rafael de la Torre

Section I. Organizational Aspects for Reliable Drug Testing

Chapter 2
General Considerations on Samples and Results 5
Manuel Repetto

Chapter 3
Legal Aspects Important for Drugs of Abuse Testing 9
Asbjørg Christophersen and Jørg Mørland

Chapter 4
Sample Collection and Chain of Custody 15
Manfred R. Moeller

Chapter 5
Chain of Custody 19
Robert E. Willette

Chapter 6
Set Up and Organization of Laboratories for Drug Abuse Testing at
the Workplace and in Therapeutics 27
Karl Verebey

Chapter 7
Organization of a Laboratory for Drug Abuse Testing in the Military 37
Paul Lafargue

Chapter 8
Considerations About Suitable Areas for Drug Testing 47
Miguel Rodamilans

Chapter 9
Concepts for Laboratory Quality Assurance 53
Francisco Hervás

Chapter 10
Forensic Constraints on Drug Abuse Testing 55
Robert V. Blanke

Chapter 11
Future Trends in Forensic Drug Testing 59
Brian S. Finkle

Chapter 12
Discussion on Organizational Aspects for Reliable Drug Testing 67

Section II. Analytical Methodology for Reliable Drug Testing

Chapter 13
Analytical Reliability: Introduction to Analytical Methods 71
Emilo Gelpí

Chapter 14
Critical Overview on Immunological and Chromatographic Analytical Methods 73
C. Edgar Cook

Chapter 15
Presumptive Analysis: Cutoff and Specificity 83
Brian Widdop

Chapter 16
In Situ Abuse Drug Detection 89
Angel L. Calvo

Chapter 17
EMIT® Enzyme Immunoassays in Testing for Drugs of Abuse 97
Kim L. Kelly

Chapter 18
Drugs of Abuse Methods for the Du Pont aca® Discret Clinical Analyzer 103
**Derek P. Lehane, Steven P. Crouse, Ricardo P. Narváez, David M. Obzansky,
Noel M. Relyea, Gerald E. Siefring, Jr., and Peter M. Tuhy**

Chapter 19
Overview of Fluorescence Polarization Immunoassay Systems in Abused Drug Testing 113
Sally P. Stewart

Chapter 20
Radioimmunoassay and Drug Measurements: The Art of the Possible 121
R. A. Moore, C. W. Hand, Dawn Carroll, and H. J. McQuay

Chapter 21
Gas Chromatography and Liquid Chromatography Coupled to Mass Spectrometry 129
Carles Barcelo

Chapter 22
Correlative Information by GC/MS in Doping Analysis 133
D. Fraisse, M. Becchi, and M. J. Bobenrieth

Chapter 23
Discussion on Analytical Methodology 145

Section III. Interpretation of Results

Chapter 24
Interpretation of Results: An Introduction 151
Jordi Camí

Chapter 25
Metabolism of Drug Abuse 153
Randall C. Baselt

Chapter 26
The Relationship between Pharmacokinetics and Pharmacodynamics 159
Gene Barnett

Chapter 27
Pharmacokinetic Approaches on Drug Testing 171
J. M. van Rossum, J. E. G. M. de Bie, and T. B. Vree

Chapter 28
Relevance of Pharmacogenetics and Drug-Drug Interactions 183
Rafael de la Torre

Chapter 29
Technical Issues To Be Potentially Standardized at International Level:
Interpretation and Reporting of Results 193
Robert Wennig

Chapter 30
Interpretation of Results of Urine Drug Testing in Clinical Practice 199
L. San

Chapter 31
Discussion on the Interpretation of Results 209

Section IV. Aspects for Potential International Harmonization

Chapter 32
Quality Control Programs 213
Jordi Segura

Chapter 33
Spanish Proficiency Testing Program (1986–1989) 219
R. de la Torre, J. Segura, A. Artola, J. Marrugat, F. Manaut, and M. Milessi

Chapter 34
Accreditation and Reaccreditation of Laboratories by the IOC Medical Commission 225
Manfred Donike

Chapter 35
Possibilities and Achievements of the BCR Program 239
B. Griepink

Chapter 36
Remarks from the Spanish National Plan on Drugs 257
Santiago de Torres

Chapter 37
Remarks from the Commission of the European Communities 259
Alex Berlin

Chapter 38
Discussion on Aspects for Harmonization 261

Section V. Final Considerations

Chapter 39
Epilogue 267
Irving Sunshine

Index

Index 275

Chapter 1

INTRODUCTION

Jordi Segura and Rafael de la Torre

An important increase on drugs of abuse consumption in western countries has appeared in the last few years. A large number of care centers for the treatment of drug addicts have been created. Drug analysis in body fluids as a tool for therapy is being used in most of these centers. Likewise, and even controversial,[1] there is an increasing number of companies implementing drug testing at the workplace to screen drug abuse among their workers. This is a trend not only in the private sector, but also in the public one, especially in the United States.[2]

The Ministries of Health of the European Community approved a resolution[3] regarding the reliability of analysis in body fluids for the detection of the abuse of illegal drugs. A proposal for the study of individual consequences when a positive result is informed, the existence of quality control programs and the circumstances, and goals and frequency of urinalysis in individuals for the detection of illegal drug consumption have been included in this resolution.

The Spanish National Plan on Drugs of Abuse has been supporting, since 1986, a Program on Quality Control for Analysis of Drugs of Abuse in order to improve the analytical reliability in those different laboratories involved in such a kind of activity. The program has been coordinated from the Municipal Institute for Medical Research of Barcelona by the editors of this monograph.

Educative aspects in drug testing are of paramount importance. As a logical extension of the Spanish program and the EEC resolution cited above,[3] it was considered highly interesting to promote an international symposium on this topic in order to revise the background information available and to identify major important points applicable to the immediate future. It was felt that joining together American and European experts would be an ideal means to stimulate exchange of mutual experiences. Thus, the "First International Symposium on Drugs of Abuse Testing" took place in Lloret de Mar (Girona, Spain) on March 28–30, 1990.

This book is an elaborated version of the proceedings of that symposium, including also some of the more interesting questions raised during the respective discussion periods. The monograph is addressed to all professionals involved in the set-up, performance, and interpretation of results for drug analysis programs in biological fluids (specifically urine):

> Organizational aspects for reliability of drug testing is deeply discussed from sample collection, chain of custody and laboratory strategies to legal and regulatory aspects.
> Analytical methodology reviews involve description and critical issues for the major presumptive and confirmatory techniques, including many immunological methodologies and reports on gas chromatographic-mass spectrometric techniques.
> The interpretation of results becomes an important part of the book and takes into account metabolic, pharmacokinetics, pharmacodynamic, pharmacogenetic, and clinical aspects.
> Final chapters on aspects for potential international harmonization include quality control and accreditation compared to international experiences in doping control and other analytes. Remarks from two administrations involved in national and multinational policies on drug testing further expands the overall interest of this text.

Concerns about ethical grounds for developing testing programs at the workplace have not been covered as they are taken up in other monographs. The major concern of this book is to afford enough information to assure reliability in all steps of drug testing when it has been decided to perform it. The editors hope to modestly contribute to reach this goal. They are also deeply grateful to other people not appearing in this volume for their collaboration, specially to Dr. Richard Hawks (U.S.), Dr. Michael Peat (U.S.), and Dr. Dominguez Gil (Spain). The assistance of Mrs. Pilar Benitez and Mr. Miquel Regalés is also acknowledged.

REFERENCES

1. **Greenblatt, D. J. and Shader, R.,** Say "no" to drug testing, *J. Clin. Psychopharmacol.,* 10, 157–159, 1990.
2. 51 *Fed. Reg.,* 32889, 1986.
3. Conclusions du Conseil et des ministres de la santé des États membres, réunis au sein du Conseil du 16 mai 1989 concernant la fiabilité des analyses de liquides corporels pour déceler l'usage de drogues illicites, *Journal officiel des Communautés Européennes,* 89/C, 185/2, 22 Juillet 1989.

Section I
Organizational Aspects for Reliable Drug Testing

Chapter 2

GENERAL CONSIDERATIONS ON SAMPLES AND RESULTS

Manuel Repetto

TABLE OF CONTENTS

I.	Introduction	6
II.	Type of Sample	6
III.	Time of Obtaining the Samples	7
IV.	Identification, Packaging, Conservation, and Transport	7
V.	Contamination and Interferences	7
	Acknowledgments	7
	References	8

I. INTRODUCTION

Over the last decade, controversy has arisen over the reliability of analytical results in positive tested subjects who denied the consumption of drugs of abuse. The problem is particularly acute when as a result of positive testing the door to promotion in the army or the civil service is closed, job applications are turned down, or the subject is dismissed from school or his/her place of work. The European Council is entirely justified in manifesting its concern on this point and in recommending that the scientific community study and improve the reliability of analytical results in an attempt to prevent the occurrence of false positives.[1]

Frequently, errors occur because only one method is used to carry out tests and results. The results are not checked using a second method. Errors also arise as a result of faulty samples.[2] The following aspects in terms of the sample should be considered when assessing the reliability of analytical results: (1) type of sample, (2) when obtained, (3) identification, packaging, conservation, and transport, and (4) contamination and interferences. Each factor will be considered briefly.

II. TYPE OF SAMPLE

Although this symposium will deal with the analysis of samples of biologic origin, we would like to draw attention to the problem of representativeness of the sample and reliability of results, i.e., the need to standardize samples taken from drug hauls. These include different kinds of substances which range in form from fine powder to granules and pieces of tablets or vegetable remains. Occasionally, the person preparing the sample to be sent to the laboratory does not obtain the sample in the correct fashion, taking small amounts of powder or granules at random from haul. Therefore, without an adequate homogenization each sample has a different composition and successive analyses to confirm or rule out results will never coincide.

The most frequently analyzed biologic samples in toxicology and particularly in the control of drugs of abuse are blood and urine. Saliva and hair have been proposed by several authors. Each specimen has its advantages and disadvantages from the legal and analytical point of view, as well as that of pharmacokinetic interpretation. It is therefore a question of choosing the *indicator sample* in the most appropriate fashion.[3]

According to Marquis,[4] selection criteria are based on the following: ease in collection (low invasive potential), amount that can be obtained, and likelihood of detecting the presence of the xenobiotic or its metabolites in the specimen and determining their relative proportions, i.e., on the toxicokinetic characteristics of the substance.

Despite its limitations, the most representative body fluid, as far as bioavailability if a drug is concerned, is blood. Blood drawing may be regarded as an aggression to the physical integrity of the subject who cannot be legally obliged to undergo venipuncture. Moreover, our laws protect citizens from self-incrimination. However, the characteristics of blood drawing provide important guarantees when identifying samples and correctly safeguarding them.

On the other hand, blood is a multicompartment fluid consisting of solid, liquid, and solute components, such as three types of cells, lipids, proteins, lipoproteins, etc., with very different affinities for drugs. These affinities should be recognized before determining drug concentrations in serum, plasma, or whole blood, since each of these should be tested in different ways.[5] It should be remembered that errors of interpretation can be made when referring to results reported by different authors in relation to concentrations in whole blood, serum, or plasma (these may present marked differences), as in the latter, xenobiotics may be present at concentrations 15% higher than those in blood. Finally, coagulation (and subsequent fractioning) of blood, as well as processes of fermentation and putrefaction, may influence analysis results.

Urine collection is not an invasive procedure but different methods may be used to falsify results, even when voiding is conducted in front of the observer. From a toxicokinetic point of view, the behavior of xenobiotics in urine differs from their behavior in blood. Some toxic agents are not excreted in urine or only in small amounts. Alternatively, other compounds or their metabolites may be found in urine for a longer period than in blood. The elimination of substances is also influenced by the circadian rhythm, volume of voided urine, its density, pH, etc. Urine concentrations of xenobiotics are therefore increasingly referred to as proportional to creatinine present instead of being expressed in units of volume. This reference has been shown to be particularly useful for interpreting values of tetrahydrocannabinol carboxylic acid in urine when evaluating periods of abstinence.[6]

On the other hand, urine is a homogeneous dissolution, i.e., monocompartment, and conservation and processing are simple. Urine may therefore be conserved with no additives, at most with an antiseptic agent, and even without the need for refrigeration. The great advantage of urine specimens is that they can be used directly in immunoassays, and preparation and purification is minimal in other analytical techniques.

For these and other reasons, urine samples are preferred in drug testing,[7] although for the purposes of legally establishing a "probable cause", analyses of blood samples collected at the time of an incident should be used to determine whether or not the concentration of the toxic substance in the blood is sufficient to apply the legal qualification of a subject being "under the influence" of the drug.

Some authors have suggested the use of saliva specimens[8] and hair specimens[9] to control the consumption of drugs of abuse. Certainly, different substances circulating in the blood may also be found in saliva. Thus, after intravenous injections, cocaine has been found in saliva at the same concentration as in plasma.[10] However, tetrahydrocannabinol (THC) in saliva seems to come from direct contact. This would seem logical given the liposolubility and low saliva/blood distribution ratio of THC. Although a saliva specimen may be obtained with relative ease and little cooperation on the part of the subject, the amount collected is small and variations occur between the volume obtained. Therefore, differences in concentrations present can be very great.

Obtaining hair specimens may be regarded as a low invasive procedure although it may be totally rejected by some subjects. Hair analysis has allowed the periods of addiction and abstinence, coinciding with hair growth to be identified, but it is not possible to detect recent consumption of drugs of abuse (24 to 48 hours).

III. TIME OF OBTAINING THE SAMPLES

The biological half-life of xenobiotics is frequently overlooked when interpreting results, since the representativeness of an analytical result of a specimen obtained at an unspecified point of time after consumption of the drug cannnot be guaranteed, although increased sensitivity in analytical techniques has permitted an increase in this period. Drugs with a short half-life, particularly acidic and neutral compounds (barbiturates, etc.), show a sharp peak effect of short duration and are not present in significant concentrations in urine. In contrast, basic compounds are easily excreted in urine and are present in higher concentrations than in blood.

It is thus accepted that although the presence of xenobiotics in blood samples may be useful to determine the degree to which the subject was affected at the time of sampling, provided an epidemiologic basis exists to establish the concentration-effect relationship for a given substance, the results of urinalysis only allows us to assume that the subject has consumed the substance, whether it be voluntarily or involuntarily.

IV. IDENTIFICATION, PACKAGING, CONSERVATION, AND TRANSPORT

Despite reiteration of recommendations, these are often sadly neglected and this fact may lead to invalidation of samples or to errors in identification.

Most drugs of abuse, including benzoylecgonine but not cocaine, are stable in blood and urine for weeks in a refrigerator and for months in a freezer. Cocaine is rapidly hydrolyzed in alkaline urine, but is stable for several weeks at pH 5. After addition of sodium fluoride as an inhibitor of plasma esterases, cocaine is maintained in blood for 8 days.[7]

V. CONTAMINATION AND INTERFERENCES

Occasionally, gas chromatography detects the presence of a substance which in certain programs appears with identical retention time as a drug such as codeine. This fact may lead to false positive results.[11] The substances detected are usually artifacts released by the plastic container into the specimen such as tri-2-butoxyethyl phosphate and certain phthalates. Confusion may even extend to techniques as safe as mass spectrometry and can only be prevented by the use of glass materials as containers. On the other hand, when radioimmunoassays are used, false positive results for cannabinoids, amphetamines, barbiturates, benzodiazepines, methaqualone, etc. may be obtained in the urine of subjects taking nonsteroidal anti-inflammtory agents, such as ibuprofen or phenylpropionic acid derivatives.[12]

In conclusion, results may be guaranteed by correct selection, identification, preparation, and conservation of specimens as, despite continuous development of analytical methodology, the statement "the quality of an analytical result can never be better than that of the specimen" continues to be valid.

ACKNOWLEDGMENTS

Thanks to Marta Pulido, M.D., for editorial assistance, supported in part by the Institut Municipal d'Investigació Mèdica, Barcelona.

REFERENCES

1. **Consejo Comunidad Europea,** Conclusiones sobre fiabilidad de los análisis de líquidos corporales destinados a detectar el uso de drogas ilícitas, 89/C, 185/02, *Diario Oficial C. E.*, July 22, 1989.
2. **McBay, A. J.,** Pitfalls and problems of drug testing, in *Analytical Aspects of Drug Testing,* Deutsch, D. G., Ed., John Wiley & Son, New York, 1989.
3. **Berlin, A., Wolff, A. H., and Hasegawa, Y.,** The use of biological specimens for the assessment of human exposure to environmental pollutants, Martinus Nijhoff Publishers, The Hague, 1979.
4. **Marquis, J.,** *A Guide to General Toxicology,* 2nd ed., S. Karger, Basel, 1989.
5. **Repetto, M.,** Toxicología fundamental, *Editorial Científico-Médica,* Barcelona, 1988.
6. **Bell, R., Taylor, E. H., Ackerman, B., and Pappas, A. A.,** Interpretation of urine quantitive 11-nor-delta-9-tetrahydrocannabinol-9-carboxylic acid to determine abstinence from marijuana smoking, *Clin. Toxicol.,* 27, 109–15, 1989.
7. **Jenny, R. W.,** Quality assurance, in *Analytical Aspects of Drug Testing,* Deutsch, D. G., Ed., John Wiley & Son, New York, 1989.
8. **Idowu, O. R. and Caddy, B.,** A review of the use of saliva in the forensic detection of drugs and other chemicals, *J. Forensic Sci. Soc.,* 22, 123–35, 1982.
9. **Baumgartner, W. A.,** Preliminary proposal: employee drug screening by hair analysis, IANUS Foundation, Los Angeles, 1986, 1–4.
10. **Thompson, L. K., Yousefnejad, D., Kumor, K., Sherer, M., and Cone, E. J.,** Confirmation of cocaine in human saliva after intravenous use, *J. Anal. Toxicol.,* 11, 36–8, 1987.
11. **Chamberlain, J.,** *Analysis of Drugs in Biological Fluids,* CRC Press, Boca Raton, FL, 1985.
12. **Lorenzen, D.,** SYVA Letters, February–July, 1986.

Chapter 3

LEGAL ASPECTS IMPORTANT FOR DRUGS OF ABUSE TESTING[*]

Asbjørg Christophersen and Jørg Mørland

TABLE OF CONTENTS

I.	Introduction	10
II.	The Main Issue	10
	A. Drug Use	10
	B. Drug Influence	10
III.	Drug Testing in Forensic Toxicology	11
	A. Selection of Biological Material	11
	B. Specimen Collection Procedures	11
	C. Legal Background	11
	D. Information to the Individuals Involved	11
	E. Information of Legal and Illegal Drug Use	11
	F. Procedures at the Institute of Forensic Toxicology	11
	G. Drug Analyses	12
	H. Analytical Control Program	12
	I. Interpretation of Results and Reports	13
IV.	Conclusions	13
	References	14

---

[*] Contributions from forensic toxicology in Norway.

I. INTRODUCTION

Drugs of abuse testing has a long tradition within the field of forensic toxicology. Quantification of alcohol in biological fluids has been performed for decades. Several drugs, also drugs of abuse, have been measured in biological samples, and the results have been interpreted for courts and police. In such cases, the consequences of the analysis and interpretation might be critical. This has hopefully provoked the development of reliable routines, chains of custody, use of analytical methods with known specificity and sensitivity, sound principles of interpretation, and scientifically based pharmacological interpretation of the results with regard to the forensic toxicological problems involved.

During the last few years, there has been an increasing demand for drug testing in other cases, including drug abuse or drug influence at the workplace, in therapy, child welfare, and other possible settings. We feel that guidelines established in forensic toxicology concerning analytical work and interpretations are important in these cases if the test results might cause negative sanctions to the individuals involved.

In the following, we will present some important aspects of forensic toxicological drug testing in Norway and discuss these in relation to workplace and therapy testing.

II. THE MAIN ISSUE

Testing for drugs of abuse in forensic toxicological cases can be summarized to answer one or both of the following questions:

1. Have illegal drugs been used by the suspect? (Drug use)
2. Has the subject been under influence of drugs of abuse at a certain time? (Drug influence)

A. DRUG USE

In the first case, it is the task to state beyond a doubt that the suspect, one or more times, has used illegal drugs. If the drug in question has been demonstrated by reliable analytical methods in some biological fluid, interpretation of these results should try to state how the drug has gained access to the body, e.g., by passive (passive inhalation, adulterated drinks/food, etc.) or active intake. In some instances, interpretation might be given with regard to time of intake and dose taken. To answer these points, information of legal drug use from prescribed medications might be useful.

B. DRUG INFLUENCE

In the second case, the degree of influence, impairment, or intoxication at a certain point of time (e.g., during car driving, the performance of some criminal act, or at the time of death) should be stated. Interpretation should be based on the concentration of drugs in blood, information on drug intake (time, dosage), and pharmacokinetic and pharmacodynamic knowledge. In such cases, it is not important whether the drug of abuse is illegal or not, since the point of interest is the *effect* of the drug. Alcohol and medicinal drugs with abuse potential (e.g., benzodiazepines) are examples of legal drugs that are of interest in this regard.

Both these questions may also be relevant with respect to drug of abuse testing at the workplace. In the United States, urine analyses, with regard to illicit drug use, involve a substantial number of private and public employees.[1] The decisions to implement drug testing programs include evidence of a growing drug use at the workplace, increasing health care costs, absenteeism, safety concerns, and as a tool for weeding out unwanted employees.[1] Another rationale is that the use of illicit drugs (even only during weekend or holidays) is considered incompatible with the employment in certain jobs. On the other hand, it has been claimed that recreational use of illicit drugs, although per se criminal, has little relevance to a person's suitability for a job, as long as the drug use does not interfere with his job capacity and performance.[2] In Norway, such views have considerable support and have to some extent counteracted the development of drug testing programs based on urine analyses at the workplace.

From a safety point of view, drug testing to show possible impairment while on the job might seem more important. However, this aspect is, to our surprise, discussed rather seldom in the international literature. Such testing would comprise both illegal drugs, as well as legal drugs of abuse (alcohol), and legal drugs with abuse potential (e.g., benzodiazepines) that could cause drowsiness, sleepiness, impaired performance, and reduced judgement in critical situations. To us, it seems important that testing for such effects is brought more actively into the discussion.

Also in a therapeutic setting, drug testing would be of interest, e.g., to state the degree of influence besides the confirmation of drug use. The need for information in cases concerning drugs of abuse overdose is obvious. Also in less dramatic cases, determination of drug influence supported by measuring blood drug concentration can be the only way to detect drug abuse or prescribed drugs. In such cases, the detection of much higher drug concentrations than suspected might be the only evidence for drug abuse.

III. DRUG TESTING IN FORENSIC TOXICOLOGY

In Norway, most drugs of abuse analyses are requested by the authorities for the following main reasons:

1. Detection of drug influence during driving
2. Detection of drug influence during criminal acts (murder, rape, violent behavior, etc.)
3. Discovery of drug use or influence in autopsy cases
4. Detection of illicit drug use in suspected drug addicts, among prison inmates, and in military personnel

Most of these samples are sent to the National Institute of Forensic Toxicology in Oslo for analyses. For these cases, special guidelines, routines, and procedures have been developed. Some of these will be briefly described and discussed in relation to the workplace and therapeutic testing.

A. SELECTION OF BIOLOGICAL MATERIAL

The most common medium for drug abuse testing is blood or urine. For cases concerning drug use, urine samples are usually analyzed. The collection of urine is noninvasive to the individual, compared to blood sampling, and relatively large volumes can be obtained. Owing to less concentrated matrix, sample preparation and analysis are simple. The concentration of drugs and metabolites in urine is relatively high as compared with blood, and drugs may be detected for a longer time period after intake. In general, test results only indicate the presence or absence of drugs and cannot be used in interpretation of impairment or influence. Another problem is that urine samples can easily be tampered with by dilution, substitution, or adulteration.

Blood samples have to be collected for cases concerning drug influence for the measurement of drug concentrations. The concentration at the critical time may be estimated from this value, the amount of drug intake, and the time when it was taken. Since there is some correlation between drug concentration and effect, the degree of impairment can be roughly outlined by such calculation. The collection of blood samples is invasive, requiring qualified personnel to draw the specimen. Concentrated matrix often makes the sample preparation complicated.

B. SPECIMEN COLLECTION PROCEDURES

Important aspects are

1. The reason for drug testing has to be clarified to secure the correct medium for testing (drug use or drug influence).
2. A medical examination must accompany the blood sampling in cases concerning drug influence.
3. Only containers checked by the institute should be used for sample collections. The institute is responsible for the selection of containers based upon experiments on the drug stability in biological samples when stored in the recommended containers.
4. The containers are labeled with the name of the suspects, time of sampling, and identity of the person responsible for the sample collection.
5. The containers must be sealed properly before registered mailing.

C. LEGAL BACKGROUND

According to the Norwegian Traffic Act, it is prohibited to drive influenced by alcohol (legal limit 0.05% [w/w]) or other drugs. For other cases concerning criminal acts, the possibility of drug influence has to be stated. The police may order blood sampling forcibly when necessary in all criminal cases. Control of drug use among prison inmates is performed according to the Norwegian Prison Act.

D. INFORMATION TO THE INDIVIDUALS INVOLVED

The reason for drug testing and the consequence of positive results should be explained to the subjects being tested. Their possible rights to deny testing should be mentioned, as well as the lack of such rights.

E. INFORMATION OF LEGAL AND ILLEGAL DRUG USE

If possible, information on legal drug use, doses, and time should be available. Informations on drugs which are suspected should also be given by those requesting the tests.

F. PROCEDURES AT THE INSTITUTE OF FORENSIC TOXICOLOGY

1. Before opening of the sample containers, the sealings are inspected for evidence of possible tampering. To assure the integrity of the specimens, urine samples are always inspected for color characteristics and signs of contaminants. Specific gravity, pH, and creatinine are measured before drug analyses.
2. The registration of samples and sample information is done by at least two persons to insure the sample identity.

3. The samples are always handled, tested, and controlled by more than one person. All these persons must sign the documents following the sample results.
4. All persons working at the institute must sign a promise of secrecy. Unauthorized persons have no admission to the institute.
5. Samples which are not tested within 1 to 2 days are stored at –20°C until the analyses are performed.
6. The technical records on sample information, results, reference standards, and control samples are stored securely and are sufficiently complete to permit scientific review of the analytical process. Only authorized persons at the institute are allowed to correct or add new information to the computer file if necessary.
7. After finished analyses, all samples are stored securely at –20°C for at least 1 year in case of reanalyses.

G. DRUG ANALYSES

The methods used for drug screening, confirmation, and quantification are important parts of the drug testing process.

Screening

In our institute, both blood and urine samples are routinely first screened by Enzyme Multiplied Immunoassay Technique (EMIT®) d.a.u.[3,4] for detection of the most common drugs that are abused in Norway. These drugs are amphetamines, benzodiazepines (doses above therapeutic levels), cannabinoids, opiates, and cocaine. On request, barbiturates and propoxyphene are looked for since they can be detected by the same screening procedure.

Concerning other drugs not covered by the primary screening procedure, alkalinized or acidified extracts of the samples are screened by gas chromatography (GC), according to special requests and information.

Confirmation and Quantification

All positive results are confirmed by alternative methods which are different in technique and chemical principle from that of the initial screening method. Gas chromatography/mass spectrometry (GC/MS) is used for the confirmation/quantification of opiates (6-monoacetylmorphine, morphine, codeine, ethylmorphine) tetrahydrocannabinol, cocaine, and benzoylecgonine. Other compounds are confirmed by GC (column specifications different from screening columns) or HPLC. For the identification of unknown compounds, full scan mass spectra combined with library search and known reference standards analyzed at the same conditions are demanded.

Standards

Blanks and spiked reference standards containing known amounts of drugs and/or metabolites in the same medium as the real samples are analyzed as real samples for every screening and confirmation process. For quantifications, the concentration of the unknown samples must be covered by the concentration range of the reference standards. Drug concentrations are calculated by means of an internal standard which is added to all reference standards and samples. At least two separate extracts from different sample aliquots are quantified.

Evaluation of the Analytical Methods

The sensitivity, specificity, precision, accuracy, and recovery, which are critical to the generation of valid and reliable results, have been evaluated for the analytical methods. Detection limits for all compounds after screening, confirmation, and quantification have been established.

Documented analytical methods are available in sufficient detail so that a trained technician in another laboratory can reproduce the results.

H. ANALYTICAL CONTROL PROGRAM

Control Samples

For the testing of day-to-day variation of the analytical methods and instruments, control samples are always included. In addition, freshly prepared control samples, from stock solutions different from reference standards, are also included. These control samples are not prepared by the same technician running the analyses.

Instruments

The quality of the analytical instruments is controlled regularly by test substances.

Interfering Substances

Special attention is given to possible interfering substances from containers, equipment, and reagents if the chromatographic conditions have to be changed.

Control of Analytical Results

All test results and samples are controlled by another technician or scientist than the analyst. The final test results are compared to the results of clinical examinations or other information being available before sanctioning.

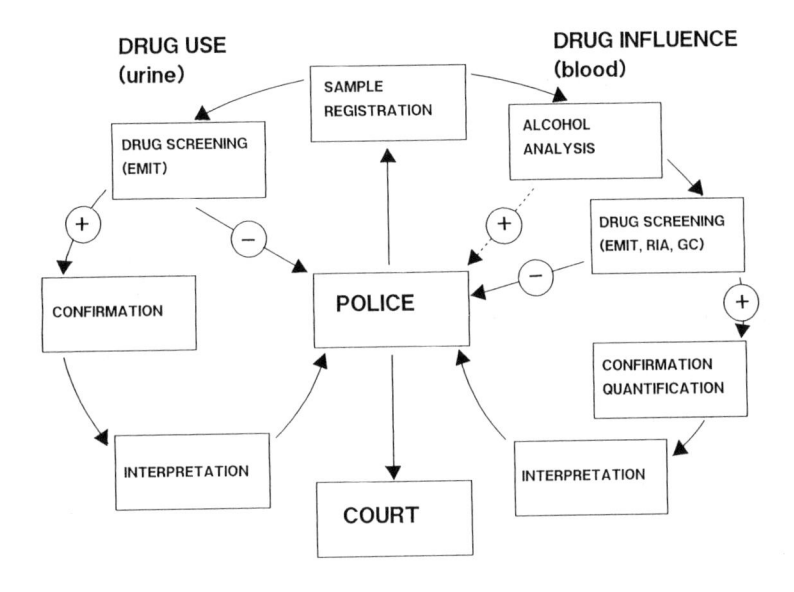

FIGURE 1. Flow diagram from the National Institute of Forensic Toxicology for sample handling, drug testing, interpretations, and reports to the police and court.

The instructions used at our institute for drug analyses are in accordance with guidelines proposed at the The International Association of Forensic Toxicologists (TIAFT) meeting in 1989.[5]

I. INTERPRETATION OF RESULTS AND REPORTS

To avoid misunderstanding by those who ordered the analyses, no results are reported without some type of interpretation. For samples concerning impairment or intoxication, this interpretation is based on blood drug concentrations and the clinical evaluations. Expert witness statements are given for several cases based on all available documents concerning the case. Positive results in urine samples from persons on frequent drug control should be evaluated preferentially according to the possibility of intake after the last urine sample. For cases concerning drug use among prisoners, the question may arise if a positive result is due to drug intake before the imprisonment. Some jails offer special agreements for favorable expiation to the prisoners when a drug-free life can be confirmed by frequent drug analyses in urine samples.

Knowledge of drug metabolism is necessary to conclude if the drug or metabolite detected in the sample is due to illegal drug use. Examples are samples containing both morphine and codeine. Here it is important to ascertain whether the morphine comes from codeine in prescribed medications or from heroin/morphine abuse.[6]

All test results, interpretations, and information concerning the samples must be given only to a contact person at the institution which ordered drug analyses. It is important that the results and interpretations are presented written in the clearest possible way. Good routines for communications between the requestor and the institute are critical to avoid misunderstanding of test results and interpretations.

An example of cases handled by the guidelines and procedures described in this paper are cases of suspected drugged driving. No fixed legal limits with regards to drugs other than alcohol have been established in Norway. Each case has to be handled individually; interpretations are given based on the final test results and the medical examinations performed at the time of apprehension. Expert witness statements with regard to possible impairment are given on several occasions

A flow diagram for sample handling, drug testing, interpretations, and reports to the police and courts are presented in Figure 1.

IV. CONCLUSIONS

Drug analyses are also performed in other Norwegian laboratories not using guidelines according to the forensic toxicological system. The prevalence of drug abuse testing in cases concerning drug control in the workplace, in therapy, in child welfare, and in other occasions is not known.

The guidelines, procedures, and chain of custody discussed in this paper seem equally important for the drug of abuse testing at the workplace. The possibility of, e.g., losing a job might be more important to a person than some sentence. An important point is the legal background which should always be recognized before starting the test process. For most Norwegian employees there exist no laws demanding participation in drug testing programs at workplaces. In spite of this lack, some testing has been performed, based on local agreements between the employee and the company. This procedure has been subject to heavy criticism. Even when such legal background exists it appears that a person's privacy should be protected in the highest possible way during sampling and analysis in workplace settings.

The guidelines and chain of custody established in forensic toxicology are not so important on all points in therapeutic drug of abuse testing. Information of legal drug use and doses from prescribed medications should be available in these cases. Confirmatory analyses should not be necessary when the results can be compared with informations from the patients. The same applies to interpretation of results in many cases. Special attention should, however, be given if negative sanctions follow positive test results. These cases should, according to our opinion, be handled according to the forensic toxicological guidelines.

In summary, the following guidelines should be followed for the different cases according to the reason for drug abuse testing.

1. All samples concerning forensic toxicology, including control of prisoners, should preferentially be analyzed in the same laboratory to insure similar treatment. The guidelines accepted in forensic toxicology should be followed in every case.

2. Control of drugs of abuse followed by sanctions (employees, child welfare, patients suspected for drug abuse, drug addicts during rehabilitations) should follow the forensic toxicological guidelines. Confirmation methods and interpretations are thus important.

3. Control of drug abuse on medical indications could be performed in laboratories operating at a somewhat less strict level. Specific controls and guidelines should preferentially exist, both for the analytical methods and interpretations. In these cases, the demands with regard to the chain of custody could be lower, and use of confirmatory methods would not always be necessary.

REFERENCES

1. **Long, K. L.,** The discovery process in drug use testing litigation, *J. Forensic Toxicol.,* 34, 1454–1470, 1989.
2. **McBay, A. J.,** Drug-analysis technology — pitfalls and problems of drug testing, *Clin. Chem.,* 33, 33B–40B, 1987.
3. **Asselin, W. M., Leslie, J. M., and McKinley, B.,** Direct detection of drugs abuse in whole hemolysed blood using EMIT d.a.u. urine assays, *J. Anal. Toxicol.,* 12, 207–215, 1988.
4. **Gjerde, H., Christophersen, A. S., Skuterud, B., Klemetsen, K., and Mørland, J.,** Screening for drugs in forensic blood samples using EMIT® urine assays, *Forensic Sci. Int.,* 44, 179–185, 1990.
5. **Moffat, A. C. and Osselton, M. D.,** Guidelines for the Performance of Quantitative Methods for the Analysis of Drugs in Blood in Forensic Toxicology, Proceedings from TIAFT, 1989, Glasgow, in press, 1989.
6. **Dutt, M. C., Lo, D. S.-T., Kheng, D. L., and Woo, S.-O.,** Gas chromatographic study of the urinary codeine-to-morphine ratios in controlled codeine consumption and in mass screening for opiate drugs, *J. Chromatog.,* 267, 117–124, 1983.

Chapter 4

SAMPLE COLLECTION AND CHAIN OF CUSTODY

Manfred R. Moeller

TABLE OF CONTENTS

I. Driving-While-Intoxicated Cases 16

II. Cases of Drug Abuse Testing 16

III. Methadone Programs, Pre-Employment and Workplace Testing 17

References 17

Sample collection, labeling, packing, and transport in an integer form to the laboratory is an essential part of urine drug testing programs.[1] The handling of the specimens in the laboratory (Good Laboratory Practices [GLP], quality control) is discussed separately.

Drug of abuse testing is done in our lab and in other forensic labs for the following sections.

I. DRIVING-WHILE-INTOXICATED CASES

In Germany, when a motorist is suspected of driving "under the influence", the police must have a physician take a blood sample. Together with the blood sampling, the physician makes a clinical statement. For urine sampling, the police use plastic containers of 50 to 200 ml volume. The policemen are ordered to optically survey the sample collection. Generally, there are no problems with the ordinary car drivers, because they usually do not try to outfox the control system. For blood or urine specimens, we have a system of four labels with one identical number. The observing policeman signs two labels. One he puts in his files and he seals the specimen with the other. The other two labels are sent together with the order to the lab. The result is sent back to the police by the lab with one of the two tags. The last label remains in the testing institution's files.

The procedure is performed identically with blood or urine samples. In cases of blood collection, *the physician* signs the labels and seals the tube. The specimens are delivered by a police courier to our lab. The fact that we always receive a blood specimen, which can be tested for individual characteristics, strongly diminishes the possibility of manipulation or mixture. We prove about 7000 to 8000 specimens per year. In less than 5 to 10 cases per year, the result or the identity of the sample are doubted. The analyzed sample is stored for 1 year, so that the analysis can be repeated and/or the identity proven by paternity tests.

II. CASES OF DRUG ABUSE TESTING

The collection of specimens in cases of drug abuse is much more difficult in large scale. Here we are dealing with "experts" in the field of sample collection and drug testing. Their inventiveness and the number of tricks that became known are nearly unlimited.

The correct sample collection, labeling procedure, package, and transportation are some of the necessary conditions for a forensic use of the analytic results. Some examples of "treatment" of the specimens during sample collection may illustrate the ingenuity of the persons concerned:

1. Household chemicals, ordinary salt, liquid soaps, and detergents available on toilets can destroy the substance to be tested or obviate the urine analysis when added to the specimen.
2. From women in jail, we detected that they had small plastic tubes with such substances in the vagina to empty them into the sample collector during urination.
3. Different body areas (e.g., the armpit, the space between the legs, or the region of the abdomen) serve as hiding places for bottles containing "clean urine".
4. The urine sample is extremely diluted with water.

Therefore it is necessary to collect the urine samples while the individual is under observation. Eventually, the tested person has to undress and must be examined physically. There should be no liquid soap, detergents, or faucet available in the room of sample collection. Toilet water can possibly be tinted to avoid an addition to urine.

The collection pot has to be transparent, unbreakable, and easy to handle. It has to have a capacity of at least 30 to 50 ml and must cover both the male and female needs during urine collection.

Containers which fulfill all these conditions are available in a broad variety in the United States.[3] The tube comes with a label which is filled out to identify the tested person. It is placed inside the bottle, printed side out. After having taken the sample, the container is to be closed with the matching cap. To open it, the destroying of the cap is unavoidable. An added plug can be used during the analysis in the lab. If the tube has to be transported, it can be closed again with a cap that can only be opened by destroying it.

The container has a temperature control strip. It discolors to green if the temperature of the sample should correspond to body temperature. Otherwise it changes its color to blue, brown, or black. The collection pot is transported in a plastic bag containing an absorbent piece of cellulose. In case of violent destruction of this very stable container, the urine will be absorbed by the cellulose and can possibly be analyzed. The necessary documents can be placed in a separate part of the same plastic bag. The bag is closed with an added seal. The tested person and the supervisor have to sign the chain of custody label.

A promising alternative to urine drug testing programs is the hair drug testing. Although no actual drug use can be detected, a chronically long-term exposure can be determined. The collection of hair samples and also the transport and storage of these specimens is much easier than collecting, transporting, or storing blood or urine samples. In cases where the results are doubted, a second, identical hair sample can be taken and analyzed. Besides, hair is stable indefinitely and is not subject to bacterial decomposition or degradation. Hair analysis can, depending on hair length or source, be used to evaluate exposure for several months up to years. Segmental analysis of hair may be used to provide a "timeline" of exposure.

On the other hand, there is still not enough experience with hair testing for all kinds of drugs of abuse. The mechanisms by which drugs are incorporated into hair have not been studied. The question of passive contamination as a source for false positives has to be investigated. We use hair testing to distinguish codeine misuse from heroin/morphine abuse.

The delivery system from prisons to our laboratory is much simpler. In the presence of the prisoner, the sample tube is placed into a wooden box. This box is closed with a wire and protected with a metal seal that contains an imprinted number. This number is unique and is additionally printed on the wooden transport box and into the file. Only by breaking the wire shielding the container can the urine box be taken out. These metal seals exist in every prison in Germany. They are used to seal the personal belongings of the prisoners when entering the jail.

Two identical specimens (split samples) with different numbers are taken in the same manner in presence of the convict. One specimen is delivered to the laboratory for drug testing. The second one is conserved under specific conditions for confirmation analysis. If the first specimen is positive, the second one can be tested as well, on the prisoner's costs.

In all cases it is important that the examined persons neither have access to the labels or containers, nor are involved in the transport of the samples. They should, however, be present when the container is sealed and sign the label exactly like the supervisor.

The documentation of the sampling process is just as important as the correct sampling itself. There must be no doubt about the tested person's identity or date and time of sampling. Furthermore, specialities of the sampling (abnormal color of the urine, volume of the collected material, especially in case of few material, etc.) have to be documented.

To exclude a manipulation of the samples in any way, the necessity of a chain of custody arises. The transport of the specimens to our lab is made exclusively by couriers because the catchment area is quite small. However, the courts have up to now not complained about mailing the specimens that came from customers not so close by. With the specimen, there should come a protocol containing the signatures and names of all persons who dealt with the sample. By this method, everyone, who could have possibly manipulated the sample directly, can be tracked down.

III. METHADONE PROGRAMS, PRE-EMPLOYMENT AND WORKPLACE TESTING

Driving while intoxicated and drug of abuse cases are the reason for more than 90% of the testing in Germany and probably the other European countries as well. These samples are collected by health authorities or by the police. Nr III is a testing procedure on a more private basis.

Guidelines are worked out for sample collection, identification, and transportation of the specimens to the laboratory and also for the procedure used for testing. A container sealed in the presence of the tested person and protected against unauthorized manipulation is indispensable for the whole procedure. Clear relation of the collected sample to the tested person has to be guaranteed. The regulations concerning the NIDA guidelines,[1] the chain of custody,[9] future trends in forensic drug testing,[4] the American point of view, and actual treatment of the problems in European countries[2,6,8] have already been discussed at this conference. The possibility of a second specimen (split samples), taken under the same conditions and stored for confirmation analysis, seems to be the most inexpensive and simple way to solve the problem, if the amount of specimens will stay in the order of less than a few hundred per week.

REFERENCES

1. **Blanke, R.,** Overview on Issues that Impact the Legal Defensibility of a Sample and Its Reported Results in Drug Abuse Testing, International Symposium on Current Issues of Drugs of Abuse Testing, Lloret de Mar, Spain, March 28–30, 1990.
2. **Cristophersen, A. S.,** Legal Aspects Important for Drugs of Abuse Testing, International Symposium on Current Issues of Drugs of Abuse Testing, Lloret de Mar, Spain, March 28–30, 1990.
3. Doxtech, Inc., Fresno, CA 93727.
4. **Finkle, B. S.,** New Issues of Regulations Related with Drug Testing at the Workplace, International Symposium on Current Issues of Drugs of Abuse Testing, Lloret de Mar, Spain, March 28–30, 1990.

5. **Harkey, M. R. and Henderson, G. L.,** Hair Analysis for Drugs of Abuse: A Critical Review of the Technology, Dept. of Alcohol and Drug Programs, Sacramento, CA, Contract No. D-0053-6, 1988.
6. **Lafargue, P.,** Organization of a Laboratory for Drug Testing in the Military, International Symposium on Current Issues of Drugs of Abuse Testing, Lloret de Mar, Spain, March 28–30, 1990.
7. **Manno, J. E.,** Specimen Collection and Handling, in *Urine Testing for Drugs of Abuse,* Hawks, R. L. and Chaing, C. N., Eds., NIDA Research Monograph, 73, 24–29.
8. **Segura, J.,** Quality Control Program, International Symposium on Current Issues of Drugs of Abuse Testing, Lloret de Mar, Spain, March 28–30, 1990.
9. **Willette, R.,** Chain of Custody, International Symposium on Current Issues of Drugs of Abuse Testing, Lloret de Mar, Spain, March 28–30, 1990.

Chapter 5

CHAIN OF CUSTODY

Robert E. Willette

TABLE OF CONTENTS

I.	Introduction	20
	A. The Need for Chain of Custody	20
	B. What Chain of Custody Provides	21
	C. The Major Steps in Chain of Custody for Drug Testing	21
II.	Specimen Collection	21
	A. Custody and Control Form	21
	B. Collection and Shipping Container	22
	C. Label	22
	D. Seals for the Bottle and Box	22
	E. Packing for Shipment	22
III.	Transport to the Laboratory	22
	A. Shipping Log and Signed Receipt	22
	B. Secured Courier	22
IV.	Handling in the Laboratory	22
	A. Separate Specimen Accessioning Area	22
	B. Transfer of Specimens	23
	C. Transfer of Aliquots	23
	D. Access to Specimens and Aliquots During Processing	23
	E. Storage of Positive Specimens	23
V.	Reporting	23
	A. Control of Data Recording	24
	B. Evidence of Review	24
	C. Validation of Accuracy of Reports	24
	D. Transmission Security	24
VI.	Records	24
	A. Secure Storage	24
	B. Retrievable for Review	24
	C. Complete — to Permit Technical and Custody Review	25
	D. Litigation Presentation	25

I. INTRODUCTION

In 1981, a crash aboard a United States Navy carrier drew that nation's attention to the widespread use of illegal drugs amongst its work forces. Drug use in unemployed populations had long been recognized since the mid-1960s, spawning many federally funded drug treatment programs. The crash on the carrier, in which several of the victims were found to have been using marijuana, only dramatized what had been found in a questionnaire survey conducted in 1980, i.e., that nearly half of the sailors interviewed admitted use of marijuana and other illegal drugs within the past 30 days. Many admitted use on the job and to being intoxicated at work.

In order to enforce a "zero tolerance" policy against such drug use, the Navy launched a ten-component program that included education, counseling, treatment, searches, mail surveillance, punishment, and aggressive random drug testing. The Navy reasoned that in order to detect those personnel that could not or would not stop using drugs, it would be necessary to identify them through the use of chemical tests. They also recognized the potential effect of random testing to deter continued drug use in light of possible detection and punishment.

The Navy program has proven to be an enormous success. Following an initial urinalysis survey in 1981, in which 48% of the sailors tested positive for cannabinoids, the positive rate for all seven drug classes for which the Navy tests had dropped to below 2% in early 1990. And over the past 12 months, the Navy has collected and tested over two million urine specimens. Two million specimens! The idea of correctly identifying and handling even two dozen specimens could easily stress many testing systems, let alone many laboratories, especially when it was recognized that each specimen and its accompanying documents must be treated as evidence.

Traditionally, drug testing in the United States was conducted either in clinical laboratories, as part of their general toxicological services, or in special drug testing laboratories that had been created to service the needs of the federally funded drug treatment programs in the 1970s. In general, both types of laboratories operated under the usual standards of care in the processing of biological specimens, with adequate identification and tracking procedures, reasonable precautions against contamination and tampering, levels of review, and routine reporting practices. Results reported back to drug treatment programs were used more or less in the same manner as any medical diagnostic result was used, e.g., for counseling and referral purposes. But, even under these circumstances, positive drug results could be used to remove patients from treatment, supposedly a form of punishment. However, few legal challenges arose, and the status quo remained.

Following the United States Navy example, many private and public sector employers began to use drug testing for employment purposes. Thus, the consequences of a positive drug test result took on an entirely different significance. Persons could be denied employment and suspended or discharged from their jobs. In the early 1980s, drug testing had developed a questionable reputation, with serious problems surfacing in the military testing programs and with other employers that started programs in a naive manner. This led to many challenges of positive results and the imposition of forensic practices.

Crime laboratories had developed procedures for the handling of evidence, including the actual physical specimen and the documents that are generated in the course of testing it. Forensic principles require that the evidence be available for court scrutiny and establish the authenticity of the specimen and its affiliated records. Such records must document from whom the specimen was collected, who handled it, who had access to it, and how the results were generated.

Usually, such forensic laboratories handled and tested one or a few specimens at a time, treating it or them as a separate case. The problem faced in the early 1980s by the United States Navy and drug testing laboratories was how to "wed" the clinical techniques of processing large numbers of specimens to the forensic practices of evidence handling. Nowhere was this task more ominous and critical than with chain of custody. The concept applied to the establishment of total accountability for every specimen collected and tested.

A. THE NEED FOR CHAIN OF CUSTODY

A lesson learned very early in the United States Navy program was that an aggressive defense attorney could easily create an aura of doubt and suspicion about the authenticity of a specimen. The government's burden was to prove that the testing results came from the specimen that had actually been produced by the accused. Although it was not uncommon to establish a trail of custody through live testimony, the idea of having all personnel involved with specimen collection, transfer, accessioning, and testing testify that, "Yes, indeed, I remember handling that specific specimen", was untenable, especially when millions of specimens were being processed. Thus, it became necessary to adopt burdensome paper trails to document these activities.

Paper trails, or chain of custody documents, were not enough. Defense attorneys need only to ask the question: "And how many people did you say had access to this poor, innocent victim's specimen?". A compromise must be reached between limiting the number of people that actually have any possible access to specimens and the number of people that would have to sign a chain of custody document. Chain of custody procedures became necessary in order to minimize the number and nature of legal challenges, otherwise the entire system would spend all of its time in court. There is an even more important reason: drug testing is only viable as a tool in eliminating drug use if it is done in a manner that protects the innocent from being falsely accused or injured. The authenticity of a specimen and its test results are an essential component of any successful drug testing program.

B. WHAT CHAIN OF CUSTODY PROVIDES

Chain of custody procedures must provide a means of identifying every individual who actually handles a specimen and any aliquot, extract, or derived sample of the specimen used in its analysis. It is necessary to know what each individual did with the specimen or sample. If the individual let the specimen or sample out of his or her custody, who was it turned over to, or where was it placed? If it was placed in a secured, temporary storage area, where was that area? It is essential to know when the specimen or sample was handled. What was the date and time? Why was the specimen or sample handled? Was it to be placed in storage? Was it placed on an analyzer? In total, this documented record traces the complete history of the handling, testing, and storage of every specimen.

C. THE MAJOR STEPS IN CHAIN OF CUSTODY FOR DRUG TESTING

Chain of custody starts at the time the specimen is collected, continues with its transfer to the laboratory, documents who received it at the laboratory, who processed it, and how the results were returned to the person authorized to receive them. All of these steps require documentation, from the label on the collection container to the final report. In order to minimize the number of persons that have access to the specimen, its test samples and documentation, and to minimize or eliminate any opportunity for tampering with these items of evidence, all areas associated with the entire process must be secured with access limited only to authorized individuals.

II. SPECIMEN COLLECTION

There is an old adage that a chain is only as good as its weakest link. Experience has demonstrated that the most vulnerable link in the chain of custody in drug testing programs is specimen collection. This is due to several reasons. If the donor of the specimen is a drug user, he or she may take every opportunity to subvert the system. Authenticity of the specimen means both in content and in identity of the donor. Drug users are known to substitute specimens, add possible adulterants, add toilet water, and falsify labels. So the collector must take adequate precautions in order to preclude such activities. In addition, the collector must prevent specimen mix-ups or contamination, properly label the bottle, provide complete documentation, and secure the bottle at all times.

Other factors that make collection more vulnerable to error than in the testing process are the experience of the collector and the frequency of performing such collections. Too often, the collector has had years of experience with collecting routine clinical specimens not subject to the strict and burdensome requirements of chain of custody. It is too easy to revert to old habits. Even when the operator is trained to follow the chain of custody procedures, collections may be infrequent and the rules not remembered. Fortunately, several actions were taken to improve this situation. Elaborate collection and custody forms were developed, some under government regulations and most by the laboratories. Special collection and shipping containers were designed. A variety of labels and seals were made available. Training videos and pictorial guides were produced. Professional specimen collection companies were formed. All of these factors have contributed to a more error-free system of collection.

A. CUSTODY AND CONTROL FORM

Federal agencies in the United States are required to conduct random drug tests on employees in sensitive positions. In addition, several federal agencies have issued regulations that require certain safety and security related occupations to be subjected to such testing. Under their guidelines and regulations, specific collection and custody forms have been mandated. These forms contain elements that clearly identify who provided the specimen, who collected it, when it was collected, and how and when it was sent to the laboratory. These "federal" forms do not permit the name of the donor to appear on the copies of the form that go to the laboratory, but link the form to the specimen container through a unique identification number, which is now commonly present on the form as a barcode. The actual identity of the specimen donor is documented on the collector, agency, and medical reviewer copies. All laboratories have developed their own versions of these required forms. Typically, the forms are preprinted with the name of the client, the address of the medical reviewer, and the preselected test panel. Often the specific destination to which each barcoded form is sent is coded into the computer. This permits a cross-check on the authenticity of the form and automatically creates a datafile when the form's barcode is "read" into the computer. Many of these techniques have greatly reduced the number of errors attributed to hand-entered information.

B. COLLECTION AND SHIPPING CONTAINER

The most common collection and shipping container is a screwcap bottle. The bottle should be transparent to facilitate the physical examination of the specimen's color. The cap should be leakproof. Once properly labeled and sealed, the bottle must be placed in a shipping container that protects the bottle from damage and precludes possible leaking. United States postal regulations and private couriers have required packaging that includes an adsorbent material to be placed inside a sealed plastic bag along with the specimen.

C. LABEL

The label that is placed on the specimen container must be designed to clearly link that labeled bottle to the custody form. It must also be nonremovable, or at least tamper-evident, such that it cannot be removed, replaced, or altered. A common feature of many labels is to integrate the label into the actual seal, thus making the seal unique. The label should be preprinted with the identifying number, and provide an area for the donor's initials (which are to be inscribed *after* the bottle is sealed), the collector's signature, and the time and date of collection. The bottle must be labeled in the donor's presence.

D. SEALS FOR THE BOTTLE AND BOX

As soon as the donor has handed the bottle to the collector, the bottle should be sealed with some form of tamper-resistant or tamper-evident tape. This can be a separate item from the label, but often the label also serves as the seal, being placed from the front to the back of the bottle and over the cap. In addition to the bottle seal, it is common and strongly recommended to seal the shipping container in a similar manner. A typical laboratory collection package provides the collection and custody form, bottle, label, bottle seal, adsorbent, sealable plastic bag, shipping box, box seal, and shipping label. In the United States, private companies usually send specimens to their testing laboratories by means of overnight couriers. In such cases, the laboratory usually provides the shipping bag or box, along with pre-addressed airbills. If specimens are sent by mail, a pre-addressed shipping box is provided by the laboratory.

E. PACKING FOR SHIPMENT

All of the items described above go into the final shipping package. The sealed bottle is placed inside of the plastic bag, along with the adsorbent and one copy of the custody form. This bag is sealed. Another copy of the custody form may slip inside an external pocket of the specimen bag or be placed in the shipping container. The container or box is sealed and mailed, or placed inside of the courier bag or box. Several specimens can be shipped together, although each must be separately sealed. The shipment is then ready to be sent to the laboratory.

III. TRANSPORT TO THE LABORATORY

A. SHIPPING LOG AND SIGNED RECEIPT

It is necessary for the collector to maintain comprehensive records of all collections and shipments to the laboratory. This is best done by means of a collection and shipping log. Preferably this should be a bound notebook with prenumbered pages. Each entry should include the donor's name and signature, the collector's signature, the time and date of collection, the airbill number (if sent by courier), and the date of shipment. The courier should be required to sign either this log book or one specifically designated for that purpose. In addition, the collection site's copy of the airbill should be signed by the courier and retained as part of the official records.

B. SECURED COURIER

Although the more common form of sending specimens to the laboratory is by couriers, other systems may be available. Many clinical laboratories that offer drug testing also provide their own courier network. This should be handled in the same manner as described above. Sometimes the collector or another employee hand delivers the specimens to the laboratory, a common occurrence with military installations. The same procedures must apply. The outer shipping box must be sealed and signatures showing change in custody must be obtained. It is also wise to use a courier that is known to be reliable.

IV. HANDLING IN THE LABORATORY

A. SEPARATE SPECIMEN ACCESSIONING AREA

When specimens arrive at the testing laboratory, they should be delivered unopened to a specially designated area, often called the accessioning area. This area must be rigorously secured in a manner that either prevents unauthorized entry or shows evidence of such entry. Only those personnel specifically assigned to the tasks of receiving and accessioning specimens or appropriate supervisory personnel should be authorized to be in this area. Their entry and exit must be recorded, either in a logbook or through the use of computerized card entry systems. All visitors or unauthorized persons entering this area must sign in and be accompanied.

A critical step in the accessioning process is to properly identify the specimens with an internal "accessioning" number. Barcoded numbers have become popular as they provide additional protection against incorrect data entry. As each package is opened, the accessioning person must sign the external custody form, noting the time and date and whether the seals were intact. He or she must also verify that the information on the bottle label exactly matches that on the custody form. If discrepancies are found, these should be recorded and reported to the client. Some discrepancies may constitute "fatal" errors and breaks in the chain of custody, such as missing initials or signatures. Such specimens should not be tested, as the results could be erroneous or rejected upon challenge. Some errors may be "correctable" by contacting the collector for clarification. If so, the specimen may then proceed to testing.

B. TRANSFER OF SPECIMENS

The original specimen container should never leave the secured accessioning area until it is ready for long-term, frozen storage. Some laboratories have tried to accommodate the principles of restricted access and complete chain of custody without a separate accessioning area. While this may be possible, it places a significant burden on the staff to fully account for all activities around the specimens when they are out of secured storage. Such arrangements are also prone to security lapses and breaches in chain of custody. All efforts should be made to provide for a separate, restricted area.

The chain of custody requirements for transferring specimens is greatly minimized in a separate accessioning area. During the steps in which specimens are received, matched against their custody forms, assigned accession numbers, and aliquots removed, they must be "signed over" to the receiving individual or into a temporary storage area. If the period of testing will exceed 1 day, temporary storage should be a locked refrigerator. When all of the testing and data review is completed, all positive specimens must be signed over to long-term, frozen storage.

C. TRANSFER OF ALIQUOTS

When the accessioning person prepares the test aliquots, a separate, internal custody document for the handling of aliquots and test samples should be initiated. Laboratories have tried to use the external form for this purpose, but such practices are overly complicated and expose the original custody documents to the testing staff. (The actual testing should be conducted in an anonymous manner insofar as possible, not even identifying the client to the technical staff, let alone the specimen donor.) The internal custody form then accompanies the test aliquots as they are signed over to the receiving technician. All persons handling the aliquots or test samples must then sign the custody document, indicating why and when.

D. ACCESS TO SPECIMENS AND ALIQUOTS DURING PROCESSING

As described above, the original specimen container must be secured at all times, preferably in a limited access area. If this is not practical or possible, then locked cages, locked refrigerators, or some other means must be used for the securing of specimens during the testing period. These temporary storage areas must have a log that fully documents who entered the area, what was entered or removed, and when these actions occurred.

If the laboratory arrangement places the test samples in an area in which nonforensic personnel are working, arrangements must be made to secure these materials, whether they are on an analyzer or autoinjector, whenever the current custodian leaves the samples unattended. Custody can be turned over to another authorized person or to a properly secured area.

E. STORAGE OF POSITIVE SPECIMENS

Due to a ruling by the United States Supreme Court, it has become mandatory to store positive specimens in a manner that permits reanalysis at some later time. This can only be accomplished by placing such specimens in a secured freezer. Any other arrangement permits too much deterioration of the drug or metabolite. United States federal guidelines require such storage for at least 1 year, and longer if requested by the client or donor. The laboratory must maintain accurate records on stored specimens and be prepared to withdraw an aliquot to be sent to another laboratory for retesting.

V. REPORTING

The concept of chain of custody is not limited to the handling of specimens. It extends to the control of the data and documents generated as part of the testing. In addition to being able to establish to the satisfaction of the court that the specimen tested came from a specific individual, it is necessary to prove that the test results came from that specimen. This can be accomplished by documentation that links the specimen to the test aliquots to the generated results to the reviewer and on to the reporting mechanism.

A. CONTROL OF DATA RECORDING

When a forensic analyst handles a single specimen, the recording of critical information and test data is fairly simple. When a laboratory is processing hundreds or thousands of specimens under the same exacting conditions, control of data becomes an enormous task. Most modern drug testing laboratories have resorted, out of necessity, to computerized tracking and data management systems. Commercial "laboratory information management systems" (LIMS) have long been available. Many laboratories have adapted these to their situation or developed their own custom-tailored systems.

A common characteristic to these systems is the use of barcoded information. Thus, as specimens arrive and are accessioned, their identifying number can be "read" into the computer. The computer can be programmed to recognize it as a valid number and which client location it was assigned to. The system can print the appropriate supply of internal barcoded accession numbers, several of which are affixed to the bottle and one on the custody form. As an aliquot is withdrawn from the specimen, one of the accession labels is transferred to the test cup or test tube. One may also be placed on the aliquot custody form, or alternatively, the aliquot custody form can be generated by "reading" the barcoded labels into the computer.

Independent of the entry of specimen and aliquot identifying numbers, the external custody form must be processed. Clerical personnel are usually assigned the task of "reading" in the barcodes on the custody documents and hand entering specific identifying information. A recommended practice is to double enter this information in order to verify its accuracy.

Modern, automated immunoassay analyzers have the capability of "reading" barcodes off the test container at the time the sample is being tested. These numbers are verified by the computer and if appropriate, the computer directs the analyzer as to which tests are to be performed. The same capabilities are available on gas chromatography/mass spectrometry (GC/MS) instruments. Thus, a positive link is made between the test sample, its result, and the original specimen and its data record.

B. EVIDENCE OF REVIEW

Once the testing is complete, various levels of data review are required. The screening and confirmation results must be reviewed and "certified" as accurate by appropriate technical personnel. The various entries of information, by hand or by barcode, must be reviewed for accuracy. This can be done through double entry and printing out data for separate review. It is important at each stage of these reviews that the reviewers sign or initial the documents, indicating the time, date, and results of the review.

C. VALIDATION OF ACCURACY OF REPORTS

It is common for the final report to be transmitted to the client by some electronic means, such as teleprinter, computer modem, or facsimile. It is a common failing of laboratories to transmit such results before the final verification of the accuracy of the information that has been entered. It is strongly recommended that after all of the testing and reviews are completed, that the specific identifying information on the original specimen bottle be entered into the system, manual or computerized, to compare with the information entered from the custody documents. Also, a hard copy of the report should be printed and signed by the appropriate certifying official. This signed copy should be mailed or sent to the client concurrent with the electronic report. Under United States federal guidelines, only the signed report is considered the official result.

E. TRANSMISSION SECURITY

The chain of custody must also extend to the report itself. It is not acceptable to send drug testing results in a manner that would inadvertently disclose this information to unauthorized individuals. Whether reports are transmitted electronically or by mail or courier, they must be sent and received in a confidential manner. Elaborate security procedures have been developed for the safe transmission of electronic messages. Mailed reports must be marked "CONFIDENTIAL" and directed to the designated person.

VI. RECORDS

A. SECURE STORAGE

Drug testing records contain potentially damaging information about individuals, especially at the collection site and in areas where the final results are stored. Although personal identifiers should not be included on documents sent to the laboratory, it is a wise practice for laboratories to store all records associated with drug testing in a secure manner. Security should include fire and water protection as well as unauthorized entry. A laboratory may be required to prove that no one was able to alter the records after the fact.

B. RETRIEVABLE FOR REVIEW

Records must be stored in a manner that permits their retrievability. Frequently, collection facilities and drug testing laboratories are required to produce their records to establish the custody and test accuracy for any given result.

C. COMPLETE — TO PERMIT TECHNICAL AND CUSTODY REVIEW

Laboratories must store a complete set of records, preferably original custody documents and test printouts. If the data is stored on magnetic media, such as computer disks or tape, appropriate precautions must be taken to preserve the stored data. Magnetic media can be damaged by various means and lose their "memory" with time. Disks and tapes may have to be rerecorded periodically to maintain the integrity of the data. The legal status of photographed documents, such as on microfiche, must be determined by local court requirements.

Another major failing of laboratories has been the inability to produce a complete set of records associated with a specific specimen. This is often due in part to the manner in which records are stored. Frequently the records may actually be stored but not available as they cannot be found. Careful planning should go into how records are filed and stored in order to produce complete records for custody and technical scrutiny.

D. LITIGATION PRESENTATION

The retrievability and completeness of records is essential when a collection facility or laboratory is confronted with presenting and defending its actions in court, arbitration, or other administrative proceedings. The overall credibility of the collection process and laboratory testing is strongly reflected in the appearance of the records. First impressions occur only once and have a lasting effect on the finder of fact. All records should be impeccable as well as complete. The records should "speak for themselves" and not require long, detailed explanations as to what they purport to reveal.

Chapter 6

SET UP AND ORGANIZATION OF LABORATORIES FOR DRUG ABUSE TESTING AT THE WORKPLACE AND IN THERAPEUTICS

Karl Verebey

TABLE OF CONTENTS

I.	Brief History of Drug Testing	28
II.	Brief History of Methodology	28
III.	Clinical Drug Testing	28
	A. Emergency Toxicology	38
	B. Rehabilitation Toxicology	30
	C. Diagnostic Drugs of Abuse Testing	30
IV.	Forensic Drug Testing	20
	A. Workplace Testing	30
	B. Post-Mortem — Medical-Legal Testing	31
	C. Prison System — Parole Testing	31
V.	Licensing Agency Policies	31
	A. Forensic Testing	31
	B. Clinical Testing	32
VI.	Abused Drugs Tested	32
VII.	Laboratory Organization	32
VIII.	Personnel	33
IX.	Conclusions	35
	Acknowledgments	35
	Recommended Readings	35

I. BRIEF HISTORY OF DRUG TESTING

Reliability of drugs of abuse testing depends on three major factors: well qualified and well trained personnel, state of the art instrumentation, and logical organization of the testing laboratory.

In order to understand the modern drug abuse testing laboratory "set up" or structure, we should briefly review its developmental history. (Figure 1) Drug testing initially was exclusively part of pathology services where overdose or fatal toxicity cases were investigated for the causative agents. "Wet chemistry" procedures were based on very large analyte volumes and crude nonspecific methodology. As drugs of abuse became a major social problem, overdose cases also became more frequent. Hospital laboratories were called upon to perform emergency toxicology to identify drug classes or specific drugs.

Identified drug abusers in treatment programs needed follow-up testing to objectively monitor the subject's abstinence from drugs. Rehabilitation testing was performed in hospitals or private clinical laboratories which were not designed specifically for qualitative or quantitative identification of drugs. In the chronological development, forensic drug testing was the last to appear on the scene. Forensic accountability was principally forced upon the clinical laboratories by the legal profession. Often positive results were questioned or flatly denied and legal suits were initiated. The lawyers started to scrutinize every step of the testing process from collection to reporting of the results to protect the "due process rights" of their clients.

After losing numerous cases, clinical laboratories performing legally sensitive testing began to reorganize. First, "chain of custody" procedures were implemented to avoid potential sample mix-up and/or adulteration. This topic is described in detail by Dr. Willette in this book. Chain of custody procedures were followed by development of quality control and quality assurance procedures to promote reliability and reproducibility of the test results. This topic is covered in detail by Dr. Blanke also in this book. With all these developments, drug testing procedures and instrumentation has also become more sophisticated. This resulted in significantly more sensitivity and specificity. Thus, extremely small amounts of analytes could be determined reliably at the nanogram per milliliter range and GC/MS provided assurance of specific identification of analytes.

II. BRIEF HISTORY OF METHODOLOGY

Figure 2 shows the progression of improving methodology. At the turn of the century pathologists tasted the bitter taste of alkaloids or smelled the characteristic almond smell of cyanide. Science marched on and one of the most significant discoveries was made in analytical science by observing the differential movement of substances on a wet piece of paper. The technique, when further developed, was called paper chromatography and it is the basis for all the sophisticated chromatographic techniques used today. Dr. Barcelo discusses chromatography methods coupled with mass spectrometry in detail in this book.

Another path of analytical method development originated in the observation of antigen-antibody interactions. The tertiary structure recognition of labeled proteins provided a scientifically alternate method of analyte identification. Figure 3 shows the various immunoassays used extensively in identification of drugs of abuse among other important analytes. Drs. Gelpi, Cook, Kelly, Stewart, and Moore cover these important immunoassay methods in this book as utilized in drug detection technology.

When looking at the internal organization of drug testing laboratories, it is important to recognize the distinct purpose of testing. The purpose points to important and less important laboratory features for the different needs. Figure 4 shows the two basic areas of drug abuse testing: clinical and forensic. Some laboratories perform both functions and must appropriately respond to the different requirements of each area.

What are the different needs for clinical and forensic laboratories for drugs of abuse testing? Figure 5 lists applications of testing in these two categories. In order to understand the logistic internal organization of drug testing laboratories, we must understand the purpose of testing. Only then can the laboratory be well designed for its specific function: clinical or forensic.

III. CLINICAL DRUG TESTING

A. EMERGENCY TOXICOLOGY

Emergency toxicology requires quick analysis responding to the critical situation in overdose cases. Sometimes the clinical symptoms or leftover drug is a sufficient clue, but most often the laboratory is on its own to determine the toxic compound's identity. Thus, the laboratory involved

History of Drug Detection
I Services

Pathological Services – Wet Chemistry Laboratories

Emergency Toxicology   Rehabilitation Toxicology

Forensic Toxicology

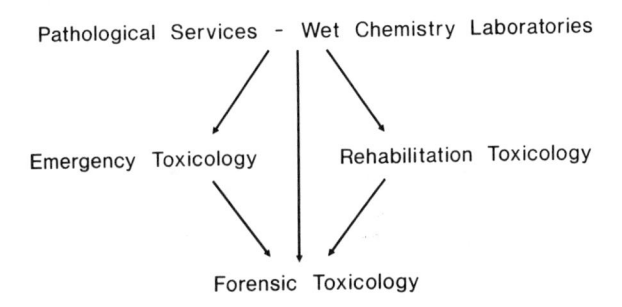

FIGURE 1. The developmental pathway from traditional toxicology to specialized areas in toxicology.

History of Drug Detection
II Chromatographic Methods

1. Isolation: Taste and Smell
2. Isolation: Color Reactions, TLC
3. GLC Packed Columns / TID, FID, ECD
4. HPLC / UV, ECD
5. GLC Capillary Column / NPD, MS, IR

FIGURE 2. Isolation and identification of chemicals by increasingly sophisticated chromatographic methods. (TLC = thin layer chromatography, GLC = gas liquid chromatography, TID = thermionic detector, FID = flame ionization detector, ECD = electron capture detector, HPLC = high pressure liquid chromatography, UV = ultraviolet detector, ECD = electrochemical detector, NPD = nitrogen phosphorous detector, MS = mass spectrometry detector, and IR = infrared detector.)

History of Drug Detection
III Immunoassays

1. Antigen – Antibody Reaction
2. Radio Immunoassay (RIA)
3. Enzyme Immunoassay (EIA)
4. Fluorescence Polarization Immunoassay (FPIA)

FIGURE 3. Development from antigen-antibody reactions to qualitative and quantitative analytical methods

Internal Laboratory Organization

Clinical   or   Forensic

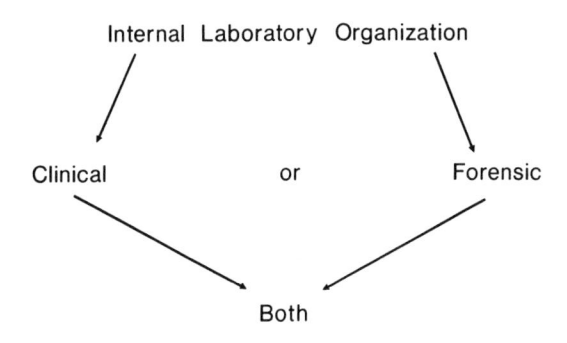

Both

FIGURE 4. Clinical laboratories either specialize or perform both types of testing.

A. **CLINICAL DRUG TESTING**

1. Emergency Toxicology
2. Rehabilitation – Drug Abuse (Adolescent, Adult)
3. Diagnostic (private or staff physicians)

B. **FORENSIC DRUG TESTING**

1. Workplace Testing (for cause, random)
2. Medical-legal, Pathology
3. Correctional Services (prisons, parole)

FIGURE 5. The subclassifications of clinical and forensic drug testing.

in emergency toxicology must be located near the emergency services and must have proven, durable methods to provide quick answers. Thin layer chromatography (TLC) used to be ideal for emergency toxicology and is still widely used. TLC is not very sensitive, but usually analyte concentrations are high in acute overdose cases. TLC's forte is that a single rapid method is able to identify a large number of analytes, based on migration and color forming or staining characteristics. Certainly more sophisticated methods can be used, such as capillary gas chromatography with a nitrogen phosphorous detector. The immunoassays are quick and practical, but they only give yes or no results for each drug or drug class tested. If the target drug is not tested, identification is not possible, and tracking down the unknown, one by one, is a slow process. However, if there is a definite clue of drug identity, immunoassays are quick to rule, in or out, the presence of a substance in question. Confirmation of positive results is required by an alternate scientific method. Confirmation of positive results is in the discretion of the physician in charge of treatment.

B. REHABILITATION TOXICOLOGY

In rehabilitation programs, drugs of abuse testing is of foremost importance. Identified ex-drug abusers need to know that the therapist or the counselor knows objectively whether or not the the subject is in good standing or in danger of relapsing to drug use. In this situation, drug abuse testing is a deterrent and an important component of the treatment process. However, from the laboratory's point of view, testing is significantly different from emergency toxicology. The urgency of test results is not hours, but days. Usually the number of samples to be analyzed for a rehabilitation clinic is more numerous than that in emergency testing. The laboratory usually performs a screening test. As discussed earlier, various methods are available for screening. The choice of methods depends on assay sensitivity, specificity, expense, and practicality. TLC or immunoassay panels are used most frequently for drugs of abuse screening when large numbers of tests must be completed at a reasonable cost.

C. DIAGNOSTIC DRUGS OF ABUSE TESTING

Diagnostic drugs of abuse testing is another important and slightly different area of drug testing. Drug abuse is defined as an addictive disorder which is characterized by paroxysmal use of a drug or drugs with almost certain relapses to drug use. Most often the drug abuser lies about his drug using habit to the physician, to his family, and often to himself. This process is commonly referred to as *denial*. Side effects of drugs of abuse often mimic various diseases or psychiatric conditions. While the physician is looking for pathological explanations, the cause of his patient's complaint is the abused drug. Astute physicians are now ordering more frequently abused drugs in their testing panels to investigate possible drug abuse of their patients. The role of the testing laboratory is different from emergency testing and from rehabilitation testing. The critical issue here is not to get false negatives if indeed a drug is being abused by the patient. Many factors affect drug detectability, including the nature of the drug, the time of last use, the size of the dose, and the pharmacokinetic nature of drug elimination. These issues are presented in detail by Dr. Barnett in this book. The essence in diagnostic testing is sensitivity. From the laboratory's perspective, the most sensitive methods must be used and a large panel screening technique must be utilized. Immunoassays and gas liquid chromatography techniques should be utilized. TLC is too insensitive for this purpose unless the abuse of the drug(s) is very recent.

IV. FORENSIC DRUG TESTING

Forensic drug testing historically developed from clinical and pathological testings. However, laboratories had to implement numerous legally acceptable security and specimen handling procedures. Testing protocols also needed improvements as prescribed in "good laboratory practices" manuals to be able to perform forensic drug testing. In other words, the laboratory must be able to produce "data packs" proving without a doubt that positive test results are accurate and reliable, and that the tests were performed on the sample from the individual listed on the requisition slip and results documented. Weak links in external or internal chain of custody, or poor standards and/or quality control in the testing process, provides the challenging expert with sufficient ammunition to contradict the validity of positive results. For this reason, the structure of the forensic drug testing laboratory must be significantly more secure and better organized than that of a clinical drug testing laboratory.

A. WORKPLACE TESTING

Workplace testing refers to tests performed on subjects at their employment. Many occupations are critical to public safety and several industries and governmental agencies mandate testing of individuals performing critical duties. These places of employment have strict drug policies in place, informing employees that drug abuse is not tolerated and that tests are performed to protect the public. Different tests performed by different agencies are pre-employment, for cause and random testing. In forensic

<u>NY City and NY State Permits
Toxicology - Drug Analysis</u>

1. Forensic Toxicology - 33C

2. Drug Analysis: Qualitative - 33

3. Emergency Toxicology - 33A

4. Rehabilitation Toxicology - 33B

FIGURE 6. Regulatory agencies license laboratories according to degrees of testing difficulty. The most difficult is forensic drug testing.

drug abuse testing, positive findings can result in loss of a job opportunity when the test is used on subjects already employed. The consequences of workplace testing are very serious and often disputed. This is the reason why the forensic laboratory has to be foolproof. People's livelihoods depend on laboratory results. There must be sufficient safeguards built into the drug testing system to provide assurance that the results of tests are totally reliable. In forensic testing, the usual testing procedure is screening with a large-volume automated immunoassay analyzer, i.e., enzyme immunoassay (EIA) or fluorescence polarization immunoassay (FPIA), Figure 3, and confirmation by GC/MS. Multiple safeguards are the multiple checkpoints built into the testing system. They are discussed under Section VII, "Laboratory Organization", of this chapter.

B. POST-MORTEM — MEDICAL-LEGAL TESTING

Other forms of forensic drug testing requiring "litigation documentation" are m*edico-legal cases* and *post-mortem analysis* of body fluids for the presence of drugs and poisons. Before workplace testing became common, even the medico-legal or post-mortem toxicology testing was less stringent. As a result of the very strict rules and regulations governing workplace testing, there is a trend toward requiring more rigorous and complete evidence documentation and use of more accurate methods in medico-legal and post-mortem testing as well.

C. PRISON SYSTEM — PAROLE TESTING

Another example of drug testing is in *correctional cases* and the prison system. A very large percentage of the prisoners' criminal activity is connected to either drug use or drug trafficking. It is not unusual to find that drug abuse continues even in the prisons. Therefore, correctional facilities have adopted a drug abuse testing policy in the prison system and also during parole. Although the consequences of testing are potentially punitive, testing of inmates requires somewhat less stringent proof of positive results than needed for workplace testing.

V. LICENSING AGENCY POLICIES

Responding to the functional distinction between clinical and forensic drugs of abuse testing, regulatory agencies defined their requirements accordingly. As an example, Figure 6 lists the various permit categories for drug analysis in the state and city of New York. The list is in order of difficulty.

A. FORENSIC TESTING

The most stringent is 33C, or forensic toxicology. This license is required for workplace testing. In order to obtain such a permit, the laboratory must satisfy an on-site inspection with on-site proficiency testing. The testing must be conducted under strict chain of custody procedure and qualitative screening and quantitative confirmation must be performed in the same laboratory. The inspector reviews the laboratory's standard operating procedure (SOP) and ascertains that what is written in the SOP is performed by the technicians routinely. The laboratory must be staffed with qualified, well-trained personnel. Acceptable Quality Control and Quality Assurance (QA-QC) practices must be in place and the laboratory must score 100% on the on-site and quarterly proficiency test samples. Some clients also require certification of the laboratory by national regulatory agencies such as the National Institute on Drug Abuse (NIDA) and the College of American Pathologists (CAP). Laboratories certified by local and national pro-

Group of Abused Drug Panels

NIDA DRUGS	OTHERS	NOT TESTED
Amphetamines	Barbiturates	LSD
Cannabinoids	Benzodiazepines	Fentanyl
Cocaine	Methadone	Psilocybin
Opioids	Propoxyphene	MDMA
Phencyclidine	Methaqualone	MDA
	Ethanol	Designer Drugs

FIGURE 7. The "5" NIDA drugs: testing required by the National Laboratory Certification Program. Other commonly abused drugs tested in a 10-drug panel and drugs not tested unless requested.

grams are considered to produce reliable, forensically acceptable test results.

B. CLINICAL TESTING

Drug Analysis Qualitative (33) and its subcategories 33A, emergency toxicology, and 33B, rehabilitation toxicology, are significantly less stringent than forensic testing. As indicated in the name "qualitative", upon confirmation no quantitative results are required. In other words, the presence of the drug in a positive sample may be confirmed by qualitative methods, i.e., TLC, and if the screening method was TLC, immunoassay is acceptable for confirmation. GC/MS confirmation is not required. In rehabilitation toxicology and emergency toxicology, confirmation of positive results is dependent on the discretion of the physician ordering the test. When confirmation is required, the results are more reliable when the screening and confirmation techniques are based on different scientific principles, i.e., chromatography confirmed by immunoassays or vice versa.

VI. ABUSED DRUGS TESTED

Epidemiological data determines the types and frequency of drug abuse by different populations in a particular geographic region or country. Effective drug abuse testing needs to utilize such information as well as new trends in drug abuse in the specific region to be effective in identifying drug abusers. Figure 7 lists the groups of drugs most frequently tested in the United States. The first panel called "NIDA" drugs are required for federal certification by NIDA. It includes amphetamines, cannabinoids, cocaine, opiates, and phencyclidine. The next column under "others" represents other commonly abused drugs, i.e., barbiturates, benzodiazapines, methaqualone, propoxyphene, and methadone. Some companies and agencies include the legal substance, ethanol. It is one of the most commonly abused substances both in the United States and the world. Interestingly, some powerful hallucinogens are seldom tested. They are listed in the third column, i.e., LSD, psilocybin, etc. These drugs are psychoactive in very low doses. Therefore, when diluted in total body volume, it is difficult to detect them unless larger than usual doses were taken or samples were collected immediately after use. Designer drugs are structural congeners of drugs of abuse often not "yet" regulated when sold and used. "Street chemists" are constantly synthesizing new, and often dangerous, drugs. They will operate as long as abusers will be willing to try new drugs and their trade remains profitable. The laboratory's role is to develop sensitive methods for the detection of designer drugs as they appear on the street.

VII. LABORATORY ORGANIZATION

A typical forensic drug testing laboratory is described. These laboratories must incorporate all the safeguards of checking and double checking needed to avoid mistakes. Figure 8 shows the sample "flow through" in the laboratory demonstrating the meticulous process that is required for accurate and reliable test results.

Forensic drugs of abuse testing starts at sample collection. At this point, several safeguards must be implemented. First, observed collection is recommended. This is important to eliminate substituting someone else's urine, diluting the urine sample with water, or adding various chemicals to try to cover up drug detection. Most adulteration methods do not work, except dilution with water and substitution of the true sample with drug-free urine. Usually, urine temperature is measured at the collection site.

Freshly voided urine is between 36 and 38°C. At some collection sites, pH and specific gravity of the urine are also measured to assure that the sample is unadulterated urine.

The external chain of custody also begins at the collection site having the signature of the donor and the collector of the sample on the requisition form. The donor also witnesses and initials the tamper-proof evidence tape as it is placed on the transport bottle cap. Modern laboratories use barcoded labels, printed on the requisition slip with an extra peel off barcoded label which is placed on the urine sample bottle. This system prevents sample mixup and errors occurring at accessioning in the laboratory.

The sample courier signs the chain of custody document when picking up the sample and signs again at the time he/she hands the sample over to the laboratory receiving staff. The laboratory receiving in turn signs the package ledger and certifies that the sample was received at the laboratory.

The next location of the sample in the laboratory is at temporary storage, which is a cold room or a large refrigerator. It is usually locked and located at or near the laboratory accessioning and aliquoting area. In fact, the original sample is never taken out of the area while the sample is being tested in the laboratory. Only aliquots of the original samples are removed for testing from the accessioning area.

When the sample is removed from the transport package, the evidence tape is checked for intactness. Testing does not proceed if the evidence tape is torn. The client is notified to send a new sample. A box on the requisition slip is checked if the evidence tape is intact. This permits testing to proceed.

The following step is accessioning. The barcode label on the sample is scanned with a scanner into the laboratory computer; it is also checked that the barcode on the requisition slip matches the barcode on the sample. An internal accessioning number is given to the sample if a barcode is not used, and the sample is placed in a rack for inclusion in the next screening batch.

The aliquoting technician, when taking a sample for screening, also checks the urine pH and specific gravity to assure that the sample is in an acceptable physiological range, indicating that the sample is urine. After screening, the sample is either negative or positive for the tested drugs. Negative samples are stored in temporary storage, while positive samples are separated for further testing. The positive samples, depending on laboratory SOP, are either rescreened by the same or similar method or accessioned for confirmation by GC/MS. First-time positives at screening and/or rescreened positives are aliquoted for GC/MS confirmation. If the confirmation method is unable to confirm the positive sample, after data review, it is reported as negative. Confirmed positives, also after data review, are entered into the computer as positives. The positive samples are moved from temporary storage to the long-term storage freezer and kept for at least 1 year.

In Figure 8, the solid squares next to each station signify checks of either sample integrity or data validity. In good laboratories, there are numerous stations where the sample and/or the results are scrutinized. The following checks are made in order to ascertain data validity. Positive results are reviewed at screening by the technician and the supervisor before rescreening or sending to GC/MS confirmation. At confirmation, the GC/MS operator and supervisor check the data. A sample which was positive by screening and confirmation is reviewed by the certifying scientist and/or the laboratory director. If all reviewers approve, the positive results are reported.

In legitimate drug testing programs, the hard copy of the results is reported to a medical review officer (MRO). This professional is specially trained in the clinical features of drug abuse and also understands the technical issues of drug testing. Any inconsistencies are discussed between the certifying scientist/director and the MRO. When necessary, the laboratory is asked to submit a "litigation package" to the MRO. This is necessary when testing results are contested. The "litigation package" contains copies of raw analytical data with standards and controls and the external and internal chain of custody documents.

The forensic laboratory organization is designed with multiple checks in mind, insuring the sample's integrity and high quality of testing. Extreme care is taken that only those results are reported to the MRO which can be supported by solid analytical data packs and unbroken chain of custody documents.

VIII. PERSONNEL

The serious nature of forensic testing requires well-trained professionals and caring technical and medical personnel. Figure 9 shows the personnel structure of a forensic laboratory. The director of the laboratory must be a seasoned professional, well versed in analytical toxicology who also understands drugs of abuse pharmacology, disposition, and pharmacokinetics. Certifying scientists and the QA-QC managers are analytical chemists who understand immunoassay and chromatography technology and are able to scrutinize raw data provided to them for review.

Supervisors and technologists in screening and GC/MS confirmation must be specialists, well qualified by education and specifically trained for the sensitive laboratory work they perform. The technical personnel is licensed by

FORENSIC LABORATORY
Sample Flow

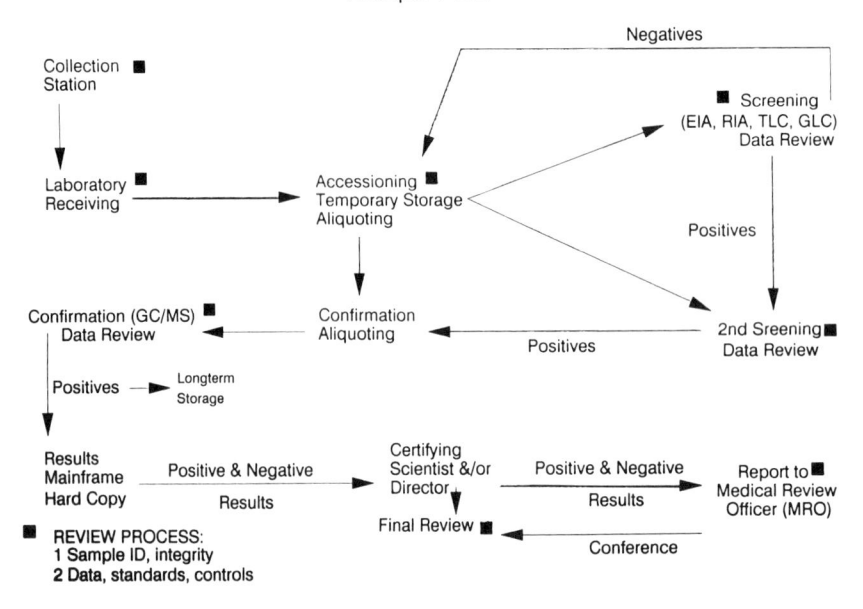

FIGURE 8. The chart traces the pathway in a forensic laboratory. The multiple "checks and balances" are marked by a solid square ■.

Forensic Laboratory Personnel

Director

General Supervisor – Certifying Scientist(s)
QA-QC Manager

Receiving   Supervisor &   Supervisor &   Data
Accessioning   Screening   Confirmation   Processing
Staff   Technician(s)   Technicians   Staff

External Certification: State and Municipal Permits

Internal Training and Continuing Education: update methodology and cross training

FIGURE 9. The personnel structure of a forensic laboratory.

the state and/or city Departments of Health for their qualification in the forensic toxicology area of laboratory specialties. Additional training must be provided by the laboratory through internal training programs and continuing education.

All other supporting staff in receiving, accessioning, and data processing must be responsible and reliable adults.

All laboratory staff must understand the critical nature of testing and sample handling. Always put samples away when not used and document every event in sample transfer. Data is confidential, no reports are given by telephone, and only the MRO may receive results. The entire staff must understand that the livelihood of human beings depends on their work.

Laboratory Testing For Drugs of Abuse
Conclusions

1. Testing is reliable in certified, well staffed well equipped, and well organized laboratories

2. Due to legal consequences, forensic testing needs stringent external and internal supervision at all phases of the operation

3. Clinical and diagnostic testing benefit from greater detection sensitivity (lower cut-offs) and needs less documentation

FIGURE 10. Essentials of drug testing in forensic and clinical settings.

IX. CONCLUSIONS

Distinction between forensic and clinical drugs of abuse testing is substantial. Clinical diagnostic testing does not require the excessive rigor in documentation and repeated data review. Clinical tests must be performed quickly for emergency toxicology, sensitively for diagnostic purposes, and cost effectively for rehabilitation toxicology. Due to legal consequences, forensic testing needs stringent external and internal supervision at all phases of testing. In certified forensic laboratories, multiple checkpoints, excellent performance with stat-of-th-art analytical technology, and well-educated and well-trained personnel instill the needed confidence in drug abuse testing results (Figure 10).

ACKNOWLEDGMENTS

The author greatly appreciates Dr. Richard Wiseman's review of the manuscript, Dr. Robert Hoffman's preparation of the tables and figures, and Debra Verebey's typing of the manuscript.

RECOMMENDED READINGS

1. **Baselt, R. C. and Cravey, R. H., Eds.,** *Disposition of Toxic Drugs and Chemicals in Man,* 3rd ed., Yearbook Medical Publishers, Chicago, 1989.
2. **Blanke, R. V.,** Accuracy in urinalysis, in *Urine Testing for Drugs of Abuse,* Hawks, R. L. and Chiang, N. C., Eds., NIDA Research Monograph, 73, 43–53, 1986.
3. **Chiang, N. C. and Hawks, R. L.,** Implications of drug levels in body fluids: basic concepts, in *Urine Testing for Drugs of Abuse,* Hawks, R. L. and Chiang, N. C., Eds., NIDA Research Monograph, 73, 62–83, 1986.
4. **Frings, C. S., Battaglio, D. J., and White, R. M.,** Status of drugs of abuse testing in urine under blind conditions: an AACC study, *Clin. Chem.,* 35(5), 891–844, 1989.
5. **Gold, M. S., Verebey, K., and Dackis, C. A.,** Diagnosis of drug abuse, drug intoxication and withdrawal states, Fair Oaks Hospital, *Psychiatry Lett.,* 3(5), 23–34, 1985.
6. **Hawks, R. L.,** Analytical methodology, in *Urine Testing for Drugs of Abuse,* Hawks, R. L. and Chiang, N. C., Eds., NIDA Research Monograph, 73, 30–42, 1986.
7. **Manno, J. E.,** Interpretation of urinalysis results in *Urine Testing for Drugs of Abuse,* Hawks, R. L. and Chiang, N. C., Eds., NIDA Research Monograph, 73, 54–61, 1986.
8. **Pottash, A. L. C., Gold, M. S., and Extein, I.,** The use of the clinical laboratory, in *Impatient Psychiatry: Diagnosis and Treatment,* Sederer, L., Ed., Williams & Wilkins, Baltimore, 1982, 205–221.
9. **Verebey, K.,** Cocaine abuse detection by laboratory methods, in *Cocaine: A Clinician's Handbook,* Washton, A. M. and Gold, M. S., Eds., The Guilford Press, New York, 1987, 214–228.
10. **Verebey, K., Martin, D., and Gold, M. S.,** Drug abuse: interpretation of laboratory tests, *Psychiatr. Med.,* 3(3), 155–167, 1986.
11. **Wadler, G. I. and Heinline, B.,** *Drugs and Athletes, Contemporary Exercise and Sports Medicine,* F. A. Davis Company, Philadelphia, 1989, chap. 18.
12. **Willette, R. E.,** Drug testing programs, in *Urine Testing for Drugs of Abuse,* Hawks, R. L. and Chiang, N. C., Eds., NIDA Research Monograph, 73, 5–12, 1986.

Chapter 7

ORGANIZATION OF A LABORATORY FOR DRUG ABUSE TESTING IN THE MILITARY

Paul Lafargue

TABLE OF CONTENTS

I.	Introduction	38
II.	Centers Participating in the Testing Program	38
III.	Materials and Methods	38
IV.	Drugs Tested For	38
V.	Tested Population	39
VI.	Aircrew	39
	A. Miltary Aviation	39
	B. Civil Aviation	40
VII.	Results on French Armed Forces in 1988	40
	A. Test Results (EMIT)	40
	B. Results of Control Examination (GC/MS)	41
VIII.	Drug Addiction Testing Procedure	41
	A. Urine Conditioning	41
	B. Treatment Program	42
IX.	Discussion	42
	A. Mono-Acetylmorphrine in Urines	42
	B. Positive Reactions in Urine Tests	42
	C. Concept of Passive Smoker	43
	D. Transformation of Codiene into Morphine	43
	References	45

I. INTRODUCTION

Considering the ever increasing drug consumption, especially of substances developing addiction and abuse, an epidemiological investigation of addictive behaviors in the military environment and a systematic detection of addiction in both military and civilian aircrew have been initiated by French authorities as early as 1986.

The Armed Forces Medical Services, common to all three branches, were tasked to run this investigation.

The author, professor of aerospace toxicology, responsible for the analytical program, presents the following:

- The organization of the procedure
- The centers participating in the testing program
- The materials and methods used
- The drugs tested
- The population tested
- The results obtained in 1988 both with immunoenzymometric method and reference method (GC/MS)
- The drug testing procedure (urine conditioning and treatment program)

Then, comes a discussion concerning the following:

- Detection of 6-mono-acetylmorphine in urines
- The complexity of positive reactions
- The concept of passive smoker
- The metabolic transformation of codeine into morphine

Air France aircrew living in the Paris area have their own medical center but it runs only screening tests. Any positive finding must be confirmed by a GC/MS analysis either in a military institution or in the F. Widal Hospital Toxicology Laboratory (Prof. Bourdon, Paris).

Personnel of other French civilian airline companies (Air Inter, U. T. A., etc.) are all systematically submitted to medical examinations and tested in Military Aircrew Medical Examination Centers.

II. CENTERS PARTICIPATING IN THE TESTING PROGRAM

Twenty-one medical centers are participating in the testing program (Figure 1).

- Navy   5 centers
- Army and Air Force   11 centers
  (except for aircrew and ATC)
- Aircrew Medical Examination Centers
  (aircrew, ATC, air defense, ...)
- Civil Aviation Personnel (hiring only) 5 centers

Of these 21 testing centers, 3 are common to several Armed Forces.

1. Toulon: Navy Air Force and Navy
2. Marseille: Aircrew Medical Examination Center and Army
3. Bordeaux: Aircrew Medical Examination Center and Army

In other words, 18 are military hospital laboratories, and 3 operate outside hospitals. They are

1. The Centre Principal d'Expertise Medicale du Personnel Navigant ((Main Aircrew Medical Examination Center) in Paris
2. The Navy Training Center in Hourtin
3. The Navy Analytical Chemistry Laboratory in Toulon

These three laboratories, which do not operate within the context of a hospital, have all the personnel and equipement necessary for drug testing.

The reference laboratory is the Toxicology Laboratory of the Centre d'Etudes et de Recherches de Médecine Aérospatiale, C.E.R.M.A., (Aerospace Medical Research Center) in Paris. Its mission is to **systematically** double-check all results found positive in the testing centers.

III. MATERIALS AND METHODS

Drugs are tested for by use of an immunoenzymatic method using automatic systems. All reagents (EMIT test) and equipments (EMIT AUTOLAB and ETS) are supplied by SYVA-Biomerieux. Considering the quantitative requirements that must be met by the reagents, a central market was contracted by the French Armed Forces Medical Service Headquarters.

Prior to running tests, SYVA-Biomerieux trained personnel and now processes all data yielded by this survey.

The reference laboratory that double-checks all result found positive by EMIT tests is equipped with two full gas chromatography/mass spectrometry (GC/MS) systems.

IV. DRUGS TESTED FOR

Drugs which are systematically tested for in the epidemiolgical survey are morphine derivates (morphine and

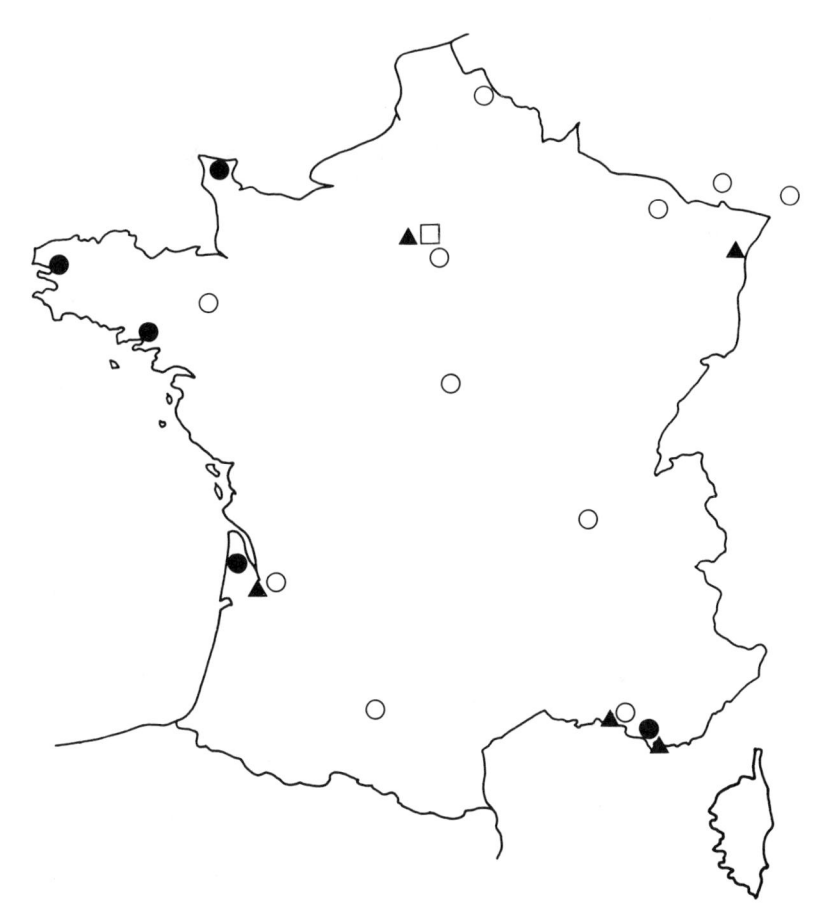

**Centers for detection of drug addict behaviors
in the French Armed Forces**

● : NAVY

○ : ARMY
  et
  AIR FORCE (except for AIRCREW, CONTROLLERS, S.S.B.S.)

▲ : AIRCREW MEDICAL EXAMINATION CENTERS
  - AIRCREW
  - ATC and AIR DEFENSE
  - S.S.B.S. FIRING OFFICERS

⊕ CIVIL AVIATION

FIGURE 1. Centers participating in the testing program.

heroine), cocaine, and cannabinoids. If addiction to other drugs (or medicines) is suspected, tests and assays are done by competent laboratories in military hospitals which, in this case, do not have to request a systematic test by GC/MS.

V. TESTED POPULATION

As it is shown in Table 1, approximately 25,000 military employees have been tested in 1989. Descriptions of tested units, the choice and distribution of personnel, the material organization of urine sampling, etc., are Command concerns. The table shows that the largest military population is made with aircrew. This situation reflects the concern of the Air Force Chief of Staff who is highly preoccupied with air safety problems.

VI. AIRCREW

A. MILITARY AVIATION
Tested personnel are

- Aircrew (pilots, copilots)
- Air traffic controllers

TABLE 1
Population Tested

DRUG ADDICTION IN THE FRENCH ARMED FORCES

TEST POPULATION

I. In French Regions

- ARMY .... 700 x 6 .... 4 200
- NAVY .... 700 x 3 = 2 100
    - Lorient maritime county .... 700 .... 3 500
    - Navy Training Center in Hourtin ... 700
- AIR FORCE .... 700 x 4 .... 2 800

        TOTAL IN FRENCH REGIONS 10 500

II. In Aircrew Medical Examination Centers

- BORDEAUX 2 200
- MARSEILLE 2 200
- STRASBOURG 2 400   14 000
- PARIS (Main Center) 6 000
- TOULON (Naval Air Force) 1 200

    TOTAL FOR AIR FORCE :
    14 000 + 2 800 = ... 16 800
    (out of 24 500)

III. Population for epidemiological study

YEAR 1989 = 24 500

- Air defense controllers
- SSBS firing officers

Tests are systematically run

- During enrollment visits
- During subsequent check-up visits, every 6 months

B. CIVIL AVIATION

Systematic testing for drugs in urines only applies to aircrew, both technical or commercial (stewards and airhostesses). Tests are run only once when these personnel are hired; however, physicians can always request a test at any moment.

VII. RESULTS ON FRENCH ARMED FORCES IN 1988

Results presented were obtained on 22,500 active military personnels, i.e., they do not take into account subjects declared unfit at the screening examination.

A. TEST RESULTS (EMIT)

- Morphine derivates: 669   (2.97%)
- Cannabinoids: 575   (2.55%)
- Cocaine: 0

TABLE 2
Drug Addiction Testing Procedure

C.E.R.M.A. : Center for Research and Studies in Aerospace Medicine

B. RESULTS OF CONTROL EXAMINATIONS (GC/MS)

- Morphine derivates
  - Morphine and/or heroine: 1   (0.004%)
  - Cough medicine: 614   (91.8% of morphine derivates)
  - Nonidentified: 54   (8.1% of morphine derivates)

- Cannabinoids
  - True cannabinoid: 537   (2.38%)
  - Non identified: 38   (6.6% of cannabinoid derivatives)

VIII. DRUG ADDICTION TESTING PROCEDURE

A. URINE CONDITIONING

Urines are collected by nurses and divided into three containers (Table 2).

- A 5 ml hemolysis tube for the EMIT test
- Two 20 ml bottles which are used only if the tube test reads positive

In this case, both bottles are sent to CERMA.

- One bottle is used for the GC/MS analysis
- The other one is kept for a potential counter-test

TABLE 3
Treatment Program

TREATMENT PROGRAM

Complete chromatographic recording

↓

Identification of internal standard on the chromatogram using its two characteristic ions (m/z = 414 and 455)

↓

Testing for various morphine compounds comparing their retention times with that of the internal standard and using their characteristic ions

MORPHINE		429 and 236
CODEINE	m/z	371 and 178
CODETHYLINE		385 and 192
PHOLCODEINE		114 and 100

↓

Display of complete fragmentmetry spectrum of each compound and identification in library using its reference spectrum

↓

Display of relative retention times and calculations of concentrations using calibration curves

TABLE 3

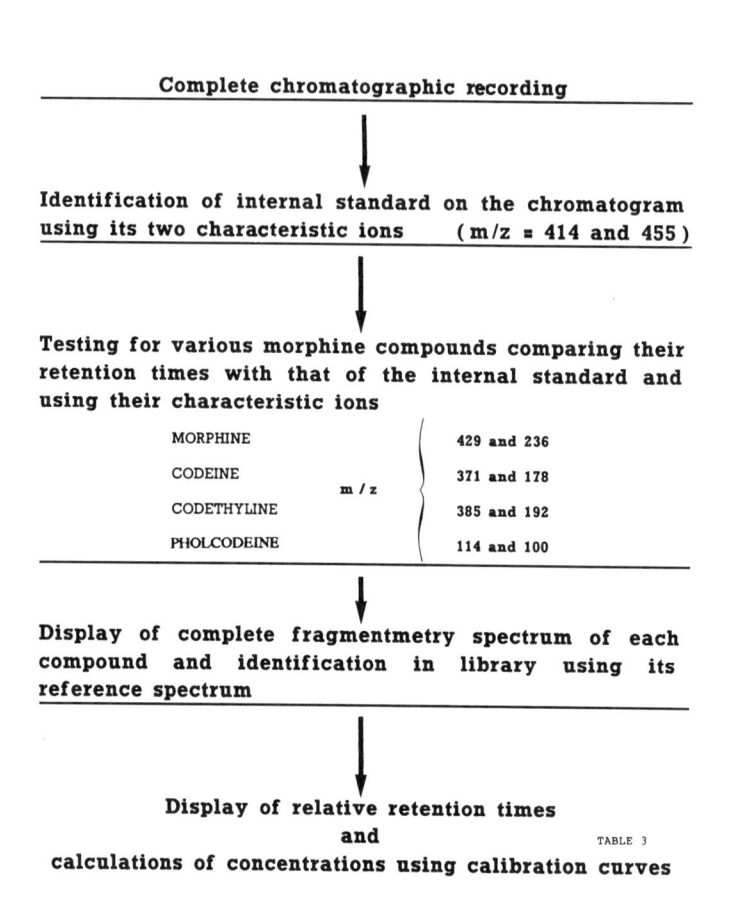

Both bottles can only be opened after tearing off the safety tab, which guarantees sample authenticity.

The label cannot be peeled off and bears a barcode number to guarantee sample anonymity, the signature of the subject who provided the urine, and the signature of the nurse who witnessed the various stages of urine collection and conditioning.

When urines arrive in C.E.R.M.A., a sample is kept at 4°C and analyzed as quickly as possible. Another sample is kept for at least 2 months at –20°C for potential subsequent counter-testing if the GC/MS analysis confirmed results of the screening test. Otherwise, urines are discarded.

B. TREATMENT PROGRAM

The GC/MS analysis done at C.E.R.M.A. is presented in the diagram shown in Table 3.

IX. DISCUSSION

A. MONO-ACETYLMORPHINE IN URINES

Only few cases of heroine consumption were identified. This may explain why, except for death by overdose, we found no systematic trace of mono-acetylmorphine derivate in urines. Our investigation therefore seems to confirm results published by many other authors who were also unable to identify 6-mono-acetylmorphine as often as some publications had suggested.

B. POSITIVE REACTIONS IN URINE TESTS

Reaction to an identification test naturally depends on several factors.

- Quantity of absorbed substance
- Whether taking the substance is a new or an old habit

TIME COURSE OF POSITIVE URINARY FINDINGS

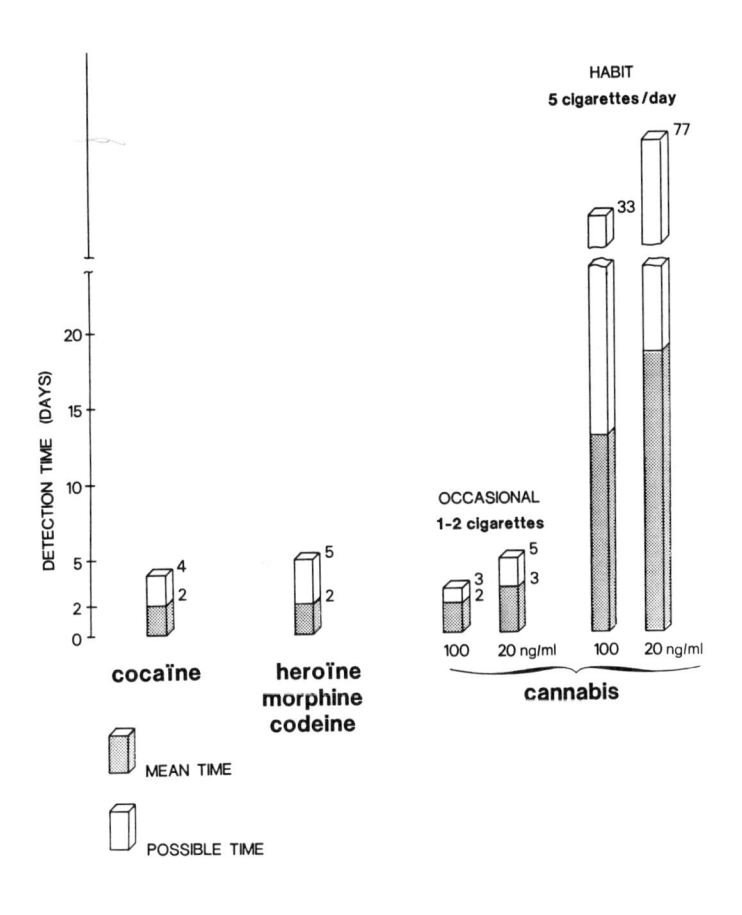

FIGURE 2. Time course of positive urinary findings.

- Sensitivity of the test
- Subject's diuresis, etc.

It thus appears that a simple response cannot be given at the question, *"How long can a test remain positive?"* Figure 2 perfectly illustrates the complexity of this problem.

C. CONCEPT OF PASSIVE SMOKER

Everyone knows that traces of 9-THC oxidation products, especially 11-nor-9carboxy-delta9-THC, may be found in the urines of a nonsmoker after passive inhalation of cannabis smoke.

This is perfectly normal since potent principles can enter the body through respiratory pathways. But the important point is to determine the threshold above which (except for very rare exceptions) only those individuals who actually smoked cannabis will be identified.

Results reported by Cone and Johnson[1] were obtained under conditions which we consider unrealistic and which bear no resemblance with what is really observed, hence the numerous positive results reported by these authors for passive smokers.

Thousands of analyses run in the laboratory showed no such positive results. We believe that a threshold of 25 ng/ml practically always keeps a passive smoker under the detection limit. However, our experience shows that the choice of a threshold value is very important for the detection of an addictive behavior. If the threshold is set at 50 ng/ml (or higher), a relatively large number of light smokers remain unidentified. Therefore, the threshold has to be selected for a specific purpose.

D. TRANSFORMATION OF CODEINE INTO MORPHINE

A study of the metabolic biotransformation patterns of codeine shows that the significant biotransformation is demethylation, which produces morphine.

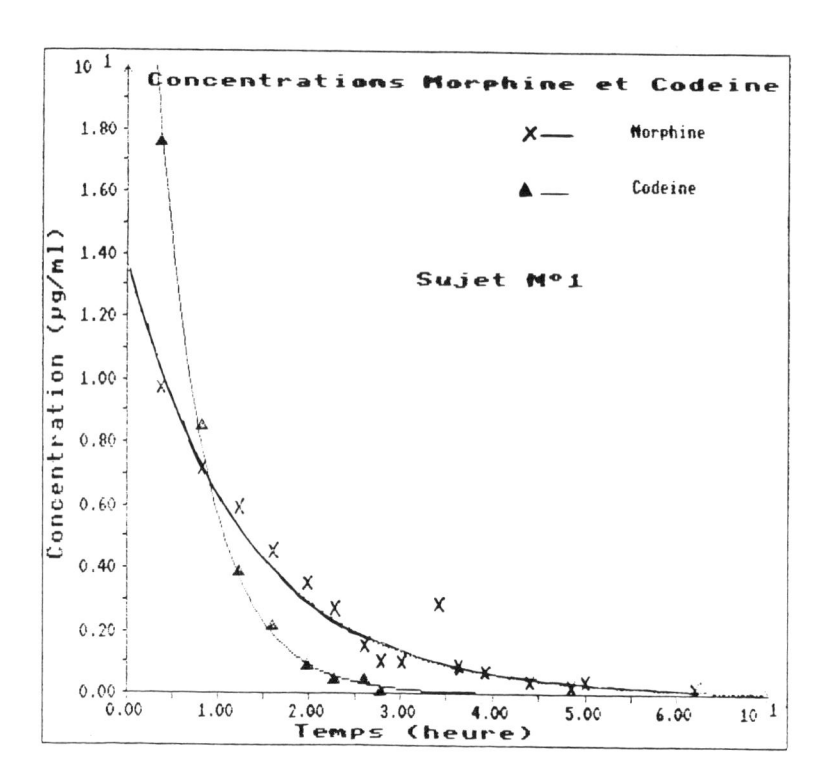

FIGURE 3. Codeine metabolism.

Figure 3 shows the changing concentrations of codeine and morphine, as a function of time, in our own urines, after absorption of a simple dose of 1mg/kg body weight of codeine (in the form of phosphate). Posey and Kimble[2] obtained similar results, which, again, pose the problem of the detection threshold.

Investigations on codeine metabolism show that after a while, morphine concentration becomes higher than codeine and may even be the only detectable compound when detection thresholds are set very low.

Consequences may be serious and preoccupying for the individual. If tests are too sensitive, a subject who took codeine, an anti-cough molecule, for therapeutic purposes may be accused of drug abuse. It is naturally impossible for the analyst to distinguish between nonmetabolized morphine and morphine resulting from the biotransformation of codeine. It is therefore crucial to set a threshold beneath which the question, *"Drug addiction or anti-cough therapy?"* cannot be honestly answered.

This is the reason why we believe that it is impossible to draw conclusions for total metabolite concentrations (morphine, codeine, normorphine, norcodeine) lower than 1 mg/l.

Table 4, however, identifies ingested substances as a function of compounds found in urines.

TABLE 4
Origin of Metabolites

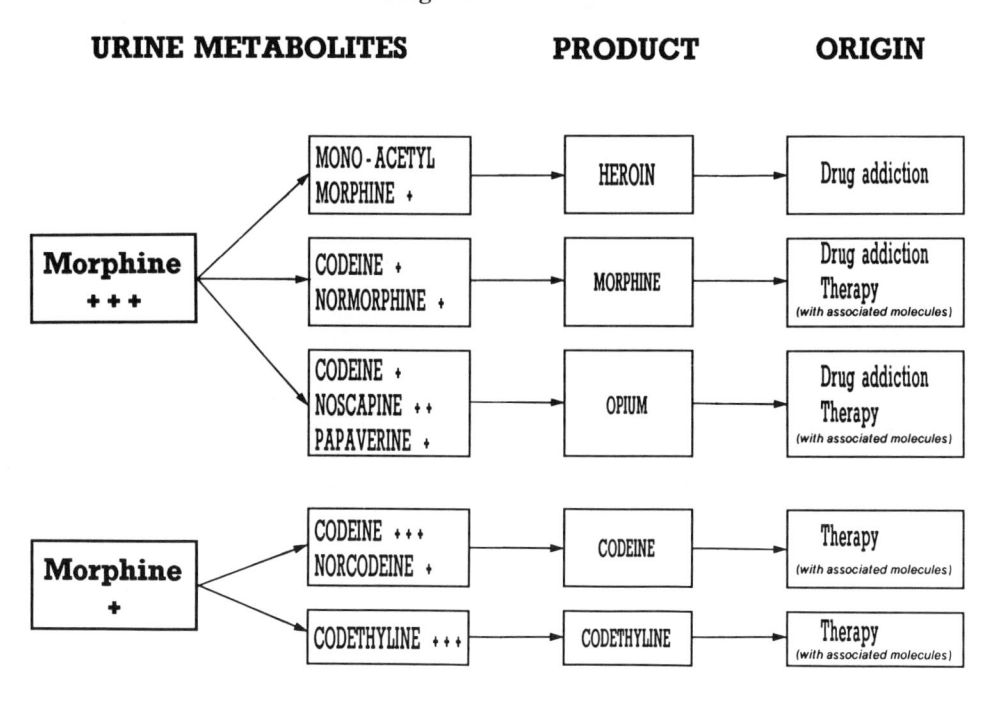

URINE METABOLITES	PRODUCT	ORIGIN
Morphine +++ → MONO-ACETYL MORPHINE +	HEROIN	Drug addiction
→ CODEINE +, NORMORPHINE +	MORPHINE	Drug addiction Therapy (with associated molecules)
→ CODEINE +, NOSCAPINE ++, PAPAVERINE +	OPIUM	Drug addiction Therapy (with associated molecules)
Morphine + → CODEINE +++, NORCODEINE +	CODEINE	Therapy (with associated molecules)
→ CODETHYLINE +++	CODETHYLINE	Therapy (with associated molecules)

REFERENCES

1. **Cone, E. and Johnson, R.**, Contact highs and urinary cannabinoid excretion after passive exposure to marijuana smoke, *Clin. Pharmacol. Ther.*, 40, 247–256, 1986.

2. **Posey, E. and Kimble, N.**, High-performance liquid chromatographic study of codeine, norcodeine and morphine as indicators of codeine ingestion, *J. Anal. Toxicol.*, 8, 68–74, 1984.

Chapter 8

CONSIDERATIONS ABOUT SUITABLE AREAS FOR DRUG TESTING

Miguel Rodamilans

Introductions are usually philosophic and try to outline the area that the various papers and reports are going to discuss. So that we do not lose ourselves, I should, perhaps, remain true to the objectives laid down for this First International Symposium. These are, quote, "The scientific objectives are centered on a revision of the legal, analytical, quality control and result interpretation aspects that affect the analysis of drugs of abuse. This is especially important in those areas where this type of analysis is becoming more popular, such as, for example, in the work or labor field."

Before continuing further in this subject, due to the quality of the speakers who will follow me in this discussion of laboratory accreditation and because of the short time available for this introduction, I would like to make some reflections on some aspects of this subject that worry me deeply.

The law in Spain for medical-health specialties, for post-graduates in the laboratory branch, which includes the specialties of clinical analysis, clinical biochemistry, hematology, and hemotherapy, immunology, microbiology, and parasitology, and genetics, clearly defines the system for the accreditation and evaluation of teaching structures and introduces control of the quality of the teaching through periodical inspections and a bilateral program for the evaluation of the different areas of the training curriculum. As for designations, the original disposition that has now become an article, establishes with the project that "in the event of the creation of new specialties, their designation will be recognized by the Spanish Ministry of Education and Science for those professionals who have been working in this area for a sufficient period of time under conditions in accordance with the regulations." When talking about training in the area of toxicology, one of the programs (that I have revised and which is close to our specialty of analytical toxicology as clinical biochemistry) mentions therapeutic drug monitoring (phenytoin, phenobarbital, digoxin, salicylates, etc.) and metals (lithium, lead, mercury, etc.). However, no consideration is given to drugs of abuse nor many other parameters which should form the area covered by the future specialty of analytical toxicology.

We see here that they do not accredit techniques or groups of techniques, rather they accredit a specialty with certain minimums as specified under present legislation. The creation of certain health structures and services is defined by an accreditation standard that requires development so that the institution can be qualified as a level one, two, or three hospital.

We should recall that laboratories, particularly the biochemistry and pharmacology services of level three hospitals, are already certified to carry out the most sophisticated analysis. My question is, within what specialty, health care or legal level, are we to demand accreditation, if this is to be granted to a certain center of service according to a wide range of requirements: staff training, number of specialists, space, equipment, files, teaching capacity, etc. I think then that we are discussing the accreditation granted to a laboratory by the Public Health Administration or some scientific association and that shows that the laboratory is capable of identifying drugs of abuse or their metabolites. We are stating that this laboratory is able to issue a medical-legal document or a forensic report. This would be required in the following cases:

- In traffic accidents, the majority of insurance companies exclude alcoholism and drug addiction as well as the practice of certain sports and/or high risk activities.
- Suspected delinquents who have broken the law because of drug deprivation in order to establish their incrimination.
- In the event of suicides or attempted suicides.
- Workers who suffer or cause an accident that results in their death or which causes serious injuries to fellow workers. The investigation is usually made at the request of a judge or forensic.

The attitude of the judge is determined by the presence of dangerous or antisocial behavior. Thus, when faced with dangerous driving, the consumption of alcohol can be determined by breathalyzer tests or by analysis of the alcohol concentration in the blood. This analysis will tell us whether the individual was, at that time, under the influence of alcohol and how much he/she was over the limits applied in the legislation. Spanish laws establish 0.8 g/l as the maximum possible limit to be able to drive safely. But the detection of drugs of abuse in urine only indicates the consumption of drugs, it does not tell us when they were ingested, or how much was consumed, or whether the individual was carrying out any activity under the effect of the drugs. What is it that we wish to establish by the detection of metabolites in urine: active consumption, passive consumption, or real drug addiction? I am afraid that it would be very difficult for the laboratories to diagnose drug addiction from only one analysis. It is necessary to carefully consider what we are going to do and why we are going to do it. What exactly do we mean when we say we are discussing "accreditation of laboratories" that carry out measurements on drugs of abuse?

As a doctor closely related to health care within a hospital, I should point out that the objective of my contribution is specifically oriented toward public health.

The question is then the following: What is the purpose behind analysis of drugs of abuse in a laboratory?

1. First and foremost, it is to establish a correct diagnosis and, through correct quantification, to begin specific therapies and/or establish a prognosis. It should be the same as the measurements made in cases of intoxications by methanol, ethylenoglycol, carboxyhemoglobin, paracetamol, amanitas, etc.
2. The second would be to provide therapeutic support. This is the case of quantitative measurements of ethanol in urine for alcohol units or abuse drugs and their metabolites for centers for the treatment of drug addicts. The purpose of both cases is the verification of abstinence in those patients who attend this type of therapeutic center of their own free will. This information is highly useful to therapeutic teams.
3. Toxicological control of the work force should be directed toward improving the health of the worker, and so this is basically preventative. This preventative aspect tends toward improving the health of the patient himself and of his fellow workers who are affected by this activity. We must ask ourselves what type of toxic products are to be controlled in these groups.

   a. Industrial products that are registered in the NIOSH-OSHA guides that could affect the normal performance of the worker and affect the work force as a whole or other persons. We should remember that many Biological Exposure Indices (BEI) have already been established and many more are being included.
   b. Medicines prescribed by General Practitioners (GPs) or specialists that could lower levels of awareness and affect the performance of risk activities.
   c. Alcohol and drugs of abuse. The problems presented by both their qualitative and quantitative detection and/or their confirmation in these groups are

   - Detection does not indicate addiction and the diagnosis should not be made by the analyst, it is rather the task of the company doctor in collaboration with an *accredited* treatment center.
   - Detection leads us to a confirmation or to the setting up of a system of more frequent controls that provide more information for both the specialist in labor medicine and the treatment team. In this case, we can see that there are two methods of approach, either analytical confirmation (GC/MS) or a qualitative analytical follow-up, both involve considerable costs. However, the information provided by the second possibility is far better than the first.

If we look closely, we find that a new element has been introduced into the picture — that of the specialist in labor medicine — a person that examines these patients, who knows their medical record, and who stays in contact with the work force through periodical medical examinations. This means that most important for the work force is the doctor that establishes a doctor-patient relationship. It is then within this area that we are going to establish the need for a certain type of analysis of drugs of abuse. This analysis should support the company doctor and confirm his suspected diagnosis; *it is a diagnosis*. The request for an analysis both for diagnostic confirmation and for preventative campaigns is to be interpreted and evaluated by the doctor making the request. A confidential doctor-patient relationship is then established, and it is the doctor who must decide whether the patient is apt or not to occupy a certain place of work. It is possible that these conclusions will not be reached on the basis of random analysis, but rather because the doctor will have noted certain traits in the worker that lead him to request complementary analyses that help to establish a diagnosis of supposed drug addiction. This diagnosis will later be confirmed by a specialized therapeutic team that then provides suitable treatment. By following this system, we see that the results of the analysis remain in the possession of the doctor-patient and form part of his personal medical record. If we study this situation, we will see that qualitative analysis is sufficient as the doctor knows very well what medication is being taken and the therapeutic team knows what medication should not be taken during the period of control of the diagnostic confirmation. When do we need to confirm a certain drug? We need to confirm only in those cases of patient-worker conflict, at the beginning of therapy, or in cases of already established conflict. The first is an example of correctly applied preventative medicine, and the second is an example of its failure.

We should not forget that the development of certain technologies allows the GP or specialist in labor medicine to use simple diagnostic tests in his own office. These tests, which are absolutely acceptable for screening and therapy control, are usually those for cholesterol using reactive strips, glucose, acetone, and many others that will be developed in the near future.

I would like to remind you that many patients with IRC (renal failure) perform dialysis in their own homes, and the doctor teaches them to carry out the analytical controls themselves. This is usually the case of patients with sufficient capacity to understand and correctly perform this type of action. After a short period of instruction, diabetic patients can control their own glucose levels and adjust the insulin dose accordingly.

Many clinics use reactive strips as a screening method for detecting dyslipemias that are later confirmed and labeled by an analytical or clinical biochemistry laboratory.

I think that we are to act on at least three levels when we speak of accrediting laboratories.

1. The first is to certify those tests that may be performed in front of the patient or in the doctor's surgery. I feel that in this case, the Public Health Administration has to validate the efficiency of the tests, and the laboratories are then to explain to the clinics involved how to perform them. Many administrations, such as those in the United States or Europe, already do this.
2. The second or health care level would be those laboratories that carry out nonconfirmative analyses and only in very special cases. At the request of the doctor, they would send the sample to a higher level laboratory with forensic or medical-legal accreditation. Their purpose is preventative and to provide therapeutical support.
3. The medical-legal level, together with the above, will be discussed here.

I would like to mention something that worries me. It is in reference to how to avoid the appearance of an open market policy, which is what would happen in Spain if a law is passed (we know how things develop in Spain: a high volume of analyses). I would like to insist on the existence of a competitive system between the different companies involved (*our laboratories*). I would like to guarantee many things, but two of them are especially important.

1. The role of the specialist in labor medicine, his association with specialists in the treatment of drug addiction, and the need for analysis levels one, two, and three.
2. Mechanisms that guarantee analytical transparency in the event that our legislation accepts what I would call *preventative* control of drugs of abuse. I would like to know why preventative programs are not established in other, more needful health care areas, especially when the resources available for health care in Spain are the lowest in Europe. The mechanisms that would improve this transparency are

   - Laboratories that perform qualitative measurements may not carry out confirmation analysis. This must be done in established centers with suitable medical-legal guarantees.
   - To avoid distrust, later samples to be taken from a patient with a positive result must be made through a center for the treatment of drug addicts, which will evaluate other clinical aspects not offered by the analysis alone.
   - In the case of workers, the results are to be made available to the company doctor and to him alone. I would like to mention here that for the company doctor and the team in the drug addiction treatment center, the follow-up on the qualitative analysis is more important than the analytical confirmation which is only of importance in the event of conflict or of criminal behavior on the part of the worker.

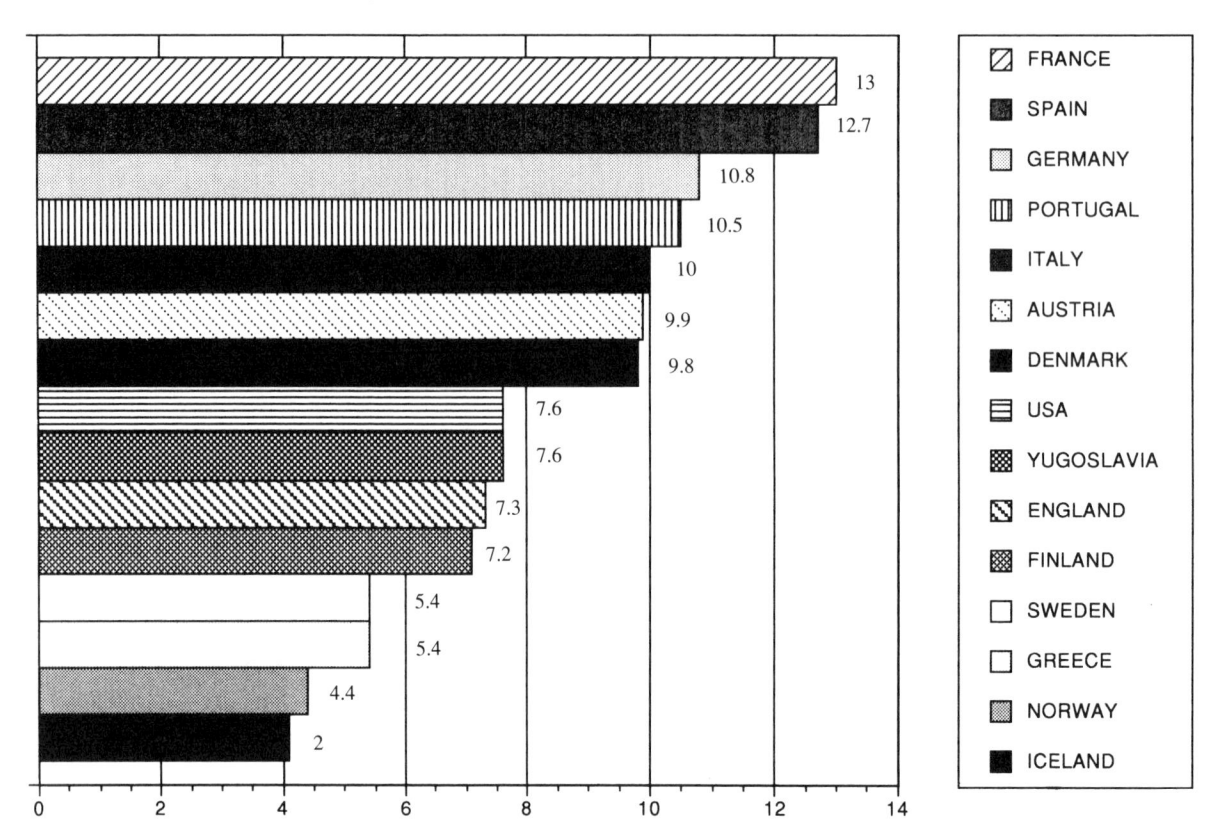

TABLE 1
Consumption of Alcohol Per Person, Per Year in Liters (1988)

Country	Liters
France	13
Spain	12.7
Germany	10.8
Portugal	10.5
Italy	10
Austria	9.9
Denmark	9.8
USA	7.6
Yugoslavia	7.6
England	7.3
Finland	7.2
Sweden	5.4
Greece	5.4
Norway	4.4
Iceland	2

In conclusion, I must say that the analysis of drugs of abuse in the work force tries to supplement the deficiencies of a correct development of labor medicine. More importance should be placed on the training and dedication of the company doctor to this field than the investment of large sums of money in the detection of drugs, which has no sense at all if the preventative aspect is ignored. If the idea behind this is preventative, then I consider that there are many other things that could be done instead of analyzing the urine of all the workers. Unless, of course, we want to make an epidemiological survey of drug consumption in the work force that would then allow a wider range of health care activities than the mere police action of detecting drug consumers that are not necessarily drug addicts. One of the many things that could be done that is more important than the control of drugs of abuse would be the control of alcohol consumption (see Table 1). In Spain, its incidence is many times greater than that of drugs of abuse. The figures for emergency admissions, as well as those for labor and traffic accidents, are all too clear.

I consider that the existence of high-level laboratories in all the countries is necessary, but they should remain as they are, and more should be created within the justice department, the body that has to officially confirm the results issued by any private or public laboratory. I must add that they should be the only ones to perform these investigations. Accreditation therefore must be at two levels: laboratories not certified for other mechanisms that perform primary measurements; and laboratories of the justice department that would be the only ones in the case of conflict, and only in the case of conflict, capable of determining the presence of drugs. By this, I do not mean that laboratories of the first level may not have advanced technology, quite the contrary, they should develop their possibilities to the utmost, but they may not make official medical-legal analysis, this lessens the possible defenselessness of the workers. The accreditation level of these laboratories would be that of qualitative tests.

Only those laboratories of the justice department that wish to identify these products at a medical-legal level are to certify their capability for correctly confirming a drug of abuse in front of the corresponding administration.

The legal limitations governing the development of

these control analyses will be imposed by legislators. Whether we like it or not, we will have to conform to what they decide.

I hope that they are very much aware of the fact that each time a new system of control is set up, it must be done with the greatest respect for the fundamental principle of individual freedom. If this individual freedom is not respected, then all the time we have spent in this conference on accreditation levels for laboratories performing analysis for drugs of abuse will have been wasted.

I also hope that the control of drugs of abuse in the work force is not carried out under the idea of policing the situation. In Spain, there is no legislation in this matter; what is legislated is the right of the worker not to allow this type of analysis to be made without his/her consent. The fact that some companies are, in fact, doing this should be the cause for an investigation by the justice department to see if this fundamental right has been violated.

In conclusion, I would like to say that I have been working in the field of labor toxicology for many years, and it would grieve me deeply if budgets were allocated to the control of drugs of abuse in the work force without previously confronting such burning issues as environmental or biological control of carcinogenic and toxic products, etc., or the consumption of alcohol, which in many countries, at the moment, represents problems that have much more serious effects on public health than the possible consumption of drugs of abuse.

If legislation is introduced to draft laws making the periodic performance of this type of control mandatory, I feel this would be a terrible injustice for this group of people who would be subjected to a police-like control of drug consumption without any solution being given to the much more serious problem of exposure to innumerable toxic products. It would seem immoral and hypocritical.

Chapter 9

CONCEPTS FOR LABORATORY QUALITY ASSURANCE

Francisco Hervás

Quality control management of laboratories where drug testing is carried out is aimed at obtaining homologated analytical results by standardizing analytical techniques, and ensuring that laboratories carrying out drug testing are officially accredited. While both aims work to the same end, they deal with different aspects of the same problem. The quality of analytical results may be controlled by standardizing analytical techniques, but official recognition of laboratories where testing takes place also requires quality control of human and economic resources.

Quality control management is carried out by internationally, nationally, autonomically, or locally accredited offices and comprises quality guarantee and quality control.

Quality guarantee ensures that minimum requirements necessary to obtain reliable analytical results are met. This is done by keeping a periodic check on accredited laboratories via questionnaires on material and human resources, continuous training courses on drug testing, and auditing.

Quality control deals with practical aspects of quality management, such as solving standard problems through the use of protocols supervised by the pertinent governing body. Quality control programs consider intralaboratory quality control, referred external quality control, and complementary interlaboratory quality control. At the International Symposium on Current Issues and Drugs of Abuse Testing, held in Spain, March 1990, we heard the speakers' views on each of these points. Quality control management should be effective in the following areas: human resources area, material resources area, and economic resources area.

Drug testing can have health care, legal, economic, social, and even ethical consequences. Effective management is therefore required of governments to ensure that the rights of the individual being tested as well as society's rights to take the necessary action to ensure compliance with the law, thereby protecting the nondrug consuming majority, should be guaranteed.

It is therefore our duty to guarantee the reliability and accuracy of our results which should not only be homologated but also accredited. To do this, routine inspection and auditing of accounts should be carried out. Techniques used in screening analyses should be normalized. These should be established by the relevant authorities. Although this might seem to be a simple procedure, it is very difficult to normalize techniques without having first catalogued the material available.

Positive results should be checked using a second technique which should also be normalized. For legal purposes, negative results should also be checked and the results of the most qualified technique should be considered valid. In case of doubt, a sample should be submitted to an accredited reference laboratory.

Clear rules should be laid down on how to collect, transport, and conserve samples. Instructions should also be given on how to safeguard samples.

Samples should be kept for an established period of time, so that if further tests are required for whatever reason to check analytical results, these may be carried out.

Authorized quality control programs should be followed up.

Rules should be laid down of how reports should be drawn up and how long they should be kept.

In the human resources area, there should be a qualified person in charge of the laboratory, as well as a trained, qualified team of laboratory assistants. There should be continuing training programs, and safety regulations should be observed.

A transition period, however, is necessary to institute these changes, particularly in Spain where no precedents exist for accrediting drug testing laboratories. Gomez Ulla Hospital has been using protocols of this kind for 4 years. In our department, we have been using a management system based on the classic PERT/CPM for 3 years now. As a result, we have been able to increase the efficiency of our drug testing laboratory. It would take too long to explain the system in detail, but suffice to say that it is a (largely computerized) double branching network of the binary type (positive and negative). This system affords the following advantages: it can be used with currently available management software, and each test is scored independently using a pre-established code. This score may reflect the overall, partial, or isolated value obtained in all, several, or only one test. This greatly facilitates error searching. It is useful in decision making as well as in the management of economic resources. It is a dynamic system that can always be improved. Because it is an open system, it can be split into several smaller systems or be linked together with systems to create a macrosystem. It is a normalized evaluation system similar to that which has been used all over the world for many years, particularly in the building industry. The system does, however, have some disadvantages: its design is somewhat complicated and requires experience in handling management techniques; to get the best from the system a larger than normal computer potential is required.

The fact is that no matter which system is used, the quality of analytical results obtained in drug testing must be controlled and guaranteed. It is, therefore, vital to establish the need to catalog and standardize materials. Cataloging is a slow and thankless task, but it is necessary to insist on the importance of including all drug testing laboratories in an accredited quality control program, institute continuous training programs for laboratory assistants involved in drug testing, standardize regulations for safeguarding samples, and check positive results obtained using screening techniques with a second normalized technique. Finally, these five points might be the basis upon which a drug testing laboratory could be accredited.

Chapter 10

FORENSIC CONSTRAINTS ON DRUG ABUSE TESTING

Robert V. Blanke

The decade of the 1980s has seen a remarkable sequence of events in the United States focused on the need to identify drug use by military and civilian workers. Urine testing for drugs was selected as the process by which drug use was to be identified. Urine is an easily obtainable body fluid in which the presence of a drug or drug metabolite implies use of the drug by the donor of the specimen. The process of urine testing has since been driven by pressures of a variety of types, inexorably expanding, constricting, defining, refining, and finally culminating in the framework of a program which permits the testing of human urine for five abused drugs with a minimum of error and a maximum of protection of individual rights. In the United States, this framework is referred to as the "NIDA Guidelines". No single event or individual can be identified as the sole contributor to this accomplishment. Rather, a combination of technological advances and management techniques were applied in a forensically credible manner to a rapidly expanding drug abuse problem of urgent concern to our society. It is useful to review the events which led to the present state of urine drug testing in the United States.

Because of concerns about the proliferation of urine drug testing laboratories, which have not generally operated under any specific professional or governmental guidelines in the United States, and at the same time recognizing the potential of drug testing to impact positively and forcefully on drug abuse in America, it was decided by the National Institute on Drug Abuse (NIDA), in August of 1986, to prepare recommendations for accreditation of laboratories engaged in such testing. The intent was to publish these "standards" and recognize laboratories meeting or exceeding these recommendations as qualified to conduct forensic urine drug testing.

Input was sought from various individual experts in the application of good laboratory practices to the testing of urine for the presence of illicit drugs. In addition to forensic toxicologists, this group included experts familiar with the Department of Defense program, with commercial laboratory operations, and with proficiency testing strategies, all applied to the management of large numbers of specimens, to be tested for drugs in a forensically credible manner.

After numerous meetings and consultations with organizations already engaged in certification efforts of other types of laboratories, the advisory panel recommended tentative guidelines. These were announced by NIDA to the scientific community in January 1987. Many individuals and professional groups took the opportunity to critique and recommend modifications of this first draft. Thereafter, the Department of Health and Human Services (DHHS) published a Notice of Proposed Guidelines in the *Federal Register* and invited comments from individuals and organizations, as required by law. After considering all of the comments and responding to them, NIDA, with the cooperation of numerous other government agencies, prepared a final version of the guidelines. This final version was published in the *Federal Register* on April 11, 1988 as the Mandatory Guidelines for Federal Workplace Drug Testing Programs. With the issuance of the President's Executive Order relating to federal agency drug programs,[1] these principles have become an integral part of the overall requirements prepared by the Department of Health and Human Services (DHHS) which are to be followed by all federal agencies when establishing drug testing programs.

These guidelines are not perfect, nor should they be considered immutable. Rather, as experience in their application is gained, they should be tuned to respond to practical needs, technological advances, and the goal of effectively identifying drug use.

In my view, the great benefit of the development and implementation of these guidelines is that they illuminate the process of testing for drugs with such brilliance and detail, that they focus the attention of analyst, lawyer, politician, and many laypersons on those aspects of nonmedical drug testing which are necessary for forensic credibility. Chain of custody, security, the use of validated methods, quality control, purity of reference material, qualified personnel, record keeping, and other factors, in addition to the methodology itself, have long been of concern to the forensic scientist. After some reluctance, nonforensic analysts have learned the value of these concepts, not only to meet accreditation standards, but because clients were demanding them.

The laboratories which conform to the NIDA Guidelines continue to demonstrate that forensically credible test results can be produced on large numbers of specimens. The technology is available and has been proven. Automated immunoassays can reliably discriminate between negative and potentially positive specimens. Microprocessor or computer controlled instruments can specifically confirm structures, resolve isomers, and quantitate concentrations at part per billion or even part per trillion levels. What has been made abundantly clear during the past decade is that almost all demands which are made on the analytical process are quickly satisfied by innovative and imaginative scientists and engineers. The necessary technology is available.

Unfortunately, the technology has outstripped our ability to interpret the results. As a result, some have boldly attempted to draw conclusions from urine drug testing which are not warranted by controlled studies. Five years ago, the National Institute on Drug Abuse sponsored a Consensus Development Panel to discuss the topic of drug concentrations and driving impairment.[2] The panel discussed many aspects of this problem and some of its conclusions are worthy of comment.

The use of urine as the specimen for analysis offers many conveniences since it can be collected relatively easily and offers a simple matrix for analytical purposes. Yet, other than showing that the drug has been used by the subject, little information relating to driving impairment can be gained.

As stated by the Consensus Development Panel,

> Testing of drugs or drug metabolites in urine is only of qualitative value in indicating some prior exposure to specified drugs. Inferences regarding the presence or systemic concentration of the drug at the time of … impairment from drug use are generally unwarranted. The presence of an illicit substance in urine that may indicate prior illegal action can, however, add a dimension to probable cause of (impaired) performance.

At this stage of our knowledge of pharmacokinetics and pharmacodynamics, the efforts of some individuals to assume impairment solely by extrapolation from quantitative amounts of drugs in the urine of the subject are invalid and lack a scientific basis. Until valid data are collected and accepted by the scientific community, great caution must be exercised when interpreting the analytical data. If a drug, or the metabolite of a drug, has been unequivocally identified in a specimen from a known individual, that individual must have been exposed to the drug at some time prior to the collection of the specimen. Whether the drug was abused or used, whether the exposure was active or passive, and whether the time of use was recent or in the more distant past, are questions which generally cannot be resolved only by the qualitative demonstration of the presence of the drug in urine. However, identifying an individual as a drug user may have far reaching consequences.

There has been considerable debate between proponents and critics of urine drug testing relative to its efficacy and appropriateness. Some of the criticisms have been legal in nature,[3] while others have drawn attention to the technical problems.[4] It is not my purpose to review these comments, other than to reinforce some concepts.[5]

> If the technology is to be applied, it must be with excellent accuracy and reliability.
> Due process for individuals must be ensured.
> Any actions taken must be with the recognition that the parties involved may end up in court.

The availability of excellent technology for the characterization and quantitation of drugs and their metabolites has already been mentioned. Many other speakers at this excellent symposium are better qualified than I for describing these features. The challenge lies in the application of the sophisticated technology available, to large numbers of specimens in a reliable manner. This becomes a complex management problem.

Even with the rigorous application of good laboratory practices, errors occur. The responsible laboratory director recognizes this fact and applies an effective quality control program to identify errors before they are reported. Quality control procedures can be designed more easily to identify machine errors than human errors. As robotics becomes more readily available, errors should tend to decrease.

Since the application of effective quality control is costly, some aggressively competitive laboratories may tend to ignore the fatigue, boredom, and distractions which plague humans carrying out routine tasks in an effort to decrease costs. Thus, the concepts of laboratory certification and performance monitoring are important to assure that "excellent accuracy" of test results is maintained. In addition to confirming the establishment of appropriate standards governing a laboratory's performance, it is necessary to ensure that the technology is used appropriately despite changes in staff or ownership, equipment depreciation, and many other factors which can influence laboratory performance.

Monitoring the laboratory performance includes two aspects: (1) inspections, both before certification and at regular intervals thereafter; and (2) proficiency testing in both an open and blind manner.

Ideally, inspections should confirm that laboratories intent upon conducting nonmedical urine drug testing meet certain minimal standards of good laboratory practices as well as the unique, forensic criteria for this activity. The required minimal standards must be clearly described. Each laboratory then adapts its facilities to meet those standards. At the same time, inspectors who are knowledgeable and experienced laboratorians themselves, should be trained to identify and evaluate all aspects of the testing process in as uniform a manner as possible. During the inspection, the procedures by which the laboratory establishes the validity of its analytical methods, calibrates measuring devices, checks the purity of standards, maintains internal chain of custody and security, conducts quality control, and all other aspects of the testing process, are assessed.

Monitoring testing proficiency is most commonly done in an open manner. Specimens containing known quantities of drugs or metabolites are distributed to the participating laboratories. The type of analyte present may, or may not, be known to the laboratory, but generally, if a substance is found to be present, the laboratory is asked to quantify it. The advantage of this open style of proficiency testing is that it compares a laboratory's performance with that of its peers. It also permits a measure of the accuracy of a laboratory's quantitative results.

Unfortunately, the style by which a laboratory conducts open proficiency testing may bear little resemblance to that applied to routine specimen testing. In order to monitor routine laboratory performance, blind proficiency testing must be done. In this type of monitoring, the laboratory is unaware that a specimen has been introduced to monitor performance. As a result, the entire process applied to a specimen, from its acquisition to reporting the test results, can be assessed. It is difficult to carry out this type of program, but the yield of useful results justifies its increased cost.[6]

All of these efforts, described here rather superficially, are directed toward the goal of producing analyses of "excellent accuracy". To add the requirement of "reliability" invokes an additional dimension.

Forensic toxicologists have long known that specimens to be examined for drugs and poisons must be treated as evidence. Post-mortem specimens collected by pathologists are placed into clean containers, sealed, and transported with appropriate chain of custody, to the laboratory where careful labeling and aliquoting are done under secure conditions. Ideally, excess specimens are preserved for re-examination if necessary. These precautions are necessary, of course, when criminal poisonings are investigated or when multimillion dollar lawsuits are under litigation. Similarly in urine testing, the reputation of prominent figures, the continued employment of a wage earner, and the establishment of liability in a major transportation accident, all may be affected by a positive test result. The forensic aspects of this testing then become obvious.

A final requirement of forensic testing is adequate documentation of all aspects of the testing process. This is frustrating and annoying to a busy laboratorian, but the only reliable proof that a test result is correct, when proof is required many months or years after the fact, is by documentation of the quality control results, calibrator results, purity of standards, and all other parameters. Storage and retrieval of these data may be the ultimate challenge of urine drug testing.

In the end, the best proof of the validity of a forensic test result is its ability to withstand a challenge in a court of law. If the analytical data are acceptable to an expert toxicologist, if the chain of custody provides an unbroken paper trail establishing responsibility for the specimen to authorized individuals from collection to reporting of results, and if all data are adequately documented, the test result is forensically acceptable.

The public is beginning to realize something any responsible laboratory director has known for some time — test results are subject to error. Fortunately, errors can be minimized, but only by applying the concepts emphasized in the NIDA Guidelines. The manner by which the concepts are implemented may vary, but the concepts must be preserved.

REFERENCES

1. **Reagan, R.,** Drug-free workplace, Executive Order, No. 12564, Sept. 15, 1986.
2. **Blanke, R. V., Caplan, Y. H., Chamberlain, R. T., Dubowski, K. M., Finkle, B. S., Forney, R. B., Hawks, R. L., Hollister, L. E., Jatlow, P. I., Maickel, R. P., and McBay, A. J.,** Drug concentrations and driving impairment, *J. Am. Med. Assoc.*, 254, 2618–2621, 1985.
3. **Curran, W. J.,** Compulsory drug testing: the legal barriers, *N. Engl. J. Med.*, 316, 318–321, 1987.
4. **Hansen, H. J., Caudill, S. D., and Boone, J.,** Crisis in drug testing, *J. Am. Med. Assoc.*, 253, 2382–2387, 1985.
5. **Lundberg, G. D.,** Mandatory unindicated urine drug screening: still chemical McCarthyism, *J. Am. Med. Assoc.*, 256, 3003–3005, 1986.
6. **Davis, K. H., Hawks, R. L., and Blanke, R. V.,** Assessment of laboratory quality in urine drug testing, *J. Am. Med. Assoc.*, 260, 1749–1754, 1988.

Chapter 11

FUTURE TRENDS IN FORENSIC DRUG TESTING

Brian S. Finkle

TABLE OF CONTENTS

I. Socio-Political Overview in the United States 60

II. Epidemiology of Drug Abuse in the Workplace 60

III. Analytical Laboratory Aspects 61

IV. HHS-NIDA Regulatory Program 61

V. Appendix I 62
    A. Overview on Legal Issues in the Development of Drug Testing at the Workplace in the United States 63

VI. Appendix II 63
    A. Summary of General Recommendations 63
    B. On-Site, Initial, Screening-Only Testing Facilities 63
    C. Additional Drugs 63
    D. Cutoff (Analytical Threshold Values) 64
    E. Laboratory Inspections and Certification 64
    F. Analytical Methods 64
    G. Specimen Collection and Reporting of Results 64
    H. The Role of the Medical Review Officer (MRO) 65
    I. Performance Testing 65
    J. Monitoring Laboratory Performance (After Certification) 65

Reference 66

I. SOCIO-POLITICAL OVERVIEW IN THE UNITED STATES

In the United States, there is a federal program devoted to the war on drugs, which is strongly supported by the President, drug czar, and both political parties in the Congress, and billions of dollars are committed to this effort. Control of drug use in the workplace is a part of this program, and therefore federal involvement is unlikely to lessen in the foreseeable future.

The federal program is intended to detect and then deter drug use in workplace. The consequences of detection are punishment and sanctions against the employee. The program is nontreatment oriented, but there are, however, growing numbers of corporate (employer) and union sponsored Employee Assistance Programs (EAPs) designed to provide treatment and maintain productive employees. This trend will certainly strengthen and grow.

Employees do not wish to work in an environment in which illegal drug use may pose a danger through industrial accidents or cause a loss of productivity and profits which would be detrimental to the financial career rewards of everyone. Urine testing has the implicit consent of employees, but not the punitive consequences such as summary dismissal that may follow for a positive test. It is likely that treatment programs will increase and will include urine analysis to monitor drug use.

The present laws require laboratory supported programs to achieve a federal drug free workplace. Regulations promulgated in order to apply these laws differ between agencies, e.g., Nuclear Regulatory Agency, Department of Transportation (including National Transport Safety Board-NTSB, Federal Aviation Authority-FAA, Federal Railroad Administration-FRA), prisons, and the Department of Defense. There is currently some movement to make a single set of uniform regulations applicable to all agencies, but this is not imminent (see Appendix I).

New bills (Hatch-Boren Bill and Bliley-Dingle Bill, see Appendix I) are intended, in part, to extend the present federal drug testing program to the private sector. This will therefore increase testing enormously and will require many more laboratories (now there are about 55 laboratories certified by NIDA), all of which will have to comply with the NIDA Guidelines and be certified.

There is a gathering movement supported by many influential businessmen, ex-government officials, and professionals in drug abuse prevention and treatment, toward some form of legalization of drug use. This movement will grow in the next few years as the cost of "the unwinnable war" becomes a burden unacceptable to the taxpayer. Even if it were to succeed, the practice of pre-employment and employee-regulated drug testing would be by then so entrenched that under the declared need for a safe and productive workplace it would continue.

II. EPIDEMIOLOGY OF DRUG ABUSE IN THE WORKPLACE

Data from the oldest programs, such as the military, strongly suggest that the percentage of positive urine tests drops dramatically when a urine testing program is instituted. Similar data from industry and particularly pre-employment testing supports this observation. Whether this truly means that there is less drug use because of a direct cause-effect relationship between urine testing and drug abuse is unclear. Drug abuse is still mainly a problem of the young; use drops after age 24 to 25 and is rare in those older than 30 to 35 years. This will not change even if the popularity of particular drugs does wax and wane. The average age for all federal employees is 38. Some logical consequences can be drawn from that.

In a recent informal survey done by J. Michael Walsh of the NIDA, results from 42 laboratories involved in drug testing at the workplace, it appears that 10% of the results obtained from specimens by screening test were reported positive. From these presumptive results, 83% were confirmed as positive with 45% marijuana, 25% cocaine, 11% opiates, 1.5% PCP, 1% amphetamines, 1.5% benzodiazepines, and 1.2% barbiturates being the drugs involved.

New drugs of abuse have rarely been predicted before they were seized by police or detected in the laboratory. Apart from designed analogs of existing drugs, and of course alcohol, misuse of new potent prescription drugs, such as sedatives, stimulants, and anxiolytics, are the easiest to predict. Concentrating on the present "Big 5" (menu of NIDA) may be misleading and will not be confined in the future.

Although the present regulations do not allow it, on-site testing is almost certain to occur in the private sector very soon. Industrial employers and unions declare that they need it. It is estimated that some form of on-site testing is done at more than 2000 sites now, some remote such as oil rigs and some airports, but the quality or performance standards are unknown. Setting operational guidelines will be a critical priority in the next few years.

There is a trend toward expanding the federal laws and regulations to include all of private industry. *De facto* extension has already occurred in transportation because the Department of Transportation (D.O.T.) has legal authority over all transport operations including trucking companies. All of these must now comply with the D.O.T. drug testing regulations. Soon, provision will be made for all employees in the United States to be tested. There are unlikely to be laws requiring random testing of employees. Labor unions and other employee representative groups are adamantly opposed, and there are legal constitutional difficulties. When it happens it will be contested in the courts. Testing will be part of a carefully defined program agreed by all parties and "for-cause".

III. ANALYTICAL LABORATORY ASPECTS

Changes and improvements in screening procedures will occur, but mass spectrometric techniques coupled to a chromatographic separation will not be superseded for confirmation analysis. A variety of different screening techniques, including use of monoclonal antibodies, fluorescence polarization, and highly efficient thin layer chromatography, are available now, but not all of them can be used under present NIDA guidelines. This will change in the near future. Laboratories will be allowed to establish their own procedures, but the methods will have to meet at least the present standards of performance criteria, not an easy undertaking.

As is well known, all immunoassays are not equivalent. Any immunoassay should have an assay specific threshold concentration based on agreement with chromatography coupled to mass spectrometry reference method. The actual cutoff levels should be reviewed and possibly revised based on operational data to date. Any changes must consider administrative needs and protect the employee from any possibility of false positive results. This is a very demanding criteria.

It has been suggested that there is enough data that screening cutoff values for cannabinoids could be reduced from 100 to 50 ng/ml with a confirmation cutoff remaining as it is now at 15 ng/ml. It has also been suggested that the cutoff value for benzoylecgonine, one of the main metabolites of cocaine detected in urine, could be reduced from 300 to 200 ng/ml and the confirmation value to 100 ng/ml.

Although blood is the best specimen from a scientific point of view, it will not be recommended because the invasive sampling is unacceptable. Some abused drugs can be detected in the hair and saliva, but much more data are needed before they could be used for mass screening. These data will be obtained in the next few years because there is a lot of political pressure to adopt, in the future, hair as a test specimen.

The triad of external proficiency testing (PT) to challenge laboratory performance, blind QC, and QA programs will remain the foundation for demonstrating competence and quality of work. Changes are likely if onsite testing and screening-only laboratories are approved. This may require analyses of split-specimens with all those which screen positive and some proportion of negatives being reanalyzed by a full service, certified laboratory.

IV. HHS-NIDA REGULATORY PROGRAM

At a recent scientific meeting, some general recommendations were proposed in order to improve the current NIDA Guidelines. Some of these recommendations have been covered in this manuscript, but full details are presented in Appendix II.

NIDA will continue to have legal, regulatory authority for laboratory certification. It may be moved to a regulatory agency such as FDA or EPA, but not soon. The certification program has come to be financially self-supporting. It is now carried out by Research Triangle Institute in North Carolina, but as it grows and becomes diversified this may change. The College of American Pathologists may well assume this responsibility under the aegis of NIDA.

Proficiency testing will remain the principal tool used by the certifying agency (NIDA) to challenge laboratory performance. After certification, these challenge specimens will be completely blind to the laboratory and will be indistinguishable from any other urine specimen submitted for test. Only in this way can the quality of the laboratory system be assessed. Assessment is difficult; for example, it remains to be defined what is the correct or incorrect quantitative result.

A set of uniform certification criteria for evaluating laboratories will eventually be developed. Much of the subjective judgments (degrees of freedom of opinion) made by inspectors will be eliminated. Frequency of inspections and the number of inspectors on a team may be reduced.

Laboratory monitoring will continue to be through open performance testing specimens, blind proficiency test specimens, and laboratory inspections. There will be a single organization charged with monitoring laboratory performance, but in the future, it will have the benefit of an advisory group which represents all appropriate professional disciplines. Better communication between the organization and certified laboratories will be developed through newsletters, electronic bulletin boards, the publication of a list of certified laboratories monthly, and regular meetings of laboratory staff and officials of the monitoring organization. There is a need for guidelines to decertify laboratories which fail.

The volume of urine specimen collected for analysis could be reduced to 25 to 30 ml. The requirements for direct observation of the specimen collection will be eliminated; it will remain optional in certain circumstances. Collection of split samples will be permitted. Temperature measurement at the time of collection will remain a requirement but pH, specific gravity, and creatinine will become optional, at the discretion of the employer.

Drugs additional to the "Big 5" should be considered in drug testing protocols when they can be justified as special problems, particularly at the workplace. Drugs that may be considered include benzodiazepines, barbiturates, and other psychoactive agents. That should be decided by the employer, but analytical procedures must meet the standards of the NIDA Guidelines.

It is certain that, in the next year or two, guidelines similar in scope and intent will be applied to post-mortem toxicology, detection of drugs in those charged with crimes, and in automobile accident investigations. The Society of Forensic Toxicologists and the American Academy of Forensic Sciences-Toxicology Section have already drafted guidelines which were approved in February 1990. How they will be enforced and monitored is not clear.

The same old drugs will remain a problem with little that is new or novel; that is predictable. Despite amphetamine analogs, MDA, MDMA, fentanyl derivatives, PCP, and some new benzodiazepines, in recent years nothing has replaced marijuana, heroin, (meth)amphetamine, cocaine, and of course alcohol. It is difficult to imagine much change in the drug products of this very profitable well-established market. I predict that Europe in the next 2 years will follow this path in some form.

V. APPENDIX I

A. OVERVIEW ON LEGAL ISSUES IN THE DEVELOPMENT OF DRUG TESTING AT THE WORKPLACE IN THE UNITED STATES

On September 15, 1986, President Reagan issued Executive Order (EO) #12564 which required all federal agencies to develop programs and policies to achieve a drug-free federal workplace. One of the requirements of the EO was that agencies institute employee drug testing under specified circumstances. The responsibility for developing technical and scientific guidelines for these drug testing programs was assigned to the secretary of Health and Human Services (HHS) and delegated to the National Institute on Drug Abuse (NIDA).

On February 19, 1987, the Secretary of Health and Human Services, Dr. Otis Bowen, issued the required set of technical and scientific guidelines for federal drug testing programs. Within weeks, legislation was proposed in the House of Representatives to prohibit the expenditure of "appropriated funds" to implement EO #12564. Several months of negotiation between the administration and the Congress resulted in the passage of a new law (PL 100-71, sec. 503).

Enacted on July 7, 1987, this law permitted the President's program to go forward only if a number of administrative prerequisites were met. Included in the list of required administrative actions was that secretary of Health and Human Services must publish the HHS technical and scientific guidelines in the *Federal Register* for notice and comment for a period of 60 days and expand the "Guidelines" to include standards for laboratory certification.

As required, the "Guidelines" were published in the *Federal Register* on August 13, 1987, and the comment period closed in October 1987. Approximately 150 comments were received during this period, some of which were extremely detailed and lengthy. Several months were required to evaluate the advice received, make the appropriate revisions, and to fully develop the standards for laboratory certification. The revised "Guidelines" and "Laboratory Certification Standards" were cleared through HHS and the Office of Management and Budget and were published in the *Federal Register* as the Final "Mandatory Guidelines for Federal Workplace Drug Testing Programs" on April 11, 1988.

In July 1988, utilizing the certification standards, a National Laboratory Certification Program was implemented by HHS/NIDA and since that time, 50 laboratories have been certified with another 100 or more applicants still in process.

During 1988 to 1989, both the Department of Transportation and the Nuclear Regulatory Commission issued regulations which require employee drug testing in their regulated industries. Furthermore, these regulations require the use of a laboratory that has been certified by HHS/NIDA, and that these private sector organizations follow the technical and scientific procedures set out in the "Mandatory Guidelines" with minor exceptions.

In 1988, 1989, and again in 1990, legislation has been proposed in both the House and the Senate which would impose federal standards for drug testing in the private sector. Congressmen Dingle (Democrat, Michigan) and Bliley (Republican, Virginia) have introduced HR33 (January 3, 1989) which would require the Secretary of Health and Human Services to establish a federal standard for test procedures and require the use of certified laboratories for all employee drug testing conducted in the United States in the same manner as the NIDA "Guidelines" treat federal agencies. Similar legislation has been introduced in the Senate by Senators Hatch (Republican, Utah) and Boren (Democrat, Oklahoma). In January 1990, a House version of the Hatch-Boren bill was introduced as HR3940. This bill would allow certification of on-site, screening-only, and confirmatory testing laboratories and defines in detail the responsibilities and limitations of private companies which undertake drug testing programs.

There appears to be general support for the concept of a single federal standard for all employee drug testing. Business is supportive of a preemptive federal statute that would eliminate the various state laws that have been enacted within the last 2 to 3 years. Since these state statutes vary considerably, businesses that have multistate operations must have a different policy for each state in which they operate. Business and industry appear ready to support federal legislation if such legislation will allow sufficient flexibility to employers. Labor is supportive of federal legislation that would provide protection for employees, guarantee due process, and place required procedural standards for collection and analysis of specimens. At this juncture, it seems reasonable to believe that if consensus can be achieved on the details of procedures and analysis a single federal standard could be developed to apply to all employees drug testing.

VII. APPENDIX II

A. SUMMARY OF GENERAL RECOMMENDATIONS[1]

The seven working groups, with significant assistance from the general audience participants, were able to reach a consensus and make many recommendations for the improvement of the present NIDA Guidelines which support employee drug testing programs. All of these consensus statements are presented in detail together with their rationale in the following sections of this report. This section presents some of the salient recommendations only.

There were some issues which were considered by multiple working groups; these included on-site testing, additional drugs, cutoff (analytical threshold) values, and laboratory inspections. It is interesting that the separate groups expressed very similar opinions on these issues and their independent assessments lend weight to their collective consensus recommendations.

B. ON-SITE, INITIAL, SCREENING-ONLY TESTING FACILITIES

- These facilities should only be allowed where safety issues demand the most rapid turnaround time, justifying the risks to the client inherent in unconfirmed test results and the considerable difficulties in achieving accurate testing that such facilities create.
- On-site urine screening can reliably identify negative specimens provided appropriate safeguards are built into the procedure. These precautions include the following:

    - Meeting the basic forensic standards for specimen collection, chain of custody documentation, and security
    - Splitting the collected urine specimen into two portions
    - Participation in open and blind proficiency testing
    - A rigorous quality assurance program
    - Being subject to site inspections
    - Using an FDA approved screening test that provides objective and documentable results
    - Use of the same cutoff concentrations as used in NIDA certified laboratories
    - Submitting all presumptive positive specimens to a NIDA certified laboratory for confirmation

- All MRO functions should remain the same as at present if laboratory testing is performed on-site. Other recommendations associated with this issue are given in the body of the report.

C. ADDITIONAL DRUGS

- Additional drugs should be considered for inclusion in urine testing protocols when they can be justified as special problems in particular workplace environments.
- Drugs that might be considered include the benzodiazepines, barbiturates, and other selected psychoactive agents.
- The option to include additional drugs should be decided by the employer, but all testing must be at a NIDA certified laboratory, and the criteria for the analytical methods and laboratory procedures must meet the present NIDA Guidelines in every respect.

D. CUTOFF (ANALYTICAL THRESHOLD VALUES)

- Any immunoassay should have an assay specific threshold concentration based on agreement with a GC/MS reference method.
- The present cutoff levels should be reviewed and possibly revised based on operational data to date, but any changes must meet program administrative needs and protect the employee from any possibility of false positive results.
- The screening cutoff value for cannabinoids (Delta-9-THC-acid) could be reduced from 100 to 50 ng/ml with the confirmation cutoff remaining at 15 ng/ml.
- The present screening cutoff value for cocaine (benzoylecgonine) could be reduced to 200 ng/ml and the confirmation to 100 ng/ml.

E. LABORATORY INSPECTIONS AND CERTIFICATION

- Beginning from the time of certification, inspection should occur as follows: at 6, 12, 18, and 24 months; following these 2 years, inspections should occur annually.
- A minimum of three inspectors should participate in the initial inspection before certification of a laboratory, and then a minimum of two inspectors for routine, maintenance inspections after certification.
- Inspectors should be carefully selected and trained to meet the same standards, and training programs should stress the critical need for inspection criteria to be applied uniformly, without bias.
- An exit summation conference between the inspection team and the person responsible for the laboratory operations should present any deficiencies and other identified problems. At the conference, the laboratory person should have the opportunity to clarify any misunderstandings.
- Supportive analytical data from the prior 60 days should be readily available for inspectors to review in the laboratory.
- The cost of laboratory inspections should be reduced to a reasonable level and reflect the shortened time, and fewer inspectors should be necessary for small laboratories.
- The Department of Health and Human Services (DHHS) should have an oversight function to monitor certification agencies, and the secretary of DHHS should rapidly establish methods to grant equivalency to acceptable accrediting agencies.
- Laboratories seeking certification should be subject to the same standards even though they may be monitored by different certification agencies.

There was only one issue on which consensus proved impossible; that was whether the Medical Review Officer (MRO) should continue to receive, review, and release all positive **and negative** drug test results. Both the MRO and the specimen collection working groups discussed this issue intensely, separately and together. It was agreed that positive results should be released by the MRO as soon as possible, but **no consensus** was reached on whether MROs should continue to receive and review all negative drug test results as at present. Serious concerns were raised about confidentiality issues caused by direct transmission results to an employer rather than sending them to the MRO. Several alternative compromise procedures were acceptable to the specimen collection working group but not to the MROs. **Consensus could not therefore be achieved.**

The principal recommendations made on issues which were considered by individual working groups are as follows, but for complete consensus statements, the appropriate section in the body of the report should be read.

F. ANALYTICAL METHODS

- Initial screening and confirmation methods must be based on different principles of analytical chemistry or different chromatographic separations.
- Laboratories should be allowed to establish their own analytical procedures, required of the present immunoassay screening methods and GC/MS confirmation procedures.
- Urine continues to be the best specimen for analysis in the context of detecting drug use in the workplace. There are insufficient data to support a recommendation for alternative specimens such as hair or saliva.

G. SPECIMEN COLLECTION AND REPORTING OF RESULTS

- A urine volume of 30 ml should be an acceptable specimen volume, provided that it does not create any technical problems for the laboratory.
- Split urine specimen should be permitted pro-

vided they are both part of the same specimen and handled with identical safeguards.
- Testing urine specimens at the collection site for acceptable pH, specific gravity, and creatinine values should be permitted, but not required, at the option of the employer. The temperature measurement requirement should be maintained, the acceptable range should be 90 to 100°F.
- Negative results should be reported to the employer promptly by direct means, but in a manner which ensures confidentiality of the information.

H. THE ROLE OF THE MEDICAL REVIEW OFFICER (MRO)

- MROs should be licensed doctors of medicine or osteopathy.
- A comprehensive continuing education program that addresses all aspects of MRO functions (not just drug abuse recognition) should be developed.
- Guidelines should be developed to define confidentiality when any new high technology electronic transmitting equipment is used in a urine drug testing program.
- Action should be taken in a drug deterrence program only after a specimen is confirmed positive and verified to be true positive by the MRO.
- In unusual circumstances, MROs should be able to request, in consultation with a laboratory director, additional tests on positive specimens that may aid in a complete identification of the drug, metabolite, or of the specimen.

I. PERFORMANCE TESTING

- Proficiency testing (PT) is necessary to establish laboratory performance before as well as after certification.
- Blind proficiency testing is the ultimate method for demonstrating the competence of a laboratory operation as applied to routine specimens.
- The specific analytes and their concentrations in the PT specimens must be prepared and verified by an independent agency unknown to the laboratory.
- Urine used for the preparation of PT specimens should be human, drug-free urine.
- For all PT challenges, a false positive result shall be cause for disqualification.
- For all PT challenges, the target concentration for each analyte should be the statistical mean of the results obtained by the laboratories
- In the initial PT series before certification, quantitative results may differ by no more than 50% from the target value. If one result differs by more than this amount, the laboratory should demonstrate that appropriate remedial action was taken and successfully complete an additional PT cycle of 20 specimens. After achieving certification, a laboratory is permitted one quantitative result differing by more than 50% from the target value within three consecutive cycles of PT.
- Methods of keeping costs to the client at a minimum while maintaining maximum proficiency monitoring should be investigated. A centralized, blind PT program may serve this purpose, but details of such a program would need to be carefully defined.

J. MONITORING LABORATORY PERFORMANCE (AFTER CERTIFICATION)

- A single agency should monitor the performance of all laboratories certified for urine drug testing. The agency should be supported by an advisory group, representing all appropriate, involved professionals, and meeting frequently at regularly scheduled intervals to provide policy advice and problem review.
- The monitoring agency should return a report which summarizes the laboratory performance as compared to the group mean result within 30 calendar days following receipt of the laboratory performance test results.
- A uniform set of specifications for blind PT specimens should be developed. These would include a mechanism for submitting the specimens and receiving, and evaluating reports of blind PT results. These specimens should be introduced proportionally over time to include a minimum of 3% of the number of client specimens.
- A variety of communication systems, such as a newsletter, electronic bulletin boards, and regularly scheduled meetings of representatives of certified laboratories and the monitoring agency, should be explored and developed in order to share information of importance in urine drug testing.
- Detection of an apparent false positive test results is of such importance that immediate action should

be initiated to investigate the cause. The investigation should be completed by the laboratory within 7 calendar days of receipt of notice.
- When certification of a laboratory is suspended, the laboratory should immediately notify all clients of the suspension; failure to do so should result in revocation of certification. If revocation occurs, then the entire initial certification process should be completed before further testing is resumed.
- The monitoring agency should publish an updated list of certified laboratories monthly.

Those laboratories which conform to the NIDA Guidelines and are certified as competent continue to demonstrate that test results which are credible in the forensic context can be produced routinely on very large numbers of urine specimens. The experience of the past 2 years has made it abundantly clear that almost all of the demands which are made on the analytical process and administrative system which supports urine drug testing in the workplace can be quickly satisfied by thoughtful, imaginative scientists and managers. Automated immunoassays can reliably discriminate between negative and potentially positive specimens. Microprocessor or computer controlled GC/MS instruments can specifically confirm structures, resolve isomers, and quantitate drugs and metabolite concentrations at parts per billion with remarkable accuracy. Conscientious application of a rigorous quality assurance program and management dedicated to the principles of fail-safe practices can insure success in detecting and deterring drug use in the workplace.

REFERENCE

1. **Finkle, B. S., Blanke, R. V., and Walsh, J. M., Eds.,** *Technical, Scientific and Procedural Issues of Employee Drug Testing Consensus Report,* HHS Pub. 90–1684, NIDA Publication, Rockville, MD, 1990.

Chapter 12

DISCUSSION ON ORGANIZATIONAL ASPECTS FOR RELIABLE DRUG TESTING

Segura: I would like to ask to any of the speakers if they can elaborate a little bit more about the split sample. This is not only a methodological problem, but also it is a conceptual problem as well. When you have only one sample, you need to have really a strict chain of custody procedure in order to certify that nothing has happened to this sample even inside the laboratory; that nobody has added something or nobody has manipulated it. The split samples procedure allows us to overcome this and if something has happened either in the beginning or at the end, you have a second sample that can be analyzed in the same laboratory or even in a different one. This is certainly a key point.

Wennig: Dr. Minty (Charing Cross Hospital, London, U.K.) has mentioned the possibility of making a chain of custody of the second sample. When there is something wrong at least in the second one you have a little bit more control over the sample and you can cut down the expenses because you only do in a few amount of samples and not in all of them.

Segura: In doping control you have the split sample, but because of the accreditation procedure for all certified laboratories, the second sample is analyzed in the same laboratory. I propose that the second sample in drugs of abuse, if you don't have a very established accreditation procedure, might be analyzed, if deemed necessary, in a different laboratory.

Wennig: I think that the second examination should be done in the same laboratory, at least at the beginning. Maybe later you can give it to another one. The laboratory should have the chance to check itself. This is being done, for instance, in Singapore where the second sample is securely stored and the individual has the right to ask for a second analysis. The laboratory itself then does the first check, which is reasonable. If there is still something wrong you can ask for confirmation in another laboratory.

Widdop: We routinely collect three samples instead of two. One of them is given to the employee, the person under test, for safe keeping. We keep two samples, under chain of custody, both sealed. The first sample is open for the preliminary testing and if that proves to be presumptively positive we then go back to the refrigerator and we take out the second sample. That sample is then analyzed by the GC/MS confirmation procedure. The reason why we are doing this is because there is always the possibility in these laboratories, specially if you are doing a lot of drug abuse, of contaminating one sample with another and I think at least if you keep your samples away from that particular area, there is a possibility that your confirmation analysis carried out on the same sample used for presumptive testing is simply confirming contamination. That is our system and that is probably better than the NIDA is using actually. I see Dr. Willette is shaking his head; they only use one. However, I think that with 4000 a day we probably would come back to a single sample.

de la Torre: I would like to ask Dr. Willette if the only reason why he prefers single sample to split sample is just a matter of space. Obviously, with two samples you need more refrigerators and more safety storage.

Willette: There is a large number of issues; complex storage is simply a part of the problem. All the procedures involved in the collection, storage, and handling of the specimens has to preclude issues like contamination. The way by which the laboratory aliquots the original specimen has to be done in a manner that it precludes that possibility, and when you take all of the steps it turns out that the results from a single specimen will be as valid as those obtained by splitting the sample. The great difficulty comes at the collection point because if collection is not done properly, splitting the samples does not really protect the individual. On the other hand, if there is a possibility of contamination in the laboratory, we would argue that procedures in the laboratory are not appropriate. I think that Dr. Segura's point is the most valid and in the United States and in those circumstances where split samples are used, it is a perception problem. It is a perception in the mind of the donor, the employer, and the applicant to guarantee some "piece of mind" to feel that there is a secured sample, sealed in their presence, and stored in the appropriate place under secure conditions that could be used to repudiate the original task, and in almost all cases, is more a perceptual than a methodological problem. The difficulty in using other laboratories and second samples is that all the rules about cutoffs change as we all know that stored specimens can lose a drug or a drug metabolite and so we have to be conscious of differences in methods, differences in cutoffs, and perhaps even the requirements use different analytical methods when retesting a stored specimen. Some drugs such as opiates do not deteriorate, but certainly in the case of the cannabinoids and in the case of cocaine positive sample, the loss of the analyte is a significant issue. So, there are a number of issues that have to be addressed and this is why, under rules in the United States that permit split specimens, the second specimen or the repeated analysis has to be done in an appropriately certified laboratory, but not using the original mandated cutoffs. Chemical presence is defined, at least in the certification system in the United States, by some agreement upon the limit of quantitation, and this is usually the cutoff on any kind of repeated analysis. Thus the security of the specimen has to be complete to begin with the analysis. The second specimen really does not add anything to the analytical answer, but I think perceptions are important there.

Moeller: You should take in mind that you are dealing with only 4% of positive samples, and after the first screening you can discard most of the specimens. On the other side, you are doubling or tripling the cost of the analysis for all these specimens that are found negative after the procedure. So I think is not a question of money to come to a solution with the split sample; it would be cheaper. You can if you handle 2000 specimens a week and you have on one side $6 or $8 for the analysis; on the other side, you have $20 for the analysis. You can buy every week ten refrigerators. But this is not necessary because you have such a low positive rate of positive cases. And what you say about the stability of drug in the stored sample, the same stability problem is if you only have one sample. Then, in my opinion there is no argument against the split sample.

Section II
Analytical Methodology
for
Reliable Drug Testing

Chapter 13

ANALYTICAL RELIABILITY: INTRODUCTION TO ANALYTICAL METHODS

Emilio Gelpí

Analytical methods for drugs, xenobiotics, endogenous compounds, and/or their metabolites in biological samples must be properly validated for the overall reliability of the results they provide. Isotope dilution GC/MS is the accepted reference method for its accuracy and precision. However, since neither the classical GC/MS nor the more recent LC-MS methods are readily available in many laboratories, data validation using different analytical methods is often given as proof of reliability even though the experimental approach leading to the data that needs to be validated may be itself at fault.[1]

The literature contains many examples of serious inconsistencies both in the design of the method and in the evaluation of previous data which are often erroneously taken as a reference basis for comparison of subsequent results. The reliability of an analytical method, be it spectroscopic, chromatographic, or immunologically based, may be dependent on factors either related to the method itself or to the nature of the samples which are being processed. Among some of these factors would be the effects of interfering compounds due to exceedingly complex matrix compositions or the possible artifactual variations of the analyte as a function of the sampling procedure. Also, the ultimate precision and accuracy defining the analytical reliability of an analytical method is directly related to the complexity of sample work up procedures, the efficiency and reproducibility of any applicable separation steps, the correct use of a suitable internal standard to compensate for volumetric errors, and the sensitivity, linearity of response, selectivity, and long-term stability of the detection system.

REFERENCES

1. **Gelpí, E.**, *Life Sci.*, 41, 849–852, 1987.

Chapter 14

CRITICAL OVERVIEW ON IMMUNOLOGICAL AND CHROMATOGRAPHIC ANALYTICAL METHODS

C. Edgar Cook

TABLE OF CONTENTS

I.	Introduction to the Problem	74
II.	General Considerations	74
	A. Extraction, Separation, and Detection	74
	B. Identification of Analyte	75
	C. Standards and Controls	76
III.	Methodologies	76
	A. Paper Chromatography or Spot Tests	76
	B. Thin Layer Chromatography	77
	C. Gas and Liquid Chromatography	77
	D. Mass Spectrometry	77
	E. Immunoassay	78
	F. Radioimmunoassay	78
	G. Enzyme Immunoassay	79
	H. Fluorescence Immunoassay	79
	I. Interferences	80
IV.	Conclusions	81
	References	81

I. INTRODUCTION TO THE PROBLEM

Analysis of body fluids is a key step in determining whether an individual has consumed an illegal drug (or excessive amount of a prescription drug) and may shed some light on the possibility of impairment from such drug use. To answer the first question, a qualitative yes or no answer may be adequate. In the latter case, not only is quantitative analysis necessary, but also an understanding of the pharmacology and pharmacodynamics of the drug is essential.

The analyst looking for evidence of an illegal drug is faced with a formidable task. The ten-millionth chemical substance[1] has recently been added to the Chemical Abstracts Service Registry System. All of the currently abused drugs, their designer analogs, and principal metabolites probably represent fewer than 100 compounds. Thus, the analyst is looking at a subset consisting of $<1/_{100,000}$ of the total register of chemical substances, and, in most cases, a single one of those.

Fortunately for the analyst, many factors combine to reduce the formidable odds against being able to locate a single drug or drug metabolite and prove its presence. Many of the ten million compounds will be too insoluble, too involatile, or too rare to present a serious interference problem. However there are still many compounds with as yet unknown structures present in biological systems, and more synthetic compounds are being prepared every day. Thus the analyst is still faced with a somewhat uphill battle. Furthermore, since the detection of an illegal drug may often have serious social, professional, or legal consequences to the individual involved, the analysis must be good enough to establish the presence of a particular substance beyond a reasonable doubt. False positive results can be exceedingly damaging.

Ironically, if as is hoped, the incidence of drug abuse is reduced by the methods, such as screening, taken to counteract it, false positive results are likely to have a more serious impact. This topic has been discussed by Spiehler et al.[2] and Root-Bernstein.[3] Consider the case in which an analytical method has 0.1% false positive and false negative rates. Suppose 10,000 urine samples are screened with this assay. If half of the samples contain the drug in question, then 5000 samples will be negative and, on the average, only 5 of the negative samples will be reported as positive. If, however, only 0.1% of the samples contain the drug in question, the false positives (10) will essentially equal the true positives. Thus, random screening of low incidence populations presents the greatest likelihood for misleading results.

One purpose of random screening is its deterrent effect on drug abuse. If, in order to avoid the problem of the false positive, the analytical procedure produces a large number of false negatives, the value of screening is greatly reduced. If the result of a false negative is that an impaired pilot is allowed to fly an airplane, the results of the false negative test may also be devastating. Thus, the analyst is forced to steer a tight course between the Scylla of false positive results and the Charybdis of false negative results. Fortunately, in most cases it has been possible to develop sufficiently sophisticated methods to meet this challenge. However, as we discuss these methods, it is well to continue to remind ourselves of the serious consequences of what we are doing when we devise, promote, and sell analytical methodology to solve a social problem.

II. GENERAL CONSIDERATIONS

Essentially all of the common chromatographic and immunological assay techniques have been proposed for use in measuring drugs of abuse. As new techniques are developed and as new drugs of abuse appear, the same types of problems will appear in making a choice of analytical methodology. What lessons can we learn from the past which will help not only in the evaluation of current methods but also in the evaluation of new methods for new drugs?

The factors which must be considered for any assay include its specificity, its sensitivity for the analyte in question, its reproducibility, its capability for giving quantitative results, the degree of skill and training required of the user, the speed or through-put of the analytical procedure, and the cost of carrying it out.

A. EXTRACTION, SEPARATION, AND DETECTION

There are usually three stages in an assay. These involve the removal of the analyte from its biological matrix, separation of the analyte from accompanying interferences, and finally detection and quantitation. There can be trade-offs among these three steps. For example, if the detector is highly selective (e.g., an antibody), it may be able to ignore the presence of numerous substances in the analyte mixture. Alternatively, a very efficient separation technique, such as high performance liquid chromatography, can sometimes permit the use of a fairly nonselective detection device such as UV or fluorescence.

Furthermore, sequential separation steps can markedly enhance the selectivity of an analysis. Thus one can envision a separation technique as having a number of defined

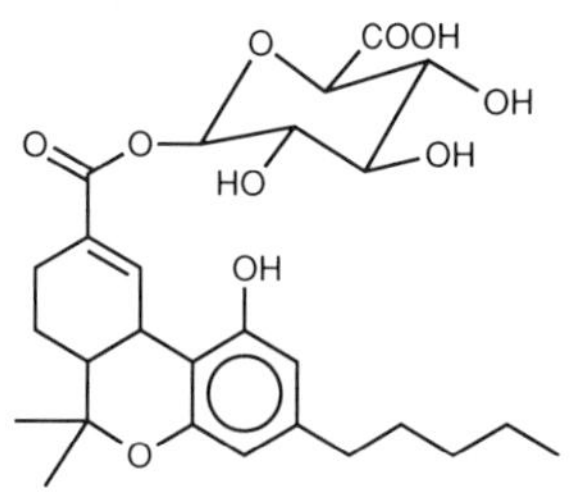

FIGURE 1. The major metabolite of Δ^9-THC, 11-nor-9-carboxy-Δ^9-THC, is excreted principally as the base sensitive glucuronate ester.

slots into which the analyte of interest may fall.[4] The actual number of slots depends on the resolution of the method. If compounds falling into a single slot are transferred to a second separation system, they can now be spread over a second set of slots with enhanced specificity and the process can be repeated. For example, one can go from solvent extraction to a peak on the gas chromatogram to an examination of the characteristic masses of ions from that peak in a mass spectrometer.[4,5]

There is often an interrelationship between sensitivity and specificity of a measurement, but ultimate instrumental sensitivity is not the only criterion. For example, mass spectrometers can detect a few hundred femtograms of Δ^9-tetrahydrocannabinol,[6] and 600 molecules of cholera toxin can be detected by an ultrasensitive enzyme radioimmunoassay;[7] but approaching such limits in a biological matrix is not usually feasible. Fluorescence can be measured with exceeding sensitivity but practical use must take into account background fluorescence. It is truly the background signal that determines the practical sensitivity of most assays. Sensitivity of detection can however sometimes be advantageous in lowering the amount of sample required and therefore the amounts of interfering substances, if the detection method is less sensitive to these impurities than it is to the analyte. Such is often the case with immunoassay methods.

B. IDENTIFICATION OF ANALYTE

The first question that must be answered in developing or assessing an analytical procedure is the very basic one of what is to be analyzed. Let us take the case of the analysis of urine for tetrahydrocannabinol metabolites. Almost 20 years ago, it was established that 11-nor-9-carboxy-Δ^9-tetrahydrocannabinol (THC-11-oic acid) could be obtained from urine.[37] Since that time, it has been shown that urine contains a wide spectrum of acidic metabolites of Δ^9-THC.[9] The 11-oic acid is however the predominant metabolite. Analytical methodology for analysis of cannabinoid metabolites in urine was therefore directed principally at detecting and measuring the 11-oic acid.

In 1980, Williams and Moffat,[10] using a combination of HPLC and radioimmunoassay, discovered that most of the 11-oic acid was excreted initially as a glucuronate ester (Figure 1). Such esters are characterized by high sensitivity to base hydrolysis. Wall and Taylor[8] examined urine samples from subjects administered THC and found that if precautions were taken to avoid the presence of base in the isolation procedure, the concentrations of free 11-oic acid were markedly diminished (Figure 2). Johansson et al.[11] and Foltz et al.[12] have also found that only trace amounts of the free carboxylic acid are excreted in urine.

Fortunately the design of most of the initial immunoassay reagents was such that considerable cross-reactivity could be expected between the glucuronate ester and the free 11-oic acid. Some hydrolysis occurs in urine on standing and most analytical methods which involved gas chromatography or gas chromatography/mass spectrometry (GC/MS) used an acid-base partition procedure as a standard cleanup method. Because of the sensitivity to basic hydrolysis of the glucuronate ester, this technique alone ensures that much of the initial metabolite will be converted to the measured analyte. However, in an early comparison of EMIT and GC/MS procedures, Peat et al.[13] found 37 samples positive by EMIT which were not confirmed by GC/MS. When three of these unconfirmed samples were hydrolyzed enzymatically (another way to

GC/MS ANALYSIS OF URINE SAMPLES FOR THC–11–OIC ACID
WITH OR WITHOUT BASE HYDROLYSIS

Route of Administration	Ng THC–11–oic Acid/mL Urine*	
	Without Hydrolysis	With Hydrolysis
IV	2	133
Smoking	11	252
Oral	17	337

* Values are mean of samples from 4 subjects
Mean ratio without/with for individual samples = 0.029 ± 0.026

FIGURE 2. Mean values of THC-11-oic acid in urine with and without base hydrolysis.(Data from Wall, M. E. and Taylor, H. L., *Marijuana '84 Proceedings of the Oxford Symposium on Cannabis,* RL Press, Oxford, England, 1985, 69–76.)

hydrolyze the glucuronate ester), they were then found to be positive by GC/MS.

The above case is one of unconfirmed positives rather than false positives. Such situations, if interpreted as showing false positive results from a screening technique, may unfairly diminish confidence in the screening procedure and result in an inaccurate assessment of its value. Thus, it is important that analysts using different methodologies should be measuring the same constituent in each case. A slightly different case of the unconfirmed positive would be the example of a designer drug which varies enough from the structure of the original drug to produce a different elution and mass spectral pattern in GC/MS but which may be sufficiently close in structure to the original drug to be detectable by immunological assay techniques. Whether such situations should be classified as false positives may depend upon the purpose for which the assay is being undertaken. However, it does emphasize that one should carefully examine the reasons for apparent false negative or false positive results.

C. STANDARDS AND CONTROLS

Another pitfall which may occur in any methodology and lead to significant problems in interpretation is the preparation of control or standard samples. Examples of this may also be drawn from the cannabinoid research field. In view of the difficulty of preparing the glucuronate ester of THC-11-oic acid, urine control samples are prepared from the acid itself. The high degree of lipophilicity even of THC-11-oic acid has been shown to enhance its nonspecific binding to many surfaces including glass. Furthermore, the compound, because of its hydrophilic carboxylic group, is a reasonable surfactant. As a result of this, vigorous shaking of urine sample containing the THC-11-oic acid can result in a marked reduction of concentration in the bulk volume with most of the drug being observed in the foam.[14] In a recent study, it was shown that under the conditions used adsorption to glass caused a 27% reduction in concentration, whereas vigorous mixing resulted in foaming and an apparent 89% reduction in concentration. The latter reduction was reversible.[15]

For immunoassay, Δ^8-THC-11-oic acid was often used as the standard in place of the much more expensive and difficult to obtain but naturally occurring Δ^9 isomer. A recent publication illustrates a significant improvement in the false negative rate for EMIT assays which were formulated using the Δ^9 compound rather than Δ^8 as standard.[16]

The matrix in which the standards are prepared may also have an influence on results. For example, Hanson et al.[17] analyzed blind control serum samples ranging from 10 to 30 ng/ml of THC. One commercial kit gave no false positives, but 33% false negatives using the serum standards provided in the kit. A high endogenous background in the serum standards provided in the kit was apparently the cause of the high false negative rate, since by making up standards in other control serum they were able to markedly reduce the false negative rate.

III. METHODOLOGIES

With this background let us look at some of the methodologies currently available and their limitations and/or problems.

A. PAPER CHROMATOGRAPHY OR SPOT TESTS

There is a demand for a test which can be carried out quickly in an on-site location with minimally trained personnel. Such a procedure is inherently difficult to produce. Methods based on paper chromatography have recently been introduced for such tests. Evaluation of these procedures has not been favorable. Thus, Schwartz et al.[18] concluded that a test purported to detect four classes of drugs of abuse was "unacceptable for use in any setting" because of its "poor sensitivity, specificity, and efficiency".[19] Similar testing of a cannabinoid paper chromatography test showed the predictive value of a positive test to be only 60% and of a negative test only 33%. Furthermore, the skilled technologist who carried out the tests stated that only 15% of the positive samples had clearly defined endpoints.[20]

B. THIN LAYER CHROMATOGRAPHY

The pros and cons of using thin layer chromatography for screening of drugs in urine have been recently summarized by Sunshine.[21] TLC utilizing high performance fine silica gel particles, a nonadsorbent layer at the bottom of the plate, and automatic spotting techniques can be a useful technique for screening of samples for drugs of abuse. Good resolution can be achieved. Commercial kits are available, and the developed chromatograms can be photographed or stored for future reference. Nevertheless, there are problems with the use of TLC — principally in its interpretation. It is important to be able to recognize the pattern of a drug and its metabolites and to distinguish the color reactions produced on the thin layer plate. The presence of impurities may have an impact on the R_f values and unusual substances may give spots and colors similar to those of the analyte. Therefore, the experience of the chromatographer is a key factor in interpreting thin layer chromatograms. Sensitivity may also be a problem, and automation is hampered by the aforementioned need for an experienced evaluator. Sunshine concludes that TLC has excellent potential where it is anticipated that there may be multidrug use at relatively high doses, in which case TLC is an excellent preliminary test procedure. It should not, however, be placed in inexperienced hands.

C. GAS AND LIQUID CHROMATOGRAPHY

Gas chromatography, like thin layer chromatography, has the capability for detecting a variety of drugs in a single run. This may be useful for screening purposes, even though samples must be run one at a time. Most GC analyses require at least a moderate amount of preliminary cleanup before injection. Most gas chromatography detectors are fairly nonselective, so the question of whether a peak on a gas chromatogram with the appropriate retention time belongs to the analyte of interest becomes a problem. Use of capillary columns has enhanced the resolution capabilities of GC markedly, and somewhat more selective detectors, such as nitrogen, phosphorus, or electron capture, may be useful in certain instances. Even these detectors, however, will respond to a wide variety of compounds and thus background interference is a significant potential problem.

One technique for enhancing the selectivity of gas chromatography is to use more than one column or detector. Thus, for example, it has been proposed that two columns of different polarity be used either one at a time[22] or in tandem.[23] Alternatively, two different detectors can be used with identical columns so that one compares the detector response for compounds of identical retention times. Using this approach and an internal standard (2-amino-5-chlorobenzo-phenone), Perrigo et al.[24] calculated detector response factors and retention times for 188 drugs. They found a cv of 3.3% for the detector response factor for 75 analyses of caffeine over a 10-month period. Combining the retention index and detector response factor showed excellent discriminative power, even when the error limits for the two parameters measured were set relatively high. Addition of a third detector, such as electron capture, is suggested by the authors.[24]

Although this type of approach will lead to better discriminative ability for drugs, it also increases the complexity of the analysis. Working with multiple columns as well as the need to maintain two or more detectors in good operating condition, while feasible in a research chromatography laboratory, may give considerably poorer results in a less favorable setting.

High performance liquid chromatography shares many of the advantages and disadvantages of gas chromatography. It does have the advantage that temperature-sensitive compounds can be analyzed. In favorable cases, direct injection of urine may be feasible. Sensitivity is sometimes a problem. Some abused drugs do not have strong chromophores except at a low wavelength where interference is likely. The use of chromophoric derivatives and electrochemical detectors may be helpful, but at the cost of additional complexity.

D. MASS SPECTROMETRY

Since the mass spectrum of a compound is generally quite characteristic, mass spectrometry as a detection system for gas (or liquid) chromatography provides a powerful means for confirming the presence of a specific analyte. Therefore GC/MS is generally considered the confirmatory technique of choice. Nevertheless, interferences do occur. To minimize this problem, general practice should be to measure multiple peaks, to use a deuterated internal standard, and to compare the ratios of the peaks for both the deuterated standard and nondeuterated analyte. When this is done, there is indeed a high probability of reaching the correct conclusion.

Other MS procedures which lend additional specificity to the methodology are the analyses of metastable ions (MS/MS) or the use of an ion trap mass spectrometer. By use of MS/MS a few hundred femtograms of THC could be detected by mass spectrometry, and the detection limit could be pushed down to 100 pg/ml for THC from rabbit serum. However, in the case of human serum, interfering substances were still present, and the limit of analysis was 1 ng/ml.[6] In contrast to this high technology approach, 100 pg/ml was measured in human plasma by a combination of careful clean up chromatography on Sephadex LH20 followed by capillary gas chromatography with mass spectrometry detection,[11] thus illustrating that careful initial cleanup can substitute for a more expensive and sophisticated detection system.

Even if the mass spectrometer were infallible, it is still necessary to remember that the mass spectrum is only the last part of a series of steps, all of which must figure into the ultimate reliability of the method. In a recent illustration of this, Brunk[26] reported on a pre-employment urine specimen that was positive by the EMIT cannabinoid assay, but appeared negative on GC/MS analysis. The subject had taken ibuprofen which was known to cause false positives with earlier formulations of the EMIT reagents but not with later versions of this test system.[27] Further testing showed, however, that ibuprofen in this case was interfering with the GC/MS assay by depleting the methyl iodide used for methylation of the THC-11-oic acid. High concentrations of ibuprofen prevented the formation of the methylated metabolite. The author points out that had he used deuterated internal standard rather than a noncannabinoid standard the interference would have been detected by the lack of internal standard peak — further impetus for the routine use of deuterated internal standards in these procedures.

E. IMMUNOASSAY

In antibodies, nature has provided a highly sensitive and selective method for detecting the presence of foreign substances, and this has been turned to great advantage in the development of analytical methodology. The development of an immunoassay requires a highly selective binding site and some means of distinguishing free from bound analyte. The immune system, with appropriate manipulation, provides the former. For the latter, usually a derivative of the analyte is labeled in some manner that permits either free and bound material to be separated or shows some change in properties upon binding.

F. RADIOIMMUNOASSAY

Radioimmunoassay has occupied a prominent role in the immunoassay repertoire and for good reason. In contrast to other sensitive physical measurements, such as fluorescence, radioactivity has a very low natural background and interference of this type is essentially nonexistent. Because high specific activity competing ligands can be readily synthesized, radioimmunoassay also provides excellent sensitivity. The major drawbacks to RIA are the need for using radioactive materials, which can introduce problems of waste disposal and (to a much lesser extent) personnel safety, and its resistance to automation, the latter being due to the general need to separate free and bound radioligand before measurement of the fraction which is bound to the antibody. Various techniques have been used to overcome this limitation. These include the coating of plastic tubes with the antibody to simplify washing and removal of unbound material and the use of magnetizable beads to aid in the separation procedure.

Recently, a method for measuring bound radioactivity without the need for separation has been introduced (Figure 3). In this technique, an yttrium scintillant is incorporated into beads to which the antibody is attached either directly or by means of an attached second antibody. The beads are then incubated with radioligand and analyte and, after equilibrium is reached, radioactivity is measured in a standard β-scintillation spectrometer. Because the effective path of a β particle is quite short, only those radioactive atoms which are bound to the beads via the antibody will be very effective in producing light. As a result, it is only the bound radioactivity which is measured by the spectrometer.[28] We have utilized this technique recently in our own laboratory for the measurement of THC and THC-11-oic acid and have found it to give results comparable to those of a double antibody solid phase radioimmunoassay.

Tritium labeled radioligands are often preferable to ^{125}I for reasons such as stability and safety of handling. Tritium ligands have fallen into disfavor, however, because of the need for use of scintillation fluids in order to measure them. With the above approach, it may be feasible to rethink the use of tritium labeled radioligands. It is also

SCINTILLATION PROXIMITY ASSAY

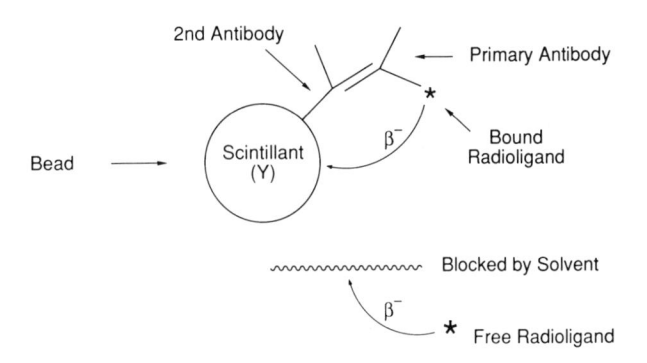

FIGURE 3. Principle of Scintillation Proximity Assay. β-Radiation from radioligand bound to antibody on beads is detected; that from radioligand in solution is not.

of interest, however, that ^{125}I is a β emitter as well as a γ emitter and can equally well be used in the THC procedure.[29]

G. ENZYME IMMUNOASSAY

Enzyme multiplied immunoassays can be carried out in homogeneous (EMIT) or heterogeneous (ELISA) fashion. The EMIT assay relies on tagging the analyte with an enzyme so that when the labeled analyte is bound to antibody enzymatic activity is diminished. This assay has been in use for many years now, and, as a result, much is known about both its positive and negative features. It is readily amenable to automated procedures. It has the disadvantage that its results are susceptible not only to interference by substances which affect the binding of analyte to antibody but can also be affected by the presence of enzyme inhibitors or promoters.

The ELISA assay has been used relatively less for analysis of abused drugs. It is capable of automation and thus can provide high through-put. Since wash steps are involved between binding to the antibody and addition of enzyme linked second antibody, it should, in principle, be less subject to interferences by enzyme inhibitors or colored substances present in the biological fluid. Recently, it has been pointed out[30] that the plate readers used for ELISA assays should be checked for reproducibility, not only by repeated measurements on the same well, but also by removing the plate and repositioning it. We have recently replicated some of Hammock's findings in our own laboratory.[31] Figure 4 shows the variation of the optical density readings from the row mean when plates containing a dye were scanned twice without moving the plate ("Normal Repeat"). As can be seen, there is very little difference between the two plate readers A and C by this test, and both show only small variations. If, however, the plate is removed and turned 180° so that the top of the plate now becomes the bottom and vice versa and this reading is repeated ("Reverse Repeat"), reader C shows much more variation than does reader A.

The importance of the percent variations is illustrated in Figure 5 in which we converted the results of a variance in the OD reading to the percent change in measured analyte for a competitive inhibition enzyme immunoassay. After the OD readings are subjected to a logit log transformation program for the calculation of analyte concentrations, the OD errors are magnified. Thus, at low analyte concentrations (88% antibody bound), an OD error of 2% translates into a measurement error of 20%. Although these tests were carried out with microplate readers, they do point out the fact that careful attention to instruments used in measurement is always essential for good quantitative results.

H. FLUORESCENCE IMMUNOASSAY

Because fluorescence can be measured with high degree of sensitivity, the use of fluorescent labeled ligands in immunoassay offers attractive possibilities. The major problem with fluorescence immunoassays is the high background of natural fluorescence which determines the actual sensitivity of an assay. In order to overcome this, two approaches have been proposed. In one, which will be described in detail in a later paper, fluorescence polarization is measured instead of fluorescence. The basic concept is that, due to slow rotation in solution of large

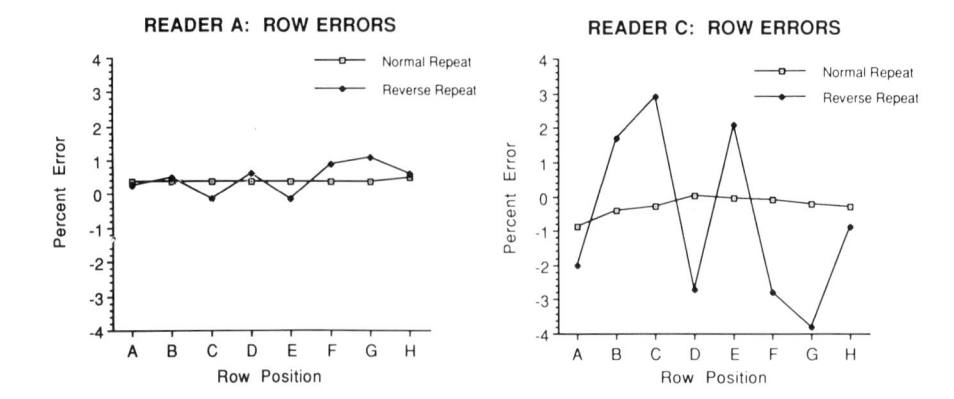

FIGURE 4. Reproducibility of two plate readers (as percentage difference from initial plate mean) for an ELISA as a function of row position. In "normal repeat" the plate was read again without moving; in "reverse repeat" the plate was turned 180° before rereading.

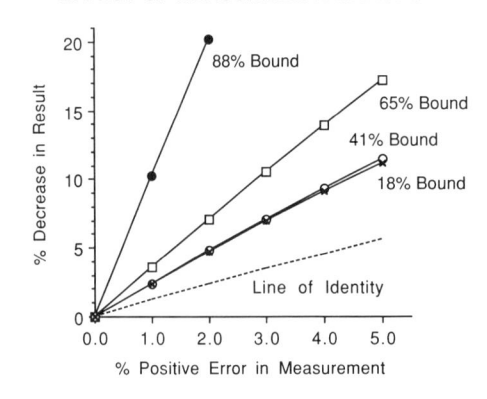

FIGURE 5. Percent error in analyte concentration as a function of error in optical density (OD) measurement. Assumptions were background OD 0.150; OD in absence of analyte 0.900; logit-log analysis of data.

molecules, fluorescent ligands which are bound to them will have increased polarization of the emitted fluorescence. The rapidly tumbling small molecules in solution will not exhibit polarization of the fluorescence.

In an alternative approach, advantage is taken of the rapid decay rate of natural fluorescence. The fluorescence of rare earth containing fluorophores is relatively slow. By intermittently pulsing with the exciting wave length, waiting for natural fluorescence to decay and then measuring the long lasting fluorescent emission, one can greatly enhance the overall sensitivity of the assay. As a final alternative, one may concentrate the fluorescent material, washing away some of the endogenous fluorescence. All of these fluorescence techniques are relatively new and undoubtedly some of their disadvantages remain to be discovered. However, they do offer promise of good selectivity and sensitivity without the problems associated with radioactivity.

I. INTERFERENCES

All of the immunoassay techniques rely ultimately on the binding of the antibody with hapten. As such, they are all susceptible to anything which interferes with this binding. A list of some recent reports of interfering substances is given in Figure 6. Most deal with immunoassays although GC and MS are also included. Many of these are adulterants which would not be present in the usual urine sample and, therefore, are more a problem of sample integrity than a true analytical problem. Others, such as the previously reported false positive results caused

INTERFERENCES IN ASSAYS

Interferent	Assay[a]	Result[b]	Reference
Ibuprofen	C	+	Syva, 1986
Ibuprofen	C	−	Brunk, 1988
Ranitidine	C	+	Grinstead, 1989
H_2O_2	Bd	−	Warner, 1989
	Bd	+	Warner, 1989
Detergent	C, Bd, P	−	Warner, 1989
	A, B, C, Bd	+	Warner, 1989
NaOCl	Ao, P, C, Bd	−	Warner, 1989
NaHCO₃	O, P	−	Warner, 1989
Visine	C	−	Pearson et al., 1989
Diphenhydramine	Antidepressants	+	Sorisky and Watson, 1986
Labetalol	A	+	Apple et al., 1986
Doxylamine	O	+	Hausmann et al., 1983
Doxylamine	P	+	Schaldenbrand et al., 1981

[a] Assays are: C - cannabinoid; B - barbiturate; Bd - benzodiazepine; A - amphetamine; O - opiate; P - phencyclidine

FIGURE 6. Some reported interferences in assays for drugs of abuse. A "+" in the result column indicates a false positive; a "−" indicates a false negative.

by ibuprofen with earlier EMIT reagents for cannabinoid assay and the interference of phenylpropanolamine with various amphetamine assays, represent potentially more serious situations. The possible interference of phenylpropanolamine, ephedrine, etc. in amphetamine assays is foreseeable on structural grounds. However, a recent report[32] that ranitidine cross-reacts in the EMIT monoclonal antibody assay for amphetamine would have been difficult to predict. Thus, there is always the possibility of an unforeseen and unpredicted interference.

IV. CONCLUSIONS

The array of potential problems which can beset either chromatographic or immunological assays does present a real problem to the analyst and very strongly suggests that a confirmatory test is essential if consequences to an individual are to flow from a positive result. Fortunately, the simple statistical analysis presented earlier in this paper indicates that a screening test which deletes most of the negative samples leads to a highly favorable situation with regard to the confirmatory test. Screening tests should be rapid and permit the determination of large numbers of samples. The confirmatory test can then be a more expensive, time-consuming procedure. This author believes that the most specific procedure available should be used for confirmatory tests. Of the current methods, gas chromatography/mass spectrometry appears best for this purpose. All tests for drugs of abuse should be looked at with a skeptical and critical eye, and apparent negative results of the confirmatory tests should be examined critically as well.

REFERENCES

1. **Anon.,** CAS registers 10 millionth substance, *Chem. Eng. News,* February 26, 30, 1990.
2. **Spiehler, V. R., O'Donnell, C. M., and Gokhale, D. V.,** Confirmation and certainty in toxicology screening, *Clin. Chem.,* 34(8), 1535–1539, 1988.
3. **Root-Bernstein, R. S.,** Misleading reliability, *Sciences N.Y.,* 30(2), 6–8, 1990.
4. **Cook, C. E.,** Analytical methodology for Δ^9-tetrahydrocannabinol and its metabolites, *Alcohol, Drugs, Driving: Abstr. and Rev.,* 2(3–4), 79–91, 1986.
5. **McBay, A. J.,** Cannabinoid testing: forensic and analytical aspects, *Lab. Manag.,* 23, 36–43, 1985.
6. **Harvey, D. J., Leuschner, J. T. A., and Paton, W. D. M.,** Measurement of Δ^1-tetrahydrocannabinol in plasma to the low picogram range by gas chromatography/mass spectrometry using metastable ion detection, *J. Chromatogr.,* 202, 83–92, 1980.
7. **Harris, C. C., Yolken, R. H., Krokan, H., Hsu, I. C.,** Ultrasensitive enzymatic radioimmunoassay: application to detection of cholera toxin and rotavirus, *Proc. Natl. Acad. Sci.,* 76, 5336–5339, 1979.

8. **Wall, M. E. and Taylor, H. L.,** Conjugation of acidic metabolites of Δ^8 and Δ^9-THC in man, in *Marijuana '84, Proceedings of the Oxford Symposium on Cannabis,* Harvey, D. J., Ed., IRL Press Ltd., Oxford, England, 1985, 69–76.
9. **Agurell, S., Halldin, M., Lindgren, J. E., Ohlsson, A., Widman, M., Gillespie, H., and Hollister, L.,** Pharmacokinetics and metabolism of Δ^1-tetrahydrocannabinol and other cannabinoids with emphasis on man, *Pharmacol. Rev.,* 38(1), 21–43, 1986.
10. **Williams, P. I. and Moffat, A. C.,** Identification in human urine of Δ^9-tetrahydrocannabinol-11-oic acid glucuronide: a tetrahydrocannabinol metabolite, *J. Pharm. Pharmacol.,* 32, 445–448, 1980.
11. **Johansson, E., Agurell, S., Hollister, L. E., and Halldin, M. M.,** Prolonged apparent half-life of Δ^1-tetrahydrocannabinol in plasma of chronic marijuana users, *J. Pharm. Pharmacol.,* 40, 374–375, 1988.
12. **Foltz, R. L., McGinnis, K. M., and Chinn, D. M.,** Quantitative measurement of Δ^9-tetrahydrocannabinol and two major metabolites in physiological specimens using capillary column gas chromatography negative ion chemical ionization mass spectrometry, *Biomed. Mass Spectrom.,* 10, 316–323, 1983.
13. **Peat, M. A., Finkle, B. S., and Deyman, M. E.,** Laboratory evaluation of immunoassay kits for the detection of cannabinoids in biological fluids, NIDA Research Monograph, 42, 85–98, 1982.
14. **Wall, M. E.,** personal communication.
15. **Dextraze, P., Griffiths, W. C., Camara, P., Audette, L., and Rosner, M.,** Comparison of fluorescence polarization immunoassay, enzyme immunoassay, and thin-layer chromatography for urine cannabinoid screening. Effects of analyte adsorption and vigorous mixing of specimen on detectability, *Annals Clin. Lab. Sci.,* 19(2), 133–138, 1989.
16. **Lehrer, M. and Meenan, G. M.,** More on the false negative rate for emit cannabinoids, *J. Anal. Toxicol.,* 14, 62, 1990.
17. **Hanson, V. W., Buonarati, M. H., Baseit, R. C., Wade, N. A., Yap, C., Biasotti, A. A., Reeve, V. C., Wong, A. S., and Orbanowsky, M. W.,** Comparison of ^{3}H-and ^{125}I-radioimmunoassay and gas chromatography/mass spectrometry for the determination of Δ^9-tetrahydrocannabinol and cannabinoids in blood and serum, *J. Anal. Toxicol.,* 7, 96–102, 1983.
18. **Schwartz, R. H., Bogema, S., and Thorne, M. M.,** Evaluation of the keystone diagnostic quik test: a paper chromatography test for drugs of abuse in urine, *Arch. Pathol. Lab. Med.,* 113, 363–364, 1989.
19. **Cone, E. J., Menchen, S. L., Paul, B. D., Mell, L. D., and Mitchell, J.,** Validity testing of commercial urine cocaine metabolite assays. I. Assay detection times, individual excretion patterns, and kinetics after cocaine administration to humans, *J. Forensic Sci.,* 34(1), 15–31, 1989.
20. **Schwartz, R. H., Bogema, S., and Thorne, M. M.,** Evaluation of instascreen cannabinoid drug screen test, *Arch. Pathol. Lab. Med.,* 113, 1204, 1989.
21. **Sunshine I.,** Preliminary tests for drugs of abuse. *Clin. Chem.,* 34(2), 331–334, 1988.
22. **Moffat, A. C., Stead, A. H., and Smalldon, K. W.,** *J. Chromatogr.,* 90, 19, 1974.
23. **Fenimore, D. C., Freeman, R. R., and Loy, P. R.,** Determination of Δ^9-tetrahydrocannabinol in blood by electron capture gas chromatography, *Anal. Chem.,* 45, 2331–2335, 1973.
24. **Perrigo, B. J., Peel, H. W., and Ballantyne, D. J.,** Use of dual-column fused-silica capillary gas chromatography in combination with detector response factors for analytical toxicology, *J. Chromatogr.,* 341, 81–88, 1985.
25. **Johansson, E. and Halldin, M. M.,** Urinary excretion half-life of Δ^1-tetrahydrocannabinol-7-oic acid in heavy marijuana users after smoking, *J. Anal. Toxicol.,* 13, 218–223, 1989.
26. **Brunk, S. D.,** False negative GC/MS assay for carboxy THC due to ibuprofen interference, *J. Anal. Toxicol.,* 12, 290–291, 1988.
27. **Anon.,** *Syva Monitor,* Syva Company, Palo Alto, CA, 4(3), 7–8, 1986.
28. **Amersham Corporation** (technical note), Scintillation proximity assay, *Amersham Research News,* 49, 8–9, December, 1989.
29. **Cook, C. E. and Schindler, V. H.,** unpublished.
30. **Harrison, R. O. and Hammock, B. D.,** Location dependent biases in automatic 96-well microplate readers, *J. Assoc. Off. Anal. Chem.,* 71, 981–987, 1988.
31. **Whisnant, C. C.,** personal communication.
32. **Grinstead, G. F.,** Ranitidine and high concentrations of phenylpropanolamine crossreact in the emit monoclonal amphetamine/methamphetamine assay, *Clin. Chem.,* 35(9), 1998–1999, 1989.
33. **Apple, F. S., Googins, M. K., Kastner, S., Nevala, K., Edmondson, S., and Kloss, J.,** Labetalol: false-positive indices by emit-d.a.u. assay and toxi-lab a urine screen, *Clin. Chem.,* 31(7), 1250–1251, 1985.
34. **Pearson, S. D., Ash, K. O., and Urry, F. M.,** Mechanism of false-negative urine cannabinoid immunoassay screens by visine eyedrops, *Clin. Chem.,* 35(4), 636–638, 1989.
35. **Schaldenbrand, J. D., McClatchey, K. D., Patel, J. A., and Muilenberg, M. J.,** Doxylamine: a cause for false-positive gas chromatographic assay for phencyclidine, *Ther. Drug Monitoring,* 3(2), 181–183, 1981.
36. **Sorisky, A. and Watson, D. C.,** Positive diphenhydramine interference in the emit-st assay for tricyclic antidepressants in serum, *Clin. Chem.,* 32(4), 715, 1986.
37. **Wall, M. E. and Brine, D.R.,** Applications of Mass Spectrometry to the Structure of Metabolites of Δ^9-Tetrahydrocannabinol, International Symposium on Mass Spectrometry in Biochemistry and Medicine, Milan, Italy, 1973.
38. **Warner, A.,** Interference of common household chemicals in immunoassay methods for drugs of abuse, *Clin. Chem.,* 35(4), 648–651, 1989.
39. **Hausmann, E., Kohl, B., von Boehmer, H., and Wellhoner, H. H.,** False-positive emit indication of opiates and methadone in a doxylamine intoxication. *J. Clin. Chem. Clin. Biochem.,* 21(10), 599–600, 1983.

Chapter 15

PRESUMPTIVE ANALYSIS: CUTOFF AND SPECIFICITY

Brian Widdop

TABLE OF CONTENTS

I.	Introduction	84
II.	Essential Characteristics of Presumptive Tests	84
III.	Sensitivity and Threshold (Cutoff)	84
IV.	Precision	84
V.	Criteria for Selection of a "Cutoff" Level	85
VI.	Comparison of Assays	86
VII.	Threshold Concentrations in Common Use	87
VIII.	Specificity of Preliminary Tests	87
References		88

I. INTRODUCTION

Urine testing for abused drugs became a routine exercise in the United States when methadone maintenance programs were introduced in the early 1960s. This type of treatment regime was adopted soon afterwards by European countries, and laboratory support services were organized that continue to this day.

In this context, the laboratory results are used to establish which drugs new patients are taking and subsequently to monitor compliance with the rehabilitation program.

Very often, a single test using an immunoassay, thin layer chromatography, or gas-liquid chromatography is acceptable evidence since the treatment programs are not punitive. Some laboratories offer a more discerning service which pin-points more specifically the substance detected.[1]

In other circumstances, where the detection of an illicit or prohibited substance in the urine can lead to loss of liberty, failure to secure employment, or job dismissal, a single test is inadequate. Any positive results must be substantiated by a second test using a different analytical technique with greater sensitivity and selectivity. The first test is therefore defined as presumptive and the second is the confirmatory test.

II. ESSENTIAL CHARACTERISTICS OF PRESUMPTIVE TESTS

The incidence of drug abuse among the general European population is still quite small. The author's experience of screening various workforce populations in the U.K. indicates a presumptive positive rate of around 5%; this falls to less than 1% after confirmatory analyses. It makes sense, therefore, to apply presumptive tests which are rapid and easily performed so that the vast majority of negative samples can be disregarded. By the same token, presumptive positive samples can be referred quickly for closer scrutiny by, for example, GC/MS.

Repetitive manual testing of large numbers of samples, especially when most are negative, leads eventually to boredom and operational errors. Presumptive tests should therefore be amenable to automation. This can also facilitate the operation of internal quality control procedures if the equipment can be programmed to highlight any significant deviation from acceptable analytical performance.

Confirmatory testing, in particular GC/MS, tends to be slow, complex, and expensive. The number of samples which test positive by the initial procedure, but are not confirmed as positive should therefore be kept to a minimum. At the same time, the number of samples which give false negatives should also be minimized to reduce the risk of not detecting drug abuse.

The above criteria are best satisfied by immunological techniques (enzyme, radioactive, or fluorescence polarization immunoassays).

III. SENSITIVITY AND THRESHOLD (CUTOFF)

The sensitivity or limit of detection of an assay can be defined as the lowest concentration of the analyte which can be detected reliably in a given matrix. All analytical instrument detectors generate a certain degree of analytical noise and this is exacerbated in the presence of a complex matrix such as urine. Sensitivity is therefore limited by the magnitude of the signal produced by the drug in comparison to the background noise. It follows that as the concentration of drug approaches the detection limit, it becomes increasingly difficult to discriminate between the response due to the drug and the background noise.

To overcome this problem, a threshold or cutoff concentration is selected for a particular assay which exceeds the detection limit by several fold. Sample results are then judged against this threshold level.

Thus, all samples which yield results equal to or greater than the cutoff level are designated presumptive positives; those with results below are deemed negative. There is a slight flaw in this rule in that statistically, all samples which give results ±2 SD of the mean cutoff value should be considered presumptive positive and sent for confirmatory testing. With a small sample load, this can be instituted without difficulty. However, it is understandable that high volume laboratories, such as those serving the U.S. Armed Forces, choose to ignore this to conserve GC/MS time.

One disadvantage of adopting threshold concentrations is that a urine sample which contains a drug in lower quantities will be taken as negative. However, this must be balanced against the inevitable increase in unconfirmed (false) positive results caused by variation in the sensitivity of the assay.

IV. PRECISION

A proportion of samples will contain the analyte at a concentration near to the chosen threshold level of the

TABLE 1
Precision of Results in 10 Aliquots of a Subject's Urine

Test no.	Result (ng/ml)
1	98
2	101
3	95
4	99
5	103
6	(130)
7	100
8	97
9	96
10	102
Mean ± SD	102 ± 10.1
CV(%)	9.9
Omit result No.6	
Mean ± SD	99 ± 2.7
CV(%)	2.8

From Blanke, R. V., *Clin. Chem.*, 33/11(B), 41B–45B, 1987. With permission.

test. It then becomes difficult to assign positive or negative status to a sample of this type unless the method has good precision. An example which illustrates this point is given in Table 1 and is taken from Blanke.[2]

Dr. Blanke's data was based on a test for a metabolite of tetrahydrocannabinol using a threshold of 100 ng/ml. A specimen with an analyte concentration near the threshold was divided into ten portions and each one assayed.

Clearly the method has excellent precision, although assay number six was an outlier and can be proved to be so by statistical analysis. Repetitive testing of this type of sample can therefore yield a valid estimate of the true value; in this example the mean value of 99 ng/ml derived by omitting the outlier would assign the sample as negative.

In practice, unknown specimens are tested only once by immunoassay and those giving results over the threshold level pass onto confirmatory analysis; "negative" samples are discarded. Even with good precision, therefore, some of the samples with analyte concentrations approaching the "cutoff" will either fail the confirmatory test or be wrongly categorized as negative (negative outliers also occur). To mitigate these problems, careful monitoring of assay performance and prompt correction of defects are essential.

VI. CRITERIA FOR SELECTION OF A "CUTOFF" LEVEL

Where to set the threshold levels is a vexed question, but the following criteria are a starting point for discussion.

1. The level should be low enough to allow for detection of recent abuse.
2. The level should be high enough to minimize false positives due to analytical noise or sample matrix effects.
3. The level should be equivalent to or higher than that of the confirmation procedure to minimize the number of unconfirmed positive samples.
4. The level should be high enough to eliminate positive test results due to inadvertent exposure to the drug.

As regards criterion 1, the operative term is *recent abuse* and what exactly this means can be defined only by the aims and objectives of the testing program. If the intention is to detect as many drug users as possible, the lowest cutoff level feasible (bearing in mind the constraints of criterion 2) must be chosen and any samples which yield results –2 SD below this should be categorized presumptive positive. This will inevitably lead to a greater number of samples which have to be re-analyzed by GC/MS with a corresponding impact on the cost of the program. Surprisingly, some laboratories fail to take heed of criterion 3 and apply confirmatory tests which are less sensitive than the primary screening test. This results in a higher proportion of truly positive samples being reported as negative. This fundamental error is compounded when, as is often the case, the preliminary immunoassay cross-reacts with other metabolites in addition to that which is estimated by the confirmation technique. For example, immunoassays for cannabinoids are standardized against 11-nor-delta-9-tetrahydrocannabi-

TABLE 2
Analysis of Seven Urine Samples Positive for Cannabinoids by EMIT-dau by Alternative Methods[8]

Test	Positive	Negative	Cutoff (ng/ml) THC-COOH [a]
EMIT-dau	7	0	20
EMIT-st	0	7	100
Immunalysis (RIA)	3	3	6
Abuscreen (RIA)	0	7	100
Toxi-Lab	0	7	20
GC/MS	4	3	4

(GC/MS values: 4.9, 17.6, 9.9, 7.8)

[a] 11-nor-delta-9-tetrahydrocannabinol-9-carboxylic acid.

nol-9-carboxylic acid, but react with other cannabinoids present in urine samples. It is possible, therefore, to achieve a positive result judged against a standard of 100 ng/ml of 11-nor-delta-9-THC-COOH in a urine sample containing considerably less than this or even none at all. It follows, then, that by reducing the threshold concentration of the confirmatory method as far below that of the primary test as is technically and economically possible, fewer unconfirmed positives will ensue.

Criterion 4 is concerned with the much debated argument that passive inhalation of cannabis smoke can yield a positive urine test for cannabinoids. Several laboratory investigations of this topic have appeared in the literature.[3-6] These studies invariably involved exposing nonsmokers to high, sometimes intolerable, concentrations of cannabis smoke in unventilated small spaces for up to 3 hours at a time. Cone et al.[3] were hardest on their volunteers who at one stage were exposed to the smoke of 16 marijuana cigarettes for 1 hour each day for six consecutive days. All but one of the five subjects voided urine samples which gave positive results with the EMIT dau-20 cannabinoid assay and the reaction rates frequently exceeded those of the 75 ng/ml calibrator. With a lower exposure rate of four marijuana cigarettes for 1 hour a day, four of the volunteers were positive on at least one occasion, but the reaction rates were only slightly higher than those for the low calibrator (20 ng/ml). Nevertheless, the latter experiment, where the conditions were not that far removed from those which might exist in a social environment, suggests that higher threshold levels (e.g., 50 or 100 ng/ml) should be used to rule out passive inhalation. Raising the levels has the additional benefit of reducing the number of tests which cannot be confirmed by GC/MS.[7]

VI. COMPARISON OF ASSAYS

Several publications have appeared which compare methods and these illustrate the wide range of cutoff levels and cross-reactivities associated with different assay systems.

Frederick et al.[8] compared the performance of four immunoassays, Toxi-Lab, and a GC/MS method in detecting the cannabinoid metabolite 11-nor-delta-9-tetrahydrocannabinol-9-carboxylic acid. Urine specimens (88) collected in an emergency room were analyzed for cannabinoids by EMIT dau-20 and Toxi-Lab. EMIT dau-20 gave positive results with 42 specimens, 7 of which were negative by Toxi-Lab. The discrepant samples were reanalyzed by the remaining four assay systems and the results are summarized in Table 2.

Failure of the EMIT-st and Abuscreen RIA systems to detect cannabinoids in these specimens is a reflection of the fivefold difference in cutoff levels compared to EMIT-dau.

The immunalysis RIA and GC/MS results were in complete agreement, but three of the EMIT-dau positive samples could not be confirmed by GC/MS. This can most probably be ascribed to the wider cross-reactivity of the EMIT-dau antibodies toward other cannabinoid metabolites; note that in the four specimens confirmed as positive by GC/MS all had THC-COOH concentrations below the EMIT-dau cutoff level of 20 ng/ml.

This type of investigation again emphasizes the need first to define the objectives of a drug screening program and then to select that preliminary testing system which best fits the bill. Moreover, the crucial role of a highly specific and quantitative confirmation method such as GC/MS as the yardstick for interpreting results is well illustrated.

TABLE 3
Threshold Concentrations for Preliminary Tests (ng/ml)

Analyte	U.S. Military	NIDA/CAP	NPU
Amphetamines	1000	1000	300
Barbiturates	200	—	300
Benzodiazepines	—	—	300
Cannabinoids	100	100	50
Cocaine (benzoylecgonine)	300	300	300
Methadone	—	—	300
Methaqualone	—	—	300
Opiates(morphine)	300	300	75
Phenyclidine	25	25	75

VII. THRESHOLD CONCENTRATIONS IN COMMON USE

As the practice of drug abuse testing in the military forces and industry escalated in the United States, it became necessary to devise inspection and accreditation programs for laboratories working in this area. The American Association for Clinical Chemistry (AACC) and the College of American Pathologists (CAP) formulated a Forensic Urine Drug Testing (FUDT) Program aimed specifically at substance abuse testing laboratories. The Department of Health and Human Services (DHHS)[9] issued guidelines for laboratories engaged in drug testing of federal employees which included the mandatory requirement to comply with the National Institute of Drug Abuse (NIDA) accreditation program. Both these programs and the Department of Defense (DOD) specify threshold concentrations based on which laboratories have to prove proficiency in distinguishing positive and negative samples. These include threshold concentrations for both preliminary tests and confirmatory tests. Table 3 lists these preliminary testing specifications alongside the cutoff levels currently used in the author's (National Poisons Unit) laboratory for substance abuse testing in the workplace.

It will be noted from Table 3 that the American accreditation schemes encompass only five drugs at present. This probably reflects both the predominance of these substances as abused agents in the United States and the difficulties of laying down confirmation test criteria for such a diverse group of drugs as the benzodiazepines.

VIII. SPECIFICITY OF PRELIMINARY TESTS

Significant cross-reactivity of immunoassays toward unrelated substances is undesirable. Whereas manufacturers take great pains to test a wide range of drugs for cross-reactivity prior to marketing the product, absolute specificity can never be guaranteed. Several years ago reports that urine samples from people taking nonsteroidal anti-inflammatory drugs (ibuprofen, fenoprofen, and naproxen) could give positive cannabinoid tests by EMIT[7] compelled the manufacturer to modify the assay. In fairness, no one could have predicted that the cannabinoid antibodies would cross-react with simple phenylpropionic acid derivatives and the manufacturer's response was swift and effective. What is surprising, however, is how long it took to recognize interference from such a popular nonprescription drug as ibuprofen and this must imply that many "positive" samples were not referred for confirmation tests.

More recently, an EMIT assay containing two monoclonal antibodies with high specificity for d-amphetamine and d-methamphetamine was launched. This was designed to reduce the number of false positives attributable to the use of OTC preparations containing other phenylethylamine compounds such as ephedrine, phenylpropanolamine, isoxsuprine, and l-methylamphetamine. Another attraction was its increased sensitivity toward methylenedioxymethamphetamine (MDMA), a substance which has sporadic popularity amongst American and U.K. drug abusers. While no doubt an advance in these respects, when the assay was applied to samples from treatment clinics, significant cross-reactivity toward phenothiazine metabolites was disclosed; patients undergoing therapy for drug addiction are often prescribed phenothiazines for anxiety. The EMIT polyclonal antibody assay, which does not cross-react with phenothiazine metabolites, is therefore more appropriate in the clinical situation.

With the exception of the RIA developed by the Diagnostic Products Corporation (DPC), Los Angeles, CA,

TABLE 4
Relative Cross-Reactivities of Opiates Immunoassays

Supplier	Syva	Syva	Abbott	Roche	DPC
Assay	EMIT-dau opiate[a]	EMIT-st opiate[a]	TDX opiate[b]	Abuscreen morphine[c]	Coat-a-count morphine[c]
Opiate cross-reactivity					
Morphine	100%	100%	100%	100%	100%
Morphine-3-glucuronide	24%	33%	47%	80%	0.2%
Normorphine	0.5%	—	4%	—	—
Codeine	104%	100%	127%	110%	0.2%
Dihydro-codeine	93%	—	48%	—	—

[a] EMIT technique.
[b] FPIA technique.
[c] RIA technique.

immunoassays for opiates detect both free and conjugated morphine as well as other opiate drugs such as codeine and dihydrocodeine (Table 4). Other cross-reacting opiates not listed in Table 4 include hydrocodone, hydromorphine, oxycodone, and pholcodine (morpholinylethylmorphine). These drugs and codeine are present in a wide variety of proprietary analgesic or cough medicines. Codeine is metabolized to morphine and norcodeine, and after 20 hours of dosage, the urine morphine concentration exceeds that of codeine.[10] A highly specific and sensitive immunoassay for morphine has limited advantages, therefore, given the ubiquitous use of codeine preparations.

Specificity toward a group of related substances, as in the case of the amphetamines and the opiates, can be considered advantageous. Phenylethylamine derivatives such as mephentermine, phentermine, and ephedrine are often abused when amphetamine and methamphetamine are not available. High doses of codeine or dihydrocodeine are commonly used as substitutes for heroin. The value of being able to detect these congeners in samples from treatment centers has long been recognized. There is no reason why these substances should not be proscribed in the workplace, provided employees are given full opportunity to prove their legitimate use before or after testing.

Group specificity toward the barbiturates and benzodiazepines is obviously desirable. However, it is unlikely that the newer, low-dose benzodiazepine drugs, such as triazolam, will be detectable by conventional immunoassays.[11]

Immunoassays for cocaine (targeted toward the benzoylecgonine metabolite), methadone, and phencyclidine (PCP) are very specific and no reports of undesirable cross-reactivity have yet emerged.

REFERENCES

1. **Widdop, B.,** Hospital toxicology, in *Clarke's Isolation and Identification of Drugs,* Moffat, A. C., Ed., The Pharmaceutical Press, London, 1986, 3–34.
2. **Blanke, R. V.,** Quality assurance in drug-use testing, *Clin. Chem.,* 33/11(B), 41B–45B 1987.
3. **Cone, E. J., Johnson, R. E., Darvin, W. D., et al.,** Passive inhalation of marijuana smoke, urine analysis and room air levels of delta-9-tetrahydrocannabinol, *J. Anal. Toxicol.,* 11, 89–96, 1987.
4. **Cone, E. J. and Johnson, R. E.,** Contact highs and urinary cannabinoid excretion after passive exposure to marijuana smoke, *Clin. Pharmacol. Ther.,* 40, 247–256, 1986.
5. **Morland, J., Bugge, A., Skuterud, B., et al.,** Cannabinoids in blood and urine after passive inhalation of cannabis smoke, *J. Forensic Sci.,* 30, 997–1002, 1985.
6. **Perez-Reyes, M., Diguiseppi, S., Davis, K. H., et al.,** Comparison of effects of marijuana cigarettes of three different potencies, *Clin. Pharmacol. Ther.,* 31, 617–624, 1982.
7. **McBay, A. J.,** Drug analysis technology — pitfalls and problems of drug testing, in *Analytical Aspects of Drug Testing,* Deutsch, D. G., Ed., John Wiley & Sons, NewYork, 1989, 273–293.
8. **Frederick, D. L., Green, J., and Fowler, M. W.,** Comparison of six cannabinoid metabolite assays, *J. Anal. Toxicol.,* 9, 116–124 1985.
9. **U.S. Department of Health and Human Services,** Scientific and technical guidelines for federal drug testing programs; standards for certification of laboratories engaged in urine drug testing for federal agencies; notice of proposed guidelines, *Fed. Reg.,* 52, 30638–30652, 1987.
10. **Posey, B. L. and Kimble, S. N.,** High performance liquid chromatographic study of codeine, norcodeine, and morphine as indicator of codeine ingestion, *J. Anal. Toxicol.,* 8, 68–73, 1984.
11. **Fraser, A. D.,** Urinary screening for alprazolam, triazolam and their metabolites with the EMIT-dau benzodiazepine metabolite assay, *J. Anal. Toxicol.,* 11, 263–266, 1987.

Chapter 16

IN SITU ABUSE DRUG DETECTION

Angel L. Calvo

TABLE OF CONTENTS

I.	Current State of Abuse Drug Detection	90
II.	The Role of *In Situ* Detection	91
III.	*In Situ* Detection Technologies	93
IV.	Critical Aspects in Drug Detection and Their Approach in the *In Situ* Mode	95
V.	Applicability of *In Situ* Detection in Companies	95
	References	96

I. CURRENT STATE OF ABUSE DRUG DETECTION

After two decades of accumulated experience in the analysis of abuse drugs, the current state of the question is still one of great imprecision and requires, above all, greater clarity and systematization. The United States offers superior experience in the matter in relation to the European countries.

We may encounter implications, not only of a legal, but also of a constitutional nature, in the definition of a drug abuse (hereinafter abbreviated to D.O.A.) detection policy. The implication is the personal right of not being investigated in aspects of private life, contained in the constitutional law of practically all countries. But almost all also include the codicil: saving the existence of a reasonable suspicion and that this interference has a useful value in the protection of the lives and property of third parties.

A typical model is the 4th Amendment to the Constitution of the U.S.[1] "The right of the people to be secure in their personal houses, papers and effects against unreasonable searches and seizures, but upon probable cause ... ."

In these circumstances, we may conclude, in an initial approach, that detecting D.O.A. should meet certain applicability requirements:

1. Have the approval of the person being checked
2. Otherwise, have the legal backing of "social protection"

The first case is not conflictive and includes drug addicts in the process of voluntary rehabilitation. They are explicitly subjected to controls. We could also explicitly include workers in professional risk groups, i.e., all those jobs that involve the use of dangerous tools or weapons or the driving and control of means of transport, such as train drivers, commercial pilots, air traffic controllers, etc., where being under the effects of drugs could entail risks for third parties or for themselves. A clause requiring submission to controls could be included in the contracts and specific ordinances. In some way, signing a contract or agreeing to belong to a group (armed forces, fire brigade, police, etc.) is a voluntary act entailing duties.

We may pinpoint yet another nonconflictive group with implicit approval: accident victims admitted to casualty departments. The physician in charge may implicitly order whatever tests he may deem necessary to guarantee the survival of the patient. Ascertaining a toxicological profile is essential for the application of emergency treatment.

The second case is really conflictive since the beneficiary of detection is not the drug addict but third parties and, in fact, society. And not only is he not the beneficiary, it may even be damaging to his interests in legal environments in which confirmed drug addiction may entail a penalty or a loss of economic or civil rights (dismissal, demotion, aggravation of criminal liability, etc.).

Examples of this application of D.O.A. detection may be persons suspected of committing an offense, private drivers behaving abnormally, or employees in not necessarily risk groups. The problem raised, in respect of which many legislators are extremely cautious, is the term "suspicion", i.e., the criterion for suspecting a person. There is an evident risk of adopting criteria based on race, social class, age, etc. But this is not all; the result of detection is often punishment. This calls for a complex mechanism for detecting D.O.A. and safeguarding the reliability of the legal decision. The problem is even greater in random detections in very large collectives, such as the personnel of big companies, etc., where trade unions' pressure does not always permit the establishment of indiscriminate detection programs.

This legal classification is supplemented with the classification of "needs", which is the one that defines the analytical needs in relation to the test conception and design. Let us say that there are two fields of detection.

1. Quick decision-making needs that will avoid the risk situation:
   - Administering methadone to a drug addict in treatment
   - Preventing a member of a professional risk group from using his tool or driving his vehicle if suspected of being under the influence of drugs
   - Crisis treatment in hospital emergencies
   - Others so requiring
2. Needs to confirm a positive result for making serious and nonurgent decisions
   - Penalizing drivers
   - Job transfer
   - Nonacceptance of job applications
   - Forensic reports in legal proceedings
   - Others that may be laid down by the law

A different detection concept emerges in each of them. In the former (quick decisions), the so-called preliminary

TEST	TECHNIQUE	NEED	SITE
Preliminary	Immunochemical	Fast decisions as a caution	Decentralized
Confirmatory	Gas chromatography/ Mass spectrometry	To make serious and definitive decisions	Specialized labs.

FIGURE 1. Concepts on drug of abuse testing.

GROUP	PURPOSE
Drug addicts under treatment	- Self-control - Monitoring drug intake during treatment
Professional groups (High risk)	- Accident prevention - To avoid weapons abuse
Emergency room in hospitals	- To make decissions for overcoming crisis after overdose - To know toxicological profile prior to surgery
Drivers	- Accident prevention
Employees (Low or no risk)	- To avoid loss of efficiency - To decrease absenteeism
Convicts and arrested individuals	- Internal control in jails - To prevent abstinence syndrome in police station

FIGURE 2. Groups and purposes for on-site testing.

test is gradually prevailing: a quick, simple detection that is inexpensive in means and personnel. It responds to the so-called "decentralized analysis" solution common to other fields of clinical analysis. The preliminary test only seeks to provide a reasonable basis for a precautionary measure: prevent anyone under the effects of drugs from assuming a situation of risk either for himself or others.

The confirmation test seeks to confirm or discount the preliminary result so as to be able to take conclusive measures. Confirmation detection is usually complex (as a counterpart to its efficacy) and requires professional means and personnel.

As is usually the case in analytical chemistry, a confirmatory method should be based on a different technology from the preliminary one, i.e., a technique is not confirmed by itself. The most widely accepted confirmatory technique and the one accepted as a universal reference is mass spectrometry combined with gas chromatography. Preliminary tests are usually based on techniques of an immunochemical type. Among these, the "decentralization" concept is beginning to be successful, both in the United States and in Europe, and it is often referred to as *in situ* detection. Figure 1 summarizes the two philosophies.

II. THE ROLE OF *IN SITU* DETECTION

In situ D.O.A. detection has its specific niche in the analytical and control effort. Needless to say, it should be regarded as a preliminary test and its most specific feature is that it permits decentralized working and the precautionary decisions that we referred to previously.

It is necessary to define what groups, what purposes, what advantages it may have, and what are the stipulations that may be required of an *in situ* detection test.

The groups (see Figure 2) would be drug addicts in disintoxication periods or protocols, in order to avoid administering methadone to one who has not given up his addiction, as well as a means of establishing a dissuasive measure, since individuals will know that they may be subjected to quick instant control. Members of professional risk groups, such as the police, professional armed servicemen (more precise regulations may be required in countries with compulsory military service), airline pilots, train and bus drivers, public works personnel, miners, merchant sailors, and an extensive etc. In these collectives, the preliminary test prevents a person, for instance, from going on duty under the effects of drugs. It is purely precautionary and in no circumstance should it

ADVANTAGE	DISADVANTAGE	WAY TO OVERCOME
* Ready to use test in any place	* Risk of missunderstanding between performers and tested persons	* Good explanations about real value of initial tests
* Visual method	* Optimal storage conditions of reagents not always achievable	* Robust design
* Good communication with tested subject		
* Adulterants addition is more difficult		

FIGURE 3. Advantages/disadvantages breakdown.

entail a final decision. This is the exclusive prerogative of the confirmative test. Another group of exceptional importance is that of the aforementioned emergency admissions.

Recently, with the entry into force of the new Traffic Act in Spain, we are spectators of a wide-ranging controversy regarding D.O.A. detection on the roads. The philosophy is similar to that already implemented for alcohol (although it presents greater operative problems, as the collection of the sample [urine] necessarily gives rise to situations of a certain discomfort). *In situ* tests therefore offer a possibility of remedying this problem.

In companies, detection may be applied generally, both at admission and on a periodic basis, or as a random selection. In the last case, it has a dissuasive purpose and for it to have due effect, a clear negotiated corporate policy has to be laid down.[2]

Finally, we should mention the police and forensic sphere as a possible target group. It is decidedly conflictive, especially in the most liberal countries in Europe. It has a variety of purposes, but two goals may be set: ascertaining whether the suspect is under the effects of drugs at the time of arrest in order to adopt the consequent measures with him, and to establish control and assistance programs in prisons.

What all these groups have in common in detection work is the need for an *in situ* test, capable of being operative in drug addict care centers, often integrated in social welfare or in town halls welfare, and far removed from hospitals or laboratories with instrumental means, police stations, military barracks, building sites, etc.

Apart from the possibility of reaching a variety of different places, the main advantages of the *in situ* test are simplification of the chain of custody or procedure to be applied to ensure the nonmanipulation of samples for fraudulent purposes. Although positive results dispatched for confirmation still require this, it guarantees the dissuasive capacity of the test as the individual being tested may observe how the test is carried through and how the result appears. It also permits dialog with the drug addict, as no more than a few minutes elapse between collection of the sample and the result.

On the other hand, the most significant drawbacks are that the declaration of a result on the part of a person not specialized in analytical tests may not always be done properly, although this may be overcome with a certain training, assuming that the result of the preliminary test is only provisional, pending the confirmative one; and the lack, at times, of reagent conservation facilities (temperature and humidity) in place calls for systems less sensitive to adverse environmental conditions.

Figure 3 analyzes the advantages and drawbacks. In spite of everything, *in situ* detection is gaining in acceptance as it is seldom possible to have sophisticated means in place that would be desirable.

Figure 4 shows the requirements that should be met by an *in situ* D.O.A. detection test. We should stress that the technique should be "open to view". In other words, the method has to be so simple as to permit "visual" follow-up of the course of the reaction, as there are no electronic control and check systems.

On the other hand, we have to point out the need for it to be a test of high analytical sensitivity (>98%) so as to prevent, or at least minimize, the possibility of a false negative occurring. This is a characteristic common to screening tests, where the strategy is to prevent a positive

```
* METHOD: AS SIMPLE AS POSSIBLE
* NO LAB. FACILITIES
* WITHOUT INVOLVING INSTRUMENTS
* NO FIGURES HANDLING IN RESULTS INTERPRETATION
* VISUAL CONTROL OF REACTION
* TO BE ROBUST AT ROOM TEMPERATURE
* TO OFFER A HIGH ANALYTICAL SENSITIVITY
```

FIGURE 4. Requirements for an on-site test.

being given as a negative (think, for instance, of the anti-HIV or AIDS virus antibody detection tests when performed on blood donors), even though specificity is lost, i.e., there is an increased risk of false positives.[3] The false positive is investigated in the confirmative test.

These characteristics are largely met by the latex agglutination systems, as we shall see later on.

III. *IN SITU* DETECTION TECHNOLOGIES

Agglutination techniques are quite old and nowadays they are regarded, often unfairly, as "low technology". A very well-known example is the classic pregnancy test, which also belongs to the *in situ* or decentralized analysis class. Figure 5 shows us the general design of the reaction. As may be seen, a latex ball covered with molecules of the metabolite of the drug to be detected is confronted with a specific antibody thereof.

This antibody will have affinity for the molecules of the drug and a molecular network will be built up (agglutination) which will precipitate. If there is a metabolite from the sample in the reaction medium, it will enter into competition with its counterpart by binding itself to the antibody, thus blocking the linkage points and inhibiting agglutination.

The immunochemical type reaction can be carried out in various supports, such as test tubes, cuvettes, strips, etc., but maximum convenience and reliability is attained on slides with the reaction medium spread over a surface. In this way we obtain the maximum reaction rate and the result is viewable in a few minutes. The macroscopic appearance of the result is (see Figure 5) either granular, which corresponds to agglutination (negative), or milky, which corresponds to nonagglutination (positive). There

may also a possibility of not being able to be define clearly whether it is one way or the other. In this case, the interpretation is that the sample contains a drug metabolite content approximately equal to the cutoff value chosen. For sample classification purposes it should be regarded as doubtful, but bearing in mind that any granulation, no matter how small, is due to the absence of the metabolite in the sample. The correct action is to repeat the test; if repeatedly negative, it is considered as such. If it remains doubtful, it has to be assumed that the sample is indeed on the borderline.

The operative method is simple (as is seen in the middle of Figure 5). Note that the reaction area is separated from the display area by a channel. The purpose of this is to prevent one of the greatest problems in agglutination techniques, which is the difficulty of display on irregular surfaces.

One of the biggest drawbacks that have been declared against agglutination tests is the lack of specificity, but this is not due to the test in itself but to the fact that in the 1950s and 1960s, when they were the only technology available, they did not demand monoclonal antibodies. It is now possible to use them and obtain specificities as good as in other techniques.

The slide arrangement, reagents, and technique described correspond to the product marketed by Roche Diagnostics Systems, Inc., Montclair, NJ, under the generic name of Abuscreen® Ontrak™.

As regards the reference method, gas chromatography/mass spectrometry (GC/MS), the Ontrak™ tests behave with good sensitivity, close on 99% on average, depending on the metabolite investigated. Figure 6 shows a correlation histogram.

The method offers a further advantage, in addition to its simplicity, and is that it is not susceptible to adultera-

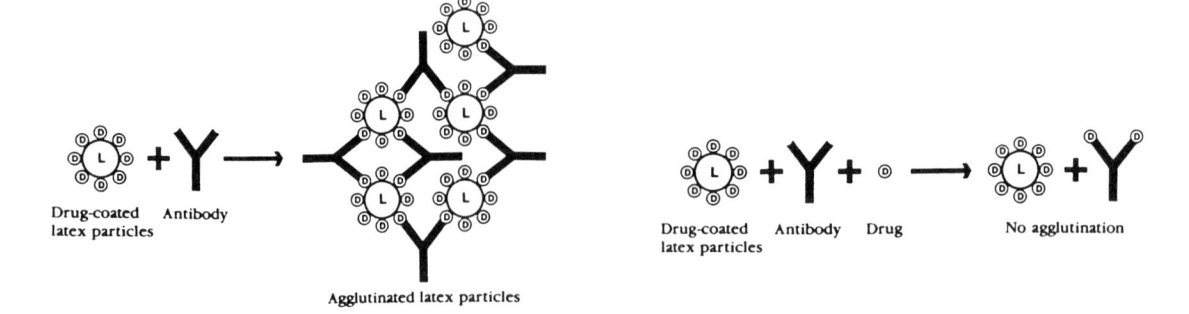

Graphic representation of a reaction with a negative urine sample

Graphic representation of a reaction with a positive urine sample

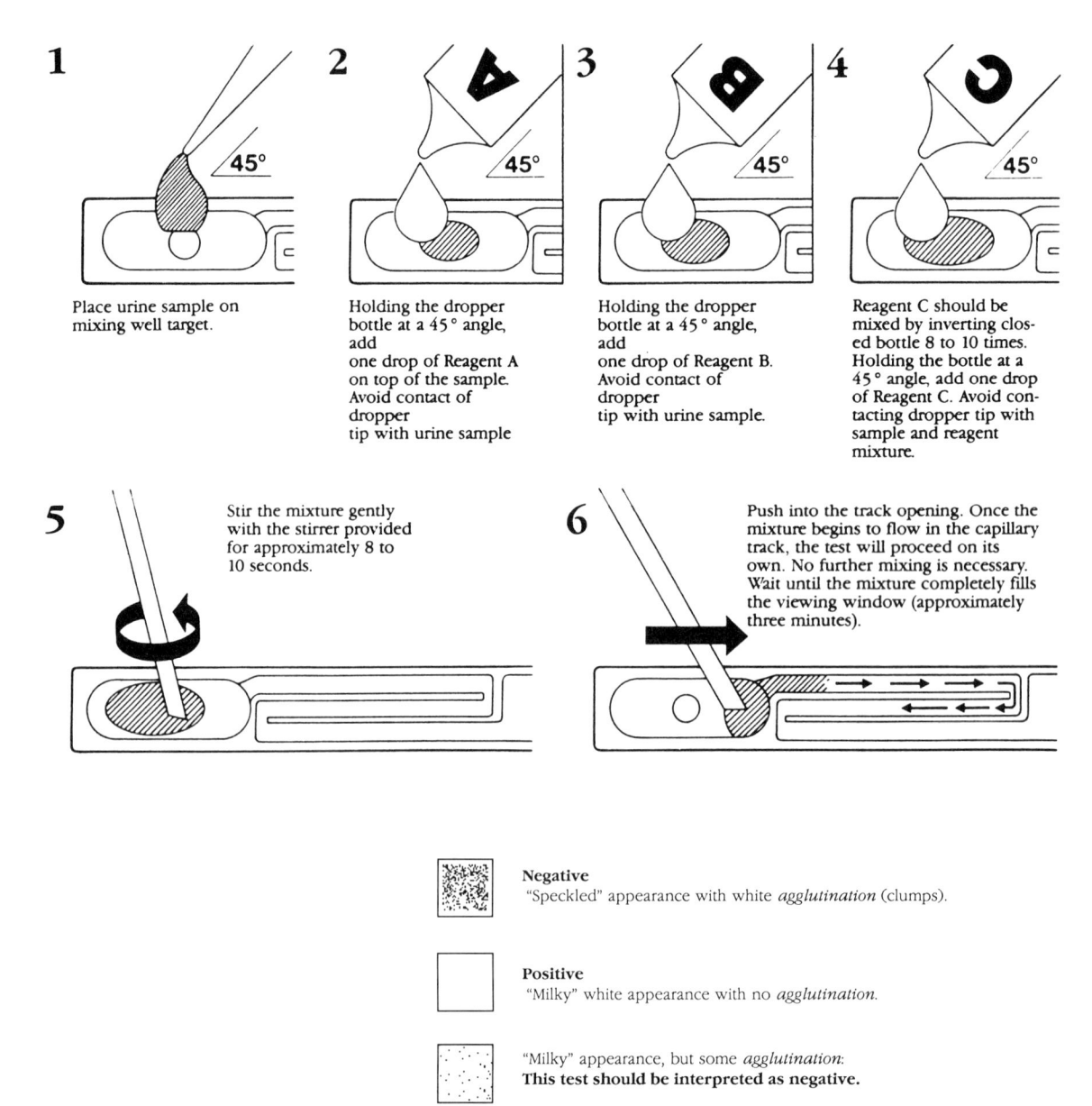

1 Place urine sample on mixing well target.

2 Holding the dropper bottle at a 45° angle, add one drop of Reagent A on top of the sample. Avoid contact of dropper tip with urine sample

3 Holding the dropper bottle at a 45° angle, add one drop of Reagent B. Avoid contact of dropper tip with urine sample.

4 Reagent C should be mixed by inverting closed bottle 8 to 10 times. Holding the bottle at a 45° angle, add one drop of Reagent C. Avoid contacting dropper tip with sample and reagent mixture.

5 Stir the mixture gently with the stirrer provided for approximately 8 to 10 seconds.

6 Push into the track opening. Once the mixture begins to flow in the capillary track, the test will proceed on its own. No further mixing is necessary. Wait until the mixture completely fills the viewing window (approximately three minutes).

Negative
"Speckled" appearance with white *agglutination* (clumps).

Positive
"Milky" white appearance with no *agglutination*.

"Milky" appearance, but some *agglutination*:
This test should be interpreted as negative.

FIGURE 5. Protocol for on-site testing.

CORRELATION ONTRAK/GC-MS

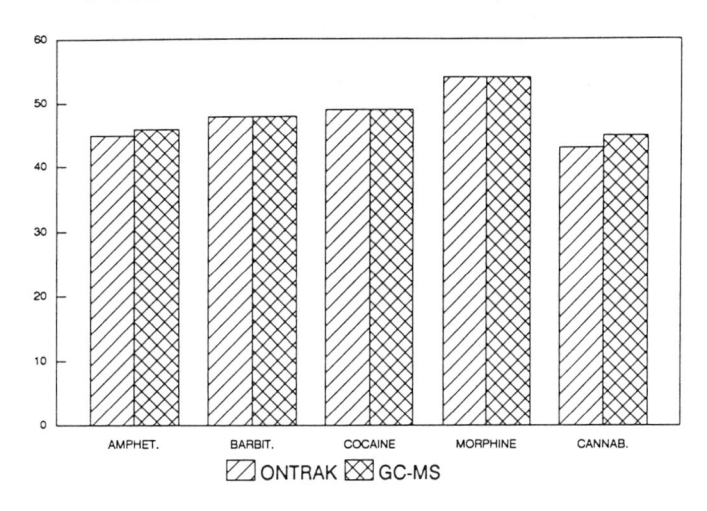

FIGURE 6. Correlation to reference method.

tions in the sample. It is common practice among drug addicts to adulterate the urine with the addition of detergents or salts, thereby inducing a false negative. In the inhibition of agglutination, this adulteration, even though the sample is negative, always leads to a positive. Furthermore, the actual philosophy of the *in situ* test makes adulteration very difficult, as sample collection may be supervised by the person conducting the test.

IV. CRITICAL ASPECTS IN DRUG DETECTION AND THEIR APPROACH IN THE *IN SITU* MODE

The *in situ* test has the same critical points as the other D.O.A. detection systems. The first of all these is the choice of cutoff or borderline, i.e., the mininum urine concentration of a given metabolite to consider a sample as positive to this drug. Reference has to be made to two facts as follows:

1. Establishment of the cutoff is a legal aspect. The sample is considered positive because it is legislated as such. This legislation is based on the fact that the formal declaration of positivity entails very serious consequences for the person so declared, as we have seen.
2. The urine concentration of a metabolite is not related to the toxicological effect of the drug (number of paranoid stimuli, greater or lesser self-esteem, loss of reflexes, etc.), since it is a multidependent variable; physiological state, weight, frequency of dose, etc.

It is therefore normal to abide by the regulation of civil institutions specialized in the subject. The Ontrak™ adheres to the standards of the NIDA (National Institute of Drug Abuse) in respect to cutoffs. These differentiate between values for the preliminary and the confirmative tests. Figure 7 summarizes these values.[4]

The initial test is purely qualitative, it only says whether the drug being investigated is present in the urine or not. The confirmative test, which is absolutely precise, can quantify and much lower cutoffs may therefore be used. In immunochemical techniques it is not desirable to use excessively low cutoffs in cannabinoids, as there is a risk of detecting passive smokers and reporting them as positive.

Another point to be considered is the differential test. Practically no immunochemical method distinguishes between the legal drug codeine and the illegal drug morphine. An excessively low cutoff would give a very high rate of false positives in morphine through detecting codeine.

In general, the *in situ* test offers a preliminary result which may be boosted in dependability terms by means of the introduction of positive and negative controls either in every series of tests or on a periodic basis.

V. APPLICABILITY OF *IN SITU* DETECTION IN COMPANIES

The work environment is one of the fields where greatest social benefit may be drawn from *in situ* detection systems. The objective is to reduce absenteeism, improve efficiency, and prevent accidents of all kinds.

DRUG	CUT-OFF (ng/ml)	
	PRELIMINARY	CONFIRMATORY
CANNABINOIDS	100	15
COCAINE	300	150
OPIATE:	300	-
MORPHINE	-	300
CODEINE	-	300
ANPHETAMINES	1.000	500

FIGURE 7. Cutoff values in D.O.A. tests (NIDA).

In view of the large number of employees that sometimes make up a single industrial group, the test to be chosen should be low cost and has to save bothersome sample transportation mechanisms (chain of custody), so that the actual medical or first aid service can perform the tests by themselves.

The greatest benefits will be reaped in medium type companies (around 500 to1000 employees), as the effects of drug addiction may be prevented in a simple fashion without resorting to the setting up or hiring of screening services.

For the detection plan that may be established to have the desired effects, it is necessary to bear in mind a number of key factors.

- Possess a defined D.O.A. detection policy, especially as to what is being looked for and why. It is evident that a punitive outlook will provoke more conflicts than it will solve.
- Explain this policy to the employees and set up and train supervision and control groups. The advantage of the *in situ* test is that, due to its simplicity, the actual workers may carry out the test, which always inspires more confidence than if it is conducted by unknown outside personnel.
- Lay down and notify the consequences of a confirmed positive.
- Discuss positives in a personalized way.
- Have planned mechanisms of assistance and aid for positive cases. For these, it is advisable to include the problem in corporate bargaining discussions and to cooperate with the trade unions in their own plans.

In short, thanks to its control capabilities within the work environment, *in situ* detection may prove a valuable aid for at least halting the advance of drug abuse among the working population.

REFERENCES

1. **Chamberlain, R. T.,** Legal issues related to drug testing in the clinical laboratory, *Clin. Chem.*, 34/3, 633–636, 1988.
2. **Marini, G.,** The corporate experience — a case history — symposium about substance abuse screening (*Clin. Chem.*, 1986). Face off with the American disease, Roche Diagnostic System Inc., Montclair, NJ, 1986.
3. **Calvo, A.,** *Curso Básico de Enzimoinmunoensayo,* Vol. 1, Roche Diagnostica, Madrid, 1989.
4. **NIDA Guidelines,** Mandatory guidelines for federal workplace drug testing programs, *Fed. Reg.*, April 11, 1988.

Chapter 17

EMIT® ENZYME IMMUNOASSAYS IN TESTING FOR DRUGS OF ABUSE

Kim L. Kelly

TABLE OF CONTENTS

I. Introduction 98
   A. History 98
   B. EMIT Assays Today 98
   C. Menu and Cutoff 98

II. Assay Principle 98
   A. Cutoff Values in Drug Screening 99

III. Applications on Chemistry Analyzers 99

IV. Accuracy and Reliability 100
   A. Scientific 100
   B. NIDA Certified Laboratories 100
   C. Legal Credibility 101

V. Summary 101

References 101

I. INTRODUCTION

A. HISTORY

The Syva Company (Palo Alto, CA) has been the leader in the field of immunoassays for drug testing for over 23 years. In the late 1960s, the Syva Company pioneered the use of immunoassays involving spin labels. This technology was called FRAT and is now obsolete, but at the time it was the first practical method for testing large numbers of urine samples. Syva assays were used in Vietnam to detect drug abuse in military personnel, and many abusers were detected and detoxified prior to returning to the states. Initial support for this effort came directly from the White House.

Over the intervening years, Syva has developed immunoassays with an enzyme label, and applied them not only to drugs of abuse, but in a quantitative fashion to therapeutic drug monitoring, hormone analysis, and infectious disease diagnostics. EMIT assays were first applied to drug testing in 1970 in an assay that detected opiates in urine samples. EMIT assays have been constantly improved over the years to increase specificity, improve the enzymes involved in the assay, and to maximize their ability to differentiate positive samples from negative samples.

B. EMIT ASSAYS TODAY

EMIT enzyme immunoassays are the most commonly used technology for drug-of-abuse testing in the world and are currently the only enzyme immunoassays for drugs of abuse. It is estimated that over 80 million EMIT assays for drugs of abuse are performed each year. Syva's enzyme immunoassay (EMIT) technology involves the use of antibodies which have been specially developed to react with a drug and its metabolites. These antibodies are engineered to react with the compounds that are most likely to be found in the urine of persons who abuse individual drugs or classes of drugs such as opiate narcotics. The proper engineering of these antibodies, optimization of polyclonal antibody preparations, and applications of new monoclonal antibody technology is the result of painstaking research into drug metabolism, patterns of drug use, and potential cross-reactivities with other non-abused compounds. The EMIT assays are regulated by the U.S. Food and Drug Administration, and each assay must be cleared by the FDA before being marketed.

C. MENU AND CUTOFF

The menu of enzyme immunoassay tests is one of the largest available, providing tests for may of the drugs commonly found in drug abusers. Not only have enzyme immunoassays been available for over two decades, but they have been constantly improved with experience as to the best substrates, antibody loading patterns, and cross-reactivity profiles. Indeed, one of the newest assays used in drug abuse testing is the result of many years experience in screening urine samples for drugs of abuse. Syva recently introduced the Monoclonal Amphetamine/Methamphetamine Assay which for the first time uses two monoclonal antibodies in the same assay resulting in a very low incidence of interference from amphetamine-like agents used in the treatment of colds and allergies. For several of the assays, different cutoffs are available depending on market demand. The subject of cutoffs will be addressed in more detail later during discussions of the assay principle.

In many cases, antibodies are produced which are relatively nonspecific so as to detect drug classes. In these cases, the level at which the assay detects the presence of drug(s) and metabolite(s) is usually set to some standard that is either a commonly abused drug (secobarbital in the barbiturate assay) or an abused drug and/or metabolite (morphine in the opiate assay and oxazepam in the benzodiazepine assay). As new drugs in a given class are developed, the antibody optimization procedures are refined or blends of new antibodies are sought so that the assay detects the drugs most likely to be abused. A list of EMIT drug of abuse assays is shown below.

EMIT® Immunoassay Menu

Assay	Cutoff
Monoclonal Amphetamine/ Methamphetamine Assay	1000 ng[a]
Amphetamine (polyclonal) Assay	300 ng
Barbiturate Assay	300 ng
Benzodiazepine Assay	300 ng
Cannabinoid Assay	20 ng, 50 ng, 100 ng[a]
Cocaine Metabolite Assay	300 ng[a]
Methaqualone Assay	300 ng
Opiate Assay	300 ng[a]
Phencyclidine Assay	25 ng[a], 75 ng
Propoxyphene Assay	300 ng

[a] National Institute on Drug Abuse recommended cutoff.

II. ASSAY PRINCIPLE

EMIT immunoassays involve a chemical reaction which occurs when the antibody produced against the drug reacts with that drug in a sample. In the EMIT reaction, known quantities of enzyme-labeled drug, specific antibodies, a substrate for the enzyme, and a coenzyme are used. When these compounds are mixed in a urine sample containing no drug, the antibody binds to the enzyme-labeled drug which sterically inhibits the enzyme. Thus, the enzyme does not react with the substrate. When the urine sample does contain the drug, the enzyme-labeled drug and the drug from the urine sample compete for binding with the antibody. As a result, some of the enzyme-labeled drug does not bind to the antibody, and some of the enzyme is free to act on its substrate. When the enzyme acts on its substrate, the reaction converts the coenzyme to a substance that absorbs ultraviolet light. Thus, the more drug present in the sample, the more enzyme-labeled drug is available, and the more that enzyme reacts with its substrate to change the coenzyme into a light absorbing compound. The instrument performing the assays reads the amount of light absorbed and compares it with the amount of light absorbed when known amounts of drug are tested. This measurement is used to determine if the light absorbtion exceeds that of the standard or calibrator. When the absorbance of light is greater than that of the calibrator the sample is positive.

Calibrators are set to contain small fixed quantities of the drug or metabolite which would most commonly be found in the urine. These so called "cutoff calibrators" assure that the client sample is compared to a sample containing some drug. This minimizes or eliminates the possibility that a drug-free sample could be positive. Syva has worked with the National Institute on Drug Abuse to develop assays with cutoffs and cutoff calibrators at the concentrations specified in the Department of Health and Human Services Guidelines. Syva was also a participant in the recent NIDA conference where new cutoffs were proposed. We understand that the EEC will be developing its own set of cutoffs. We welcome the chance to participate in those discussions and will develop assays optimized to whatever cutoff values are chosen.

A. CUTOFF VALUES IN DRUG SCREENING

EMIT enzyme immunoassays pioneered the field of therapeutic drug monitoring. Thus, these assays have a well-documented capability of detecting nanogram concentrations of drugs such as digoxin. It is clear, however, that use of EMIT immunoassays for quantitation of drugs of abuse is simply not necessary. As noted above, the use of single cutoff values has been validated by the National Institutes on Drug Abuse and the Department of Health and Human Services and is by far the predominant testing strategy in the United States. EMIT immunoassays are optimized for performance at their specified cutoff levels where their ability to discriminate positive from negative samples is maximum.

Assays are available not only for the cutoff levels approved by the U.S. Department of Health and Human Services, but also for some assays, at other levels, that are occasionally used in industrial or security settings. Selection of cutoffs that are uniform and are uniformly applied allow for the highest level of accuracy and the fundamental fairness of screening all urine samples using the same criteria.

Quantitation of drug from random urine samples gives no valuable information and may even be misleading. Many physiological variables affect urine drug concentration including fluid intake, renal impairment, and urine pH to name a few. Occasionally, a low urine concentration signifies a more calculating, sophisticated user who has tried to lower his urine level with fluid intake rather than someone who has used only small amounts of drug.

In a recent editorial on quantitation in random urine samples in the *Journal of Analytical Chemistry*,[1] Dr. Randall Baselt (an earlier speaker on this program) noted that the use of immunoassays as a quantitative tool was "inappropriate" and that reporting of quantitative immunoassay results for random urine samples, especially those with multiple metabolites "smacks of professional carelessness".

III. APPLICATIONS ON CHEMISTRY ANALYZERS

As noted above, the EMIT reaction involves measurement of light absorbance. This means that the results can be read using a spectrophotometer which is present in the vast majority of chemistry analyzers. The chemistry laboratory has a great deal of flexibility in the analyzer it chooses. This flexibility allows EMIT assays to be run in chemistry laboratories on dozens of different analyzers and on smaller instruments which can be used at the site where the urine is collected.

The flexibility of EMIT assays has facilitated their use in many areas where immediate results are vital. These areas include nuclear power plants, oil rigs, prisons, and many other sites where one cannot wait even a short time for an answer. However, while flexibility may be a benefit, it can also be problematic. In the United States, NIDA certification standards require that separate enclosed areas of the laboratory be designated as drug testing areas. If a laboratory does its drug tests on an analyzer that is also used for other tests, that lab must make the decision to either dedicate that analyzer full time to drug testing or to obtain a dedicated system to handle the drug testing workload. This situation has led Syva to develop a dedicated drug testing analyzer, the ETS System. This truly random-access analyzer is made specifically for EMIT reagents. It is currently the leading system for drug testing in small to moderately sized laboratories, in industrial settings, and in criminal justice settings such as in parole, probation, pretrial, and work release programs. However, flexibility is not enough ... you also need accuracy and consistent performance.

IV. ACCURACY AND RELIABILITY

A. SCIENTIFIC

The scientific literature contains over 200 studies involving EMIT assays. Fifteen of the larger studies in that population were reviewed in an article in 1977.[7] In that review, the total number of samples reported was 27,059 and 2883 of these (10.6%) were positive. Confirmation methods varied, but the overall confirmation rate was 98.2%. Notably, many of these studies were conducted a number of years ago with earlier versions of the EMIT assays, and in many cases with less sophisticated confirmation methods. It is reasonable to expect that if similar studies were to be performed today that the accuracy (confirmation) rates of the EMIT test would be even higher than 98+%.

In addition to scientific validation of the accuracy of these assays, several other investigations have been performed to evaluate their accuracy in everyday use. In 1985, the accuracy of EMIT assays used alone was at issue in a New York district court. In that case [*Peranzo v. Coughlin (608 F. suppl. 504 S.D.N.Y., 1985)*],[2] the court noted that the American Association of Bioanalysts had performed several thousand proficiency tests and found that the EMIT tests "have a accuracy rate of over 99.7%".

In 1988, Dr. Richard Crooks of the National Psychopharmacology Laboratory[3] updated the original observations from the American Association of Bioanalysts at a consensus conference sponsored by the National Bureau of Standards. In his presentation, Dr. Crooks noted that in testing for cocaine, cannabinoids, opiates, and phencyclidine, EMIT assays had the lowest overall incidence of false positive results of all methods including thin layer chromatography, radioimmunoassay, and fluorescence-polarization immunoassay. The incidence of unconfirmed positive results for amphetamines was higher with EMIT because at the time the amphetamine assay in common use was a polyclonal formulation and detected abuse of not only amphetamines, but also phenylpropanolamine. Phenylpropanolamine is the most common drug of abuse among commercial truck drivers in the United States.

In 1989, the Bureau of Justice Assistance[4] (an agency of the Federal Government) validated the accuracy of drug testing assays in a study comparing thin layer chromatography and several different immunoassays, including radioimmunoassay and fluorescence polarization immunoassay. In that study, samples were analyzed by gas chromatography with mass spectrometry (GC/MS) using the GC/MS cutoff values approved by the U.S. Department of Health and Human Services and NIDA for cannabinoids, cocaine, phencyclidine, amphetamines, and opiates. EMIT assays had the highest overall sensitivity and specificity.

In 1987, the American Association for Clinical Chemistry (AACC)[5] evaluated the accuracy of 47 laboratories in an open proficiency sample study. The results of 1880 analyses showed an accuracy rate of over 99%. This study was criticized for being an open study, so in 1989, the AACC extended that study in 31 laboratories using blind proficiency samples. There were no false positive results reported. False negative results occurred in only 45 out of 1486 (3.0%) samples. Ninety percent of the laboratories in that study used EMIT assays for their testing.

The U.S. Coast Guard requires a blind proficiency testing program as part of its contract with a large commercial laboratory in the United States which performs drug testing according to Coast Guard antidrug policies. During the years for which data is available[6] (1983 to 1988), blind proficiency testing of over 59,000 samples known to be drug free did not yield a single false positive result. Testing performed on over 28,000 samples that contained one or more drugs yielded a false negative rate of just over 3%. EMIT assays are the screening tests used by the U.S. Coast Guard.

B. NIDA CERTIFIED LABORATORIES

Finally, the most significant statistic relating to accuracy and reliability of EMIT enzyme immunoassays concerns laboratories certified by the National Institutes on Drug Abuse (NIDA). The standards for certification by NIDA are among the most stringent in the world. NIDA certification requires that laboratories submit to blind proficiency testing, and that at least 10% of all samples that the laboratory performs be proficiency samples. Laboratories are inspected twice a year, and all results are reviewed. If the laboratory has even a single false positive result their certification is revoked. Thus, these laboratories must use the most accurate methods available or risk the loss of certification and many thousands of dollars in revenue. In the 2 years that NIDA certification program has been in operation, only 44 laboratories have been able to pass the rigorous certification process. One hundred percent (100%) of these laboratories use EMIT assays.

Thus, enzyme immunoassays have been established in the scientific literature in everyday use by many laboratories as accurate and reliable.

C. LEGAL CREDIBILITY

Not only have the accuracy and reliability of EMIT assays been established scientifically, but they have also been established in hundreds of court cases across the United States. Most recently in a case involving the Customs Service, the United States Supreme Court made the following statement; "... the combination of EMIT and GC/MS tests required by the [Customs] Service is highly accurate assuming proper storage, handling and measurement techniques."

As many of us know, acceptance of a technology by the courts in any country is just as important as acceptance by the scientific community.

V. SUMMARY

In summary, EMIT enzyme immunoassays are accurate, reliable, and the most commonly used tests for screening for drugs of abuse. They have gained a level of acceptance in the scientific community and the court system unprecedented in the field of drug abuse testing. Syva has worked in partnership with many regulatory and laboratory agencies and associations to develop assays to meet the cutoffs required by regulatory agencies. But more than that, we have worked with those same groups to develop testing guidelines, educational programs, and legal information to assist the laboratory and industrial communities in developing drug testing programs.

REFERENCES

1. **Baselt, R. T.,** *J. Anal. Chem.*
2. *Peranzo v. Coughlen* (608 F. suppl. 504 S.D.N.Y., 1985).
3. **Crooks, R.,** Conference sponsored by the National Bureau of Standards.
4. Bureau of Justice Assistance, 1989.
5. *Am. Assoc. Clin. Chem. (AACC),* 1987.
6. U.S. Coast Guard, Data on blind proficiency testing, 1983–1989.
7. *Pharmacotherapy,* 8, 263–275, 1988.

Chapter 18

DRUGS OF ABUSE METHODS FOR THE DU PONT aca® DISCRETE CLINICAL ANALYZER

Derek P. Lehane, Steven P. Crouse, Ricardo P. Narváez, David M. Obzansky, Noel M. Relyea, Gerald E. Siefring, Jr., and Peter M. Tuhy

TABLE OF CONTENTS

Summary 104

I. Background 104
    A. Drugs of Abuse Screening Assays 104
    B. Toxicology Testing on the aca®* 104

II. Drug Screening Technology on the aca® 105
    A. EMIT®** Assay Methodology 105
    B. Principles of Instrument Operation 105
    C. Results Reporting and Cutoff Values 106

III. Quality Assurance Considerations 106
    A. Specimen Collection and Storage 107
    B. Calibration 107
    C. Quality Control (QC) 107

IV. Performance Characteristics of the Urine Cocaine
    Metabolite Screening Assay (U COC) 108
    A. Reproducibility 108
    B. Recovery 108
    C. Comparison of Methods 109
    D. Interferences 109

V. Conclusions 110
    A. Limitations of Urine Drug Screening Procedures 110
    B. Advantages of Automated Drug Screening on the aca® 110

Acknowledgments 111

References 111

---

* aca® is a registered trademark of E. I. Du Pont de Nemours & Company, Inc., Wilmington, DE 19898.
** EMIT® is a registered trademark of Syva/a Syntex Company, Palo Alto, CA 94303.

SUMMARY

Six urinary drugs of abuse methods, a single three-level calibrator, and a single two-level daily control have been developed for the aca® discrete clinical analyzer. The methods include amphetamines, cocaine metabolite (benzoylecgonine), cannabinoids, opiates, benzodiazepines, and barbiturates. The methods are adaptations of the EMIT® homogeneous enzyme immunoassay technique. Quantitative results are provided for the purpose of calibration and quality control, but the methods are recommended as a qualitative screen for unknown samples.

Within-day reproducibility ranged from 2 to 7% CV, between-day reproducibility ranged from 2 to 13% CV, and analytical recovery ranged from 95 to 113% for all six methods. Analysis of negative and positive urine samples showed excellent agreement between the aca® and three comparison methods: EMIT® reagents adapted to the COBAS-BIO®* (Roche Diagnostics), TDx®** (Abbott Laboratories), and a gas chromatographic/mass spectrometric (GC/MS) technique.

The aca® offers discrete testing capabilities and a fast turnaround of results; a six-test panel is complete in less than 15 min. Calibration is necessary at intervals of only 1 to 3 months, depending on the method. These fully automated assays are simple to perform and provide convenient, reliable, cost effective, and consistent screening for drugs of abuse.

I. BACKGROUND

A. DRUGS OF ABUSE SCREENING ASSAYS

The Du Pont drugs of abuse screening assays are sensitive, effective methods for distinguishing which urine samples have a high likelihood of containing a drug from those which have a high likelihood of being drug-free. A six-test panel for the urine drugs of abuse can be run on the aca® in less than 15 min. The fast turn-around time of the tests makes them especially well-suited to medical emergency situations in a hospital setting. However, as with all screening methods, a positive result must be confirmed by a more specific test, based on a chemical principle different from that used in the screening assay.

The commonly used methodologies for drugs of abuse screening include the immunoassay techniques of radioimmunoassay, the homogeneous enzyme immunoassay, EMIT®, fluorescence polarization assays, and thin layer chromatography. High performance liquid chromatography and gas chromatography, with or without subsequent mass spectrometry, are most often confirmatory test methods. However, GC/MS is considered to be the method of choice for confirming presumptive positive results from urine drugs of abuse screening.[1,2]

Urine specimens are the samples of choice for drugs of abuse screening because they are easy to collect and can be screened inexpensively. It should be emphasized that screening tests are not meant to be a primary diagnostic tool, but rather are to be used to define a subgroup, for which more specific confirmatory testing would be cost-effective.[2] Research also continues in assessing the efficacy of drugs of abuse testing with alternate specimens, such as hair.[3]

When screening tests for drugs of abuse are properly run, interpreted, and confirmed, they can be highly reliable.[4,5] The latter reference describes an American Association for Clinical Chemistry Special Study on Drugs of Abuse in Urine, which concluded that urine drug screens give accurate results. (The overall accuracy rate in this open study in 47 laboratories was 99.3%.) One caveat was that the laboratories must be "challenged to detect drugs at the concentrations at which they accept business", i. e., by using technologies with detection limits capable of measuring the drug levels in the study specimens. It thus becomes critical for laboratories to communicate their threshold (cutoff) concentrations for differentiating positive from negative samples. More recently, a second study conducted in 31 of the original 47 laboratories showed that the overall accuracy rate under blind conditions, at 97%, was still quite impressive.[6]

Clearly, the reporting of results from drugs of abuse testing has not only medical, but also legal, economic, and social consequences. Another survey of drug testing experts concluded that the key to designing an effective testing program is assurance that appropriate analytical and administrative controls and their documentation exist, all positive screening results are confirmed by GC/MS, and the testing laboratory performs well in a recognized proficiency testing and inspection program.[7] Quality assurance considerations for drugs of abuse testing laboratories are discussed further in Section III.

B. TOXICOLOGY TESTING ON THE aca®

The aca® was first introduced in the United States in 1970 as a clinical chemistry analyzer with a total menu of eight tests. Today the aca® provides a wide menu of available tests, which number more than 80, in clinical chemistry, clinical enzymology, therapeutic drug monitoring, and drugs of abuse screening. Over the years,

---

* COBAS-BIO® is a registered trademark of Roche Diagnostics, Nutley, NJ 07110.

** TDx® is a registered trademark of Abbott Laboratories, Diagnostics Division, Abbott Park, IL 60064.

$$Ab + BARB + BARB\text{-}G6PDH \longrightarrow Ab\text{-}BARB + Ab\text{-}BARB\text{-}G6PDH\ (\text{inhibited}) + BARB\text{-}G6PDH\ (\text{active})$$

$$Glucose\text{-}6\text{-}phosphate + NAD^+ \xrightarrow{BARB\text{-}G6PDH\ (\text{active})} 6\text{-}phospho\text{-}gluconolactone + NADH + H^+\ (\text{abs. @ 340nm})$$

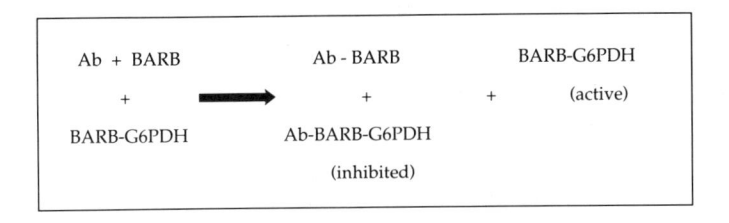

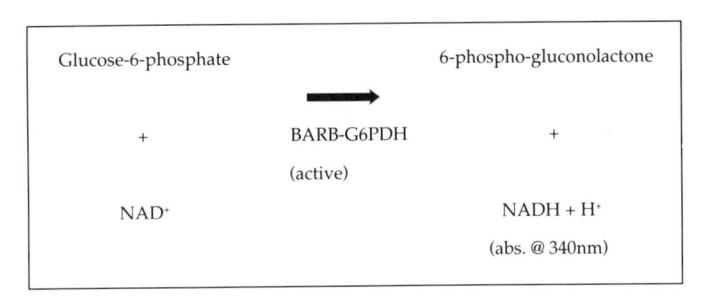

FIGURE 1. The drugs of abuse methods are adaptations of Syva's homogeneous enzyme immunoassay technique (EMIT®).

various models have been introduced that have provided greater ease of use and significantly enhanced software capabilities. Since the introduction of the aca® IV in 1983, both the calibration and problem solving routines have been improved and simplified. In addition, the display of results has been improved for ease of interpretation. All of these improvements have significantly enhanced the ease-of-use of the drugs of abuse screening methods.

Du Pont has developed a complete system for the assay of six drugs of abuse screening methods. This system includes the aca® analyzer, the aca® test packs for the individual drug methods, and a single three-level calibrator product and a single two-level level daily control product for all six methods. Assays are available for amphetamines, barbiturates, benzodiazepines, cannabinoids, the cocaine metabolite benzoylecgonine, and opiates. All of these tests are qualitative urine screening assays, which may be used either in toxicology testing or as an initial screen in drug testing and monitoring programs.

These urinary screening assays complement an existing series of toxicology assays on the aca®, including the rapid screening assays for barbiturates, benzodiazepines, and tricyclic antidepressants in serum. Quantitative assays are also available for salicylates and acetaminophen in serum, and for alcohol in both serum and urine.

II. DRUG SCREENING TECHNOLOGY ON THE aca®

A. EMIT® ASSAY METHODOLOGY

All of the drugs of abuse methods for the aca® are adaptations of the EMIT® homogeneous enzyme immunoassay technique. In the urine barbiturate screen, for example, the unique reagents consist of matched lots of secobarbital antibody and a secobarbital conjugate of the enzyme glucose-6-phosphate dehydrogenase (Figure 1). During the assay procedure, the drug-enzyme conjugate and free drug from the patient specimen compete for a limited number of antibody binding sites. Binding of the conjugate and antibody results in inhibition of the enzyme activity. The remaining free, active drug-enzyme conjugate catalyzes the oxidation of glucose-6-phosphate to 6-phosphogluconolactone and the reduction of NAD^+ to NADH. The rate of increase in absorbance due to the appearance of NADH is related to the presence of drug by a previously established calibration of the aca® system.

B. PRINCIPLES OF INSTRUMENT OPERATION

The heart of the aca® system is a plastic pack that contains all of the unique reagents needed for a single assay. The arrangement of the various reagents for the urine cannabinoids assay is depicted in Figure 2. Each liquid or tableted reagent is segregated in its own specific dimple within the plastic pack. The aca® automatically adds 320 µl of patient sample to the urine cannabinoids pack and then dilutes it with purified water.

In addition to the dimples containing the specific reagents, each pack has a rigid header. On the right side of the header is a rubber stopper, through which the urine sample and the diluent are automatically injected. In the center of the header is a mnemonic or shortened version of the test name for easy identification of the specific

**PACK DESIGN
URINE CANNABINOIDS**

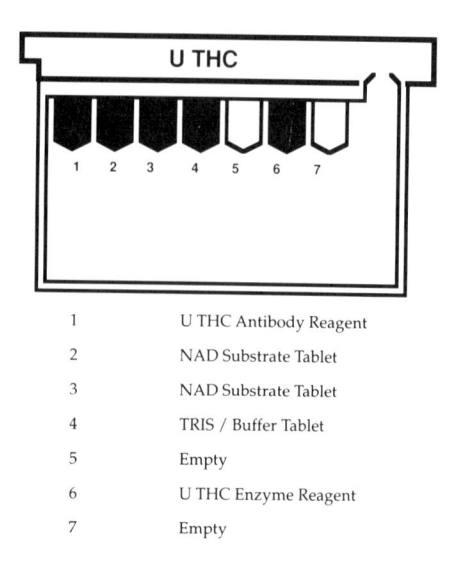

```
U THC
1  2  3  4  5  6  7
```

1	U THC Antibody Reagent
2	NAD Substrate Tablet
3	NAD Substrate Tablet
4	TRIS / Buffer Tablet
5	Empty
6	U THC Enzyme Reagent
7	Empty

FIGURE 2. The aca® pack design for the drugs of abuse methods includes both liquid and tableted reagents enclosed in dimples with breakable seals.

pack by the laboratory technologist. On the left side of the header is a unique barcode that identifies the pack to the aca®. This code sets in motion the specific mechanical and software routines necessary to process the chemical reactions and to compute the test result.

Within the aca® itself are two mechanical stations called breaker/mixers. These serve to break the temporary seals around the reagent dimples, allowing specific reagents to be added in a predetermined, timed manner to the diluted sample. At the first breaker/mixer, the antibody against cannabinoids and tablets containing substrate and buffer are added. Analyte from the patient sample is, thus, allowed to bind to the specific antibody first. The THC-glucose-6-phosphate dehydrogenase conjugate is then added in the second breaker/mixer, and the rate of increase in absorbance at 340 nm is measured. The absorbance signal is automatically related to the concentration of analyte in the sample by means of a logit function.

C. RESULTS REPORTING AND CUTOFF VALUES

At the termination of the chemical reaction, the rate of increase in absorbance in milliabsorbance units per minute is converted to arbitrary relative units, called Qualitative (QUAL) units. They are equivalent to drug concentration only when the sample is a standard containing pure drug or metabolite. The QUAL units are, in turn, compared to the positive/negative cutoff level specific for the assay, which is based on designated concentrations of pure drug standards. These cutoff values were selected based on U. S. National Institute on Drug Abuse (NIDA) recommendations,[1] U. S. Federal Guidelines, and information gathered from expert consultants. Cutoff values for all six drug screening methods are listed in Table 1.

The aca® IV prints out a report slip for each patient sample, listing the date and time, as well as a sequence number that relates the sample identification to a load list. It also includes the name of the drug test, the actual numeric result in QUAL units, and the reportable result of either positive or negative. The latter is determined automatically by an instrument software comparison of the numeric result with the designated cutoff value for the test. The numeric result is available to the laboratory technologist for a better understanding of the difference between the two values.

III. QUALITY ASSURANCE CONSIDERATIONS

A strong quality assurance program is essential for drugs of abuse testing laboratories, since the reliability of results has far-reaching consequences. Some basic requirements of a quality assurance program include adherence to sample handling, assay and quality control proce-

TABLE 1
Reproducibility and Recovery Data for the Six aca® Drugs of Abuse Screening Methods

Method	Cutoff (mg/l)	Within-day CV (%)	Between-day CV (%)	Recovery (%)
U AMP	0.30	4.1	4.5	103
UBARB	0.30	2.9	3.6	113
UBENZ	0.30	3.6	4.4	100
U COC	0.30	4.7	7.0	97
U OPI	0.30	1.7	1.9	109
U THC	0.050	7.2	12.9	95

dures, continued training of laboratory personnel, confirmation of screening assay results, participation in proficiency testing programs, and adequate documentation of the whole quality assurance effort.[8] Proficiency testing programs for drugs of abuse in urine are becoming more prevalent worldwide as their benefits are recognized.[9]

The toxicology laboratory is especially challenged to acquire reliable and verifiable standards for drugs and their metabolites.[10] Du Pont has provided well-characterized, stable calibration and quality control materials for the six drugs of abuse assays, along with sample handling and storage information.

A. SPECIMEN COLLECTION AND STORAGE

As with other human fluid and tissue specimens, urine should be handled appropriately and as potentially infectious. A recent report describes a method of heat treating urine that still allows for accurate determinations of some of the more labile, commonly abused drugs.[11] Freshly voided urine samples should be used for analysis, if possible, which are in the pH range of 5 to 8. The pH may be adjusted with 1 M HCl or 1 M NaOH in samples outside of this range. Highly turbid samples should be clarified by centrifugation before analysis.

Sample storage conditions are also an important variable to control in validating an assay. Samples not immediately tested in urine drug screens should be refrigerated and used within 3 days. If longer storage is necessary, the samples should be frozen at –20°C or colder or one of the following preservatives added: 0.1% sodium azide, 0.01% thimerosal, or 0.1% boric acid. Thawed specimens must be mixed thoroughly before analysis. Refrigerated storage of urine specimens without preservatives for longer than 3 days may result in positive samples with drug concentrations near the 0.30 mg/l cutoff value for the cocaine metabolite screen, for example, assaying as falsely negative. On the other hand, drug-free samples have not been observed to test positive after storage.[1]

B. CALIBRATION

Du Pont recommends a three-level calibration for each of the drug screening methods. The Du Pont calibrator is a single lyophilized, human urine-based product, formulated to contain appropriate levels of each of the six pure drug standards. These levels were chosen to provide an optimum separation at the cutoff values. For each of the methods, the Level 0 calibrator is, indeed, a drug-free standard, Level I contains the cutoff value of each drug, and Level II contains the upper limit for the claimed range for each method. For example, the urinary opiate screen calibrator levels are 0, 0.3, and 1.0 mg/l of morphine.

Instrument calibration has been shown to be remarkably stable for the aca® drugs of abuse assays, with a three-month stability for amphetamines, opiates, benzodiazepines, and barbiturates. The tests for the cocaine metabolite, benzoylecgonine, and cannabinoids require monthly calibration. Once hydrated, the reconstituted calibrators are stable for 15 days, when stored resealed at 2 to 8°C, allowing for cost effective use of the material.

Precision studies were done with Level I calibrator over a 20-day period. At the cutoff drug concentrations, good reproducibility was demonstrated for all six methods (Table 1). Within-day reproducibility, expressed as the coefficient of variation, varied from 2% for the opiate assay to 7% for the cannabinoid assay. Between-day coefficients of variation, not unexpectedly somewhat higher, ranged from 2% again for the opiate assay to 13% for the cannabinoid assay.

C. QUALITY CONTROL (QC)

A separate aca® urine drugs of abuse control product is available for daily QC for the six drug screening methods. Like the calibrator, it is also a lyophilized, human urine-based product, formulated at two levels — a drug-free, negative control and a positive control containing purified drugs at approximately twice the cutoff values for the assays. Constituent concentrations are verified by a GC/

TABLE 2
Reproducibility Results for the aca® Urine Cocaine Metabolite Screening Assay

		Standard deviation (%CV)	
Units	Mean	Within-run	Between-run
Level 1 Calibrator			
QUAL	0.29	0.013 (4.36)	0.015 (5.01)
MAU	374.1	2.78 (0.74)	3.20 (0.86)
Positive Control			
QUAL	0.81	0.025 (3.04)	0.026 (3.19)
MAU	465.8	3.00 (0.64)	4.39 (0.94)
Negative Pooled Urine			
QUAL	0.01	0.012 (—)	0.013 (—)
MAU	319.4	2.90 (0.91)	3.13 (0.98)
Positive Spiked Pooled Urine			
QUAL	0.85	0.043 (5.03)	0.041 (4.87)
MAU	462.7	4.39 (0.95)	4.24 (0.92)

MS procedure. Like the calibrator, the control product is stable as a hydrated solution for 15 days, when resealed and stored at 2 to 8°C.

IV. PERFORMANCE CHARACTERISTICS OF THE URINE COCAINE METABOLITE SCREENING ASSAY (U COC)

In developing a new method for the aca®, wide-ranging performance and stability studies are conducted in Du Pont laboratories at Glasgow, DE. To validate the performance of the assay under actual working conditions, field evaluations of the new assays are conducted in clinical laboratories around the world. The performance characteristics of the aca® method for urinary cocaine metabolite were validated in independent studies conducted at two major drug testing laboratories. The first study was at Allentown Hospital in Allentown, PA, and the second at Medtox Laboratories, Inc. in Minneapolis, MN. For this method, the key reagents are benzoylecgonine antibody and a benzoylecgonine conjugate of glucose-6-phosphate dehydrogenase.

A. REPRODUCIBILITY

Reproducibility of the cocaine metabolite method was tested by analyzing calibrators, control products, and pooled urine samples. One pooled urine sample had essentially a zero level of benzoylecgonine, while the second pool was spiked with benzoylecgonine to a concentration of approximately 0.85 mg/l. The specimens at each level were analyzed in duplicate for 20 days. Table 2 shows the concentration of drug both as qualitative (QUAL) units, approximately equivalent to the concentration expressed as milligrams per liter, and as unconverted instrument milliabsorbance units, shown as MAU. Results for within-run and between-run variability were determined using a standard analysis of variance technique. Reproducibility was excellent, with coefficients of variation of 5% or less for all materials containing benzoylecgonine. The assay also has ample milliabsorbance signal separation to discriminate drug levels in samples with negative, cutoff level, and positive analyte values, exceeding those separation values recommended by Blanke and Decker.[10]

B. RECOVERY

To assess the accuracy and recovery of the assay for cocaine metabolite, 20 drug-free urine samples were first tested. A histogram of the results (Figure 3) shows that the assayed values clustered quite closely around the zero level. Increasing amounts of benzoylecgonine were then spiked into the drug-free urine samples. The first spike was at a concentration, 0.15 mg/l, which is below the cutoff level. The second spike, 0.3 mg/l, was just at the cutoff, and the third, 0.75 mg/l, was well above the cutoff. Note that the assay range extends from 0 to 3.00 mg/l. All assayed values for the spiked urine samples clustered closely around their expected values.

Twenty-one positive urine samples were also tested, which contained both benzoylecgonine and other cocaine metabolites (Figure 3). As is usual with assays for cocaine, all the measured values were substantially in excess of the cutoff. Each positive sample contained greater than the equivalent of 1.0 mg/l of benzoylecgonine.

In earlier studies done in Du Pont laboratories, the

U COC RECOVERY HISTOGRAMS

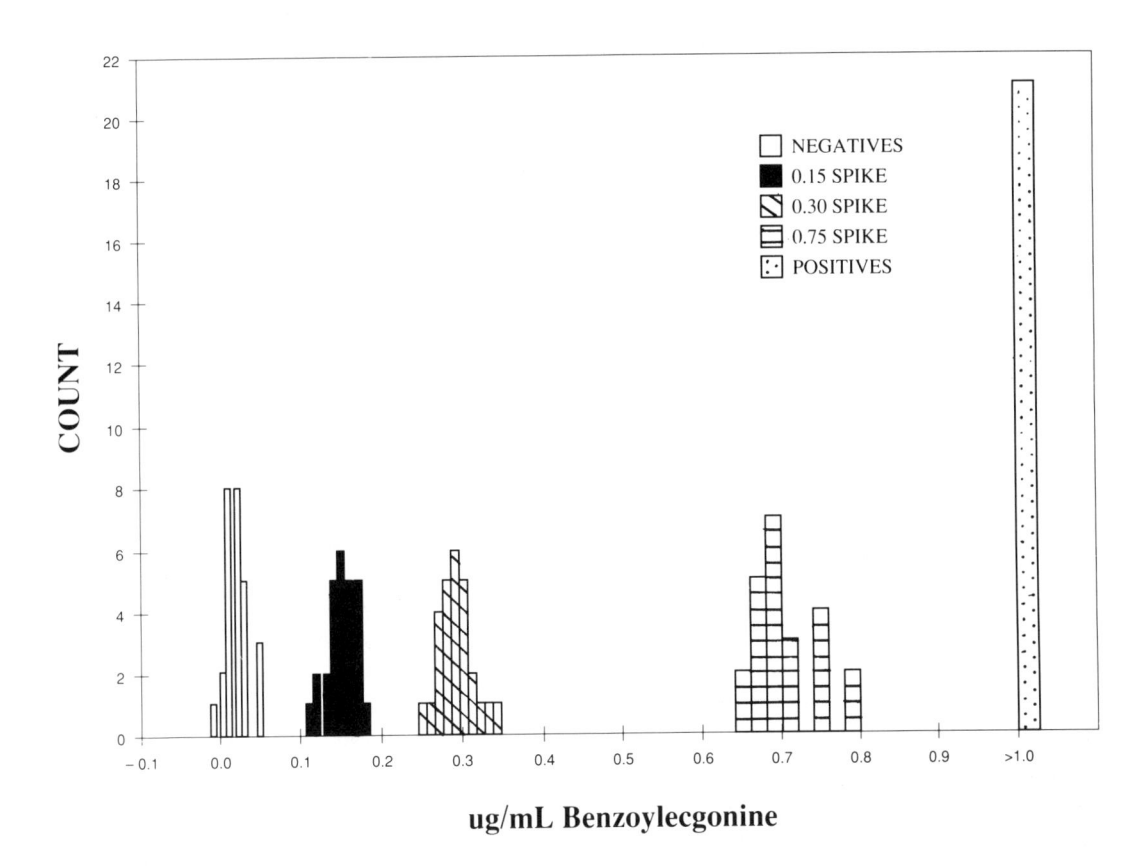

FIGURE 3. Recovery histograms for the aca® urine cocaine metabolite screening assay demonstrate that the assayed values cluster closely around their expected values.

average recovery of purified drugs spiked into 25 drug-free urine specimens ranged from 95% for the cannabinoid screen to 113% for the barbiturate screen (Table 1). Recovery of benzoylecgonine assayed by the cocaine metabolite screen was 97%. Another study of 98 drug-free urine specimens and 98 drug-free samples spiked with 0.5 mg/l of benzoylecgonine showed that all samples were properly classified as positive or negative by the aca®.

C. COMPARISION OF METHODS

The accuracy of the aca® method for urinary cocaine metabolites was determined in independent studies conducted at the two field evaluation sites. At Allentown Hospital, the aca® method was compared to the EMIT® Urine Cocaine Metabolite assay, adapted to the Roche COBAS-BIO® centrifugal analyzer, and also to a gas chromatographic/mass spectrometric (GC/MS) procedure. All 66 positive and all 99 negative urine samples, as categorized by the latter methodology, were correctly classified by both the aca® method and the EMIT® procedure (Table 3).

At Medtox Laboratories, Inc., the aca® method for urinary cocaine metabolite was evaluated against the EMIT® and GC/MS procedures, as well as the TDx® fluorescence polarization assay for cocaine metabolite. The positive or negative status of each sample was again established by the GC/MS procedure. As at the Allentown site, all 50 positive and all 100 negative urine samples were correctly classified by the aca® method, as they were by the EMIT® and TDx® assays.

In separate studies done at both evaluation sites, a total of 199 urine specimens, shown to be drug-free by GC/MS, was tested in the aca® cocaine metabolite drug screen. Again, all samples were correctly categorized as negative using this assay.

D. INTERFERENCES

A selection of other drugs, common clinical analytes, and physiological substances was added to samples of

TABLE 3
Comparison of Patient Results From the aca® Urine Cocaine
Metabolite Screening Assay and Three Other Methodologies

Allentown Hospital

GC/MS	n	aca® U COC pos/neg	Syva EMIT® pos/neg
Positive	66	66/0	66/0
Negative	99	0/99	0/99

Medtox Laboratories, Inc.

GC/MS	n	aca® U COC pos/neg	Syva EMIT® pos/neg	Abbott TDx® pos/neg
Positive	50	50/0	50/0	50/0
Negative	100	0/100	0/100	0/100

pooled human urine. In no case was there evidence of clinically significant interference in the cocaine metabolite screening assay. The drug classes tested were analgesics, tricyclic antidepressants, stimulants, and anesthetics. Common clinical analytes included albumin, ammonia, bilirubin, creatinine, glucose, and uric acid. The physiological conditions tested were hemolysis, icterus, and extremes of pH. For a complete listing of the potential interferents and their concentrations, see Crouse and Narváez.[12]

It is interesting to note that the antibenzoylecgonine antibody behaves in the assay as significantly more specific for the immunogen, benzoylecgonine, than for cocaine itself or another cocaine metabolite, ecgonine.[12] However, benzoylecgonine is an appropriate choice for the analyte, since it accounts for 35 to 54% of a single dose of cocaine in a 24-hour urine sample.[13]

V. CONCLUSIONS

A. LIMITATIONS OF URINE DRUG SCREENING PROCEDURES

As discussed in the background above, drugs of abuse screening assays provide reliable results, when properly understood and interpreted. However, all such screening assays have limitations, which must be appreciated. Drug concentrations in all biological samples are affected by complex and individually variable pharmacokinetics.[14] Urine analysis is further complicated by dilution effects, due to wide differences in urine volume, and by pH differences. It is also not generally possible to correlate urinary drug levels with physiologic and pharmacologic effects or to define specific time periods of exposure to the drug.[1]

Antibody-based screening assays must be interpreted cautiously (and confirmed), since antibodies show different cross-reactivities to drugs within a class and also to various metabolites of a given drug.[13] Thus, a positive result from an immunoassay may be obtained when a specimen contains several drugs or metabolites that produce a cumulative response in excess of the assay cutoff value. Negative results reflect either the absence of drugs or metabolites or their presence at levels below the cutoff decision value.

B. ADVANTAGES OF AUTOMATED DRUG SCREENING ON THE aca®

With its 12 toxicology methods, the aca® discrete clinical analyzer provides for convenient testing of the major categories of drugs of abuse in use today. The assays employ proven technologies, are simple to perform, give consistent results, and are fully automated, i.e., they provide one button, "walk away" operation 24 hours a day.

Since the tests are discrete, profiles can be designed to meet the needs of individual patients and laboratories. However, even a six-test panel of urine drugs of abuse screens can be run in less than 15 min. As such, the panels are especially well-adapted to emergency drug screening in suspected overdose cases.

Calibrator and daily quality control testing are conveniently done with one three-level calibrator kit and one two-level control kit for all six urine drugs of abuse.

System calibration is stable for at least 1 month, and for four of the six methods, for 3 months.

Du Pont continues to provide a comprehensive support network for aca® users through experienced personnel and continuing education materials. Training and field support specialists are readily accessible, as is a large group of technical service biochemists with clinical laboratory technical and management experience. Continuing education is available through a monthly newsletter for aca® users, technical bulletins on new methods and new applications,[12] and a concise description of the clinical significance of aca® tests.[15]

The six urinary drugs of abuse screening methods currently available on the aca® will detect a large majority of the top 20 controlled substances implicated in acute drug abuse episodes, tabulated in the U. S. Drug Enforcement Agency's DAWN database.[16] In 1991, Du Pont plans to introduce a seventh urinary drug of abuse screening method, for phencyclidine (U PCP), complete with calibrator and control products. Thus, the addition of the U PCP test to the toxicology methods already available on the aca® represents Du Pont's ongoing commitment to the worldwide drugs of abuse testing market.

ACKNOWLEDGMENTS

We gratefully acknowledge the participation of Dr. Gerald Clement at the Allentown Hospital (Allentown, PA) and Dr. Kingsley Labrosse of Medtox Laboratories, Inc. (Minneapolis, MN) in the Field Evaluations of the urine cocaine metabolite screen method. We would also like to thank Dr. Elinor L. Knodel for contributions to and preparation of the manuscript.

REFERENCES

1. **Hawks, R. L. and Chiang, C. N., Eds.,** Urine testing for drugs of abuse, *NIDA Research Monograph,* Vol. 73, 1986.
2. **Aziz, K., Staples, B., and Donlon, J.,** Drug abuse testing, *Am. Clin. Prod. Rev.,* October, 44–46, 1987.
3. **Cone, E. J.,** Testing human hair for drugs of abuse. I. Individual dose and time profiles of morphine and codeine in plasma, urine and beard compared to drug-induced effects on pupils and behavior, *J. Anal. Toxicol.,* 14, 1–7, 1990.
4. **Boone, D. J. and Walsh, J. M.,** Reliability of urine drug testing, *J. Am. Med. Assoc.,* 258, 2587–2588, 1987.
5. **Frings, C. S., White, R. M., and Battaglia, D. J.,** Status of drug-of-abuse testing in urine: an AACC study, *Clin. Chem.,* 33, 1683–1687, 1987.
6. **Frings, C. S., Battaglia, D. J., and White, R. M.,** Status of drug-of-abuse testing in urine under blind conditions: an AACC study, *Clin. Chem.,* 35, 891–894, 1989.
7. **Hoyt, D. W., Finnigan, R. E., Nee, T., Shults, T. F., and Butler, T.J.,** Drug testing in the workplace — are methods legally defensible?, *J. Am. Med. Assoc.,* 258, 504–509, 1987.
8. **Westgard, J. O. and Klee, G. G.,** Quality assurance, in *Textbook of Clinical Chemistry,* Tietz, N.W., Ed., W.B. Saunders, Philadelphia, 1986, 424–458.
9. **Segura, J., de la Torre, R., Congost, M., and Camí, J.,** Proficiency testing on drugs of abuse: one year's experience in Spain, *Clin. Chem.,* 35, 879–883, 1989.
10. **Blanke, R. V. and Decker, W. J.,** Analysis of toxic substances, in *Textbook of Clinical Chemistry,* Tietz, N.W., Ed., W.B. Saunders, Philadelphia, 1986, 1670–1744.
11. **Wolff, K., Shanab, M. A., Sanderson, M. J., and Hay, A. W. M.,** Screening for drugs of abuse: effect of heat-treating urine for safe handling of samples, *Clin. Chem.,* 36, 908–910, 1990.
12. **Crouse, S. P. and Narváez, R. P.,** *Performance characteristics of the urine cocaine metabolite screen method for the Du Pont aca® discrete clinical analyzer,* Medical Products Department, E.I. Du Pont de Nemours & Co. Inc., Wilmington, DE, 1987. A series of six technical bulletins is available, describing all of the urine drug of abuse screening assays.
13. **Baselt, R. C.,** Urine drug screening by immunoassay: interpretation of results, in *Advances in Analytical Toxicology,* Baselt, R.C., Ed., Vol. 1, Biomedical Publications, Davis, CA, 1984, 81–123.
14. **Warner, A., Hassan, F. M., and Fant, W. K.,** Drug abuse testing: pharmacokinetic and technical aspects, *Therapeutic Drug Monitoring and Emergency Toxicology Continuing Education Program,* American Association for Clinical Chemistry, 8, 1–9, December 1986
15. **Larson, F.,** *Clinical significance of urine drugs of abuse tests available on the Du Pont aca®,* Medical Products Department, E.I. Du Pont de Nemours & Co., Inc., Wilmington, DE, 1987.
16. **Frank, R. S.,** Drugs of abuse: data collection systems of DEA and recent trends, *J. Anal. Toxicol.,* 11, 237–241, 1987.

Chapter 19

OVERVIEW OF FLUORESCENCE POLARIZATION IMMUNOASSAY SYSTEMS IN ABUSED DRUG TESTING

Sally P. Stewart

TABLE OF CONTENTS

I.	Principle	114
	A. Summary	114
	B. Rotation and Polarization	114
	C. Sensitivity and Specificity	114
II.	Methodology	114
III.	Flexibility of FPIA Methodologies	116
	A. Numerical and Qualitative Results	116
	B. Cross-Reactivity	116
	C. Adjustable Threshold	117
IV.	Diversity in Testing Systems	117
	A. Instrumentation Overview	117
	1. The TDx® System	117
	2. The ADx® System	118
	3. The MTDx™ System	118
	4. The HTDx™ System	118
V.	Summary	118
	Acknowledgments	118
	References	118

I. PRINCIPLE

A. SUMMARY

Fluorescence Polarization Immunoassay (FPIA) is a competitive protein binding technology that incorporates the specificity of immunoassay with a fluorescent tracer to distinguish the bound from the free analyte.[1-3] Abbott Laboratories FPIA technology labels the analyte, a drug or drug derivative, with fluorescein. A specific antibody to the analyte (antigen) is prepared. Abbott FPIA instruments excite the fluorescein tracer with polarized light, and the fluorescent polarization of tracer is determined. The concentration of the analyte is inversely related to the amount of polarized light detected.[4]

B. ROTATION AND POLARIZATION

Molecules in solution rotate, and the rate of rotation is related to the size of the molecule.[5] The analyte from the specimen and tracer compete for binding sites on the protein antibody. The bound antibody-tracer molecule that results is larger and rotates slower than the free tracer molecule.[6]

The FPIA analyzers excite the fluorescent tracer with polarized light at 481–489 nm. The emitted polarized light is measured at 525 to 550 nm.[7] When the tracer is not bound to an antibody (free), it rotates rapidly, and the emitted light has little or no remaining polarization. When little or no drug is present in the specimen, the antibody binds with tracer. The large antibody-tracer rotates slowly and polarization of the emitted light is retained (see Figure 1).

When high concentration of analyte is present in the specimen, more tracer rotates freely resulting in a decrease in polarized light detected. Conversely, when the concentration of analyte in specimen is low, the tracer is bound and rotates slowly, resulting in the detection of more polarized light (see Figure 2).

C. SENSITIVITY AND SPECIFICITY

Sensitivity is defined as the lowest concentration of analyte that can be distinguished from zero with 95% confidence. Because of the inverse relationship between the polarized light detected by the instrument (signal output generated) and the concentration of the analyte, the Abbott Abused Drug Reagent Systems (FPIA reagents and instrumentation) are able to easily distinguish between signal and background noise. The result is improved sensitivity.[7]

The specificity of the abused drug assays has been enhanced by the use of FPIA technology. The effect of interference from sample matrix or adulterants added to the specimen has been minimized by incorporating the following four characteristics.

Nonenzyme reagent system — Urine specimens frequently contain enzyme inhibitors which decrease the rate of enzyme activity. Adulterants may also have this effect. Although adulterants and interferents may affect the integrity of the analyte, they are of less concern in systems that do not use enzymes.[9]

Small sample volume — Using sample volumes of less than 20 µl reduces the effect of turbidity and other interferences in the sample matrix.[10]

Measurement of background fluorescence — By taking a blank reading for each sample and comparing the value to a maximum background specification defined in the FPIA instrument software, correction is made for nonanalyte fluorescence.[7,10]

Specific antibody — Nonspecific protein binding is minimized by use of antibodies with high affinity for the analyte and tracer.[4,7,10] The specificity is validated by cross-reactivity analysis (see Figure 3).

II. METHODOLOGY

The Abbott FPIA technology is a homogeneous immunoassay. No manual or separation steps are necessary. The determination of fluorescence polarization as the tracer binds to the antibody allows the reaction and fluorescence polarization readings to occur in a single cuvette. Fluorescence polarization values are interpolated by the system software from fluorescence intensity readings.[7,10-12]

The Abbott FPIA methodologies employ a six point calibration curve. The calibration curve is generated from six calibrators of different concentrations. The calibration material is liquid and packaged in ready-to-use vials. The use of ready-to-use calibrators eliminates the problems that may occur when dilution is required by the operator. The software of the FPIA analyzer is designed to ensure the acceptability of the calibration readings and preclude operator and system failure.[8]

The FPIA systems measure the intensity of the light emitted by each calibrator and calculates the polarization values. Using the polarization, a calibration curve is generated (see Figure 4). The analyzer determines the validity of the curve by evaluating seven parameters. The criteria for acceptance of each parameter is determined for each assay and stored in the assay information file in the system software.[8]

Six-point calibration curve — When processing a calibration run, the Abbott FPIA Systems expect six data points for generation of a calibration curve. If six accept-

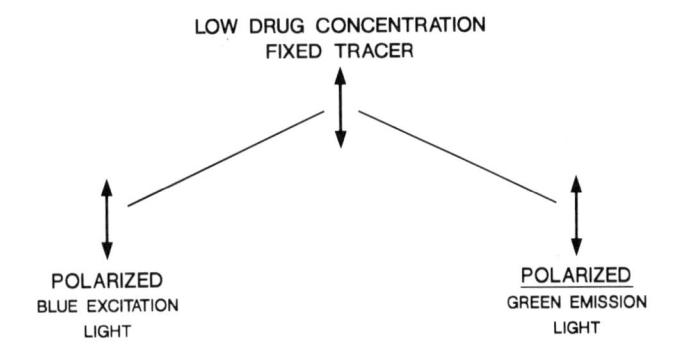

FIGURE 1. Fluorescence polarization on a low drug concentration sample.

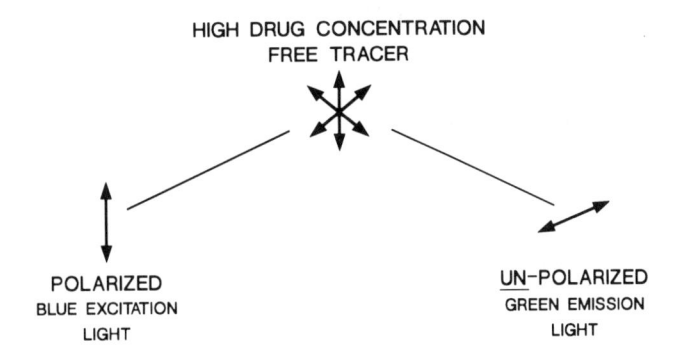

FIGURE 2. Fluorescence polarization on a high drug concentration sample.

COMPOUNDS TESTED FOR CROSS-REACTIVITY

AMPHETAMINE/METHAMPHETAMINE II	384
AMPHETAMINE CLASS	326
BARBITURATES	152
BENZODIAZEPINES	223
CANNABINOIDS	275
COCAINE METABOLITE	181
METHADONE	259
OPIATES	210
PHENCYCLIDINE (PCP)	202

FIGURE 3. Cross-reactivity analysis.

able values are not measured during the analytical process, the systems will abort the calibration run.

Background readings — A background or blank reading is taken on each sample. The maximum background fluorescence that can occur in a sample without adverse effect on the result has been determined for each assay and is stored in the FPIA System software. If the background reading of any calibrator exceeds the defined value, the calibration will not be accepted by the system. Any sample that exhibits a large background reading is identified, and an error message is reported, instead of a result. Through analysis of background readings, the operator may recognize samples that may be contaminated or adulterated.

Intensity readings—To correct for background sample

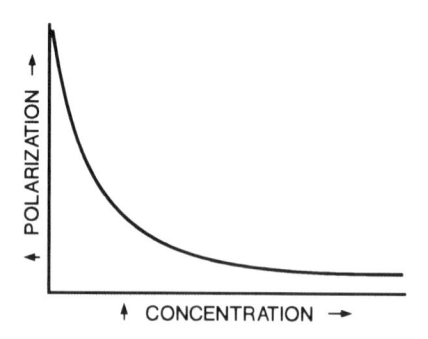

FIGURE 4. Calibration curve.

fluorescence, a net intensity value is determined by subtracting the blank intensity reading of the sample from the final intensity. The polarization values are calculated from the net intensity. The acceptable minimum intensity value is determined for each assay. If any calibrator intensity values are less than or equal to the minimum value, the calibration will not be accepted by the system. This check ensures the integrity of the fluorescein tracer and verifies that an adequate quantity of tracer has been added to the reaction cuvette.

Reproducibility — Each calibrator can be processed in duplicate. If the duplicate calibrators are used, the maximum deviation allowed between sample replicates is determined for each assay. If the difference between the calibrator pairs exceeds this value, the calibration curve will not be accepted by the system.

A to F sequence — If the polarization values of the calibrators do not decrease monotonically, the curve will not be accepted. Failure of the check on calibrator sequence indicates that the calibrators are not correctly placed in the carousel or the optical system is not functioning properly. Either operator errors or system failures are monitored by the system and will cause the calibration to be unacceptable.

Polarization of the A calibrator — The A calibrator is a zero concentration calibrator demonstrating the largest polarization values of the calibrator set. The minimum acceptable polarization value for the A calibrator is defined for each assay. If the polarization of the A calibrator is not equal to or greater than this value, the curve is not accepted. The check is one evaluation of the function of the optical system.

Polarization range from A to F — The difference in the polarization readings of the A and F calibrator is measured. The minimum, acceptable difference in the polarization values is defined for each assay. The check ensures the integrity of the reagent systems.

The system evaluates the calibration data. If it is acceptable, the calibration curve is determined, stored, and used to calculate the concentrations of unknown samples.

III. FLEXIBILITY OF FPIA METHODOLOGIES

A. NUMERICAL AND QUALITATIVE RESULTS

The use of a six-point calibration curve allows both numerical and qualitative results. Numerical results are sometimes termed semiquantitative because the results are the summation of the concentrations of the drug or drug metabolite and similar cross-reactive substances. For example, all members of the barbiturate family react with the barbiturate antibody. The standard used for the calibration of the barbiturate assay is secobarbital. Other barbiturates are evaluated relative to the secobarbital standard. Either a semiquantitative/numerical or qualitative format may be chosen for reporting results. The ability to produce numerical/semiquantitative results offers several advantages.

- Numerical results of drug screens can be more closely correlated with quantitative confirmation tests such as GC/MS.
- Numerical quality control data can be maintained to ensure and document the reliability of the analytical system.
- Numerical results provide a better research tool to aid in the evaluation of impairment and recency of use as it relates to urine screening values.

B. CROSS-REACTIVITY

The actual concentrations and cross-reactivities are listed in each Abbott FPIA Abused Drug Assay manual. The cross-reactivity lists published in the assay manual inserts are periodically updated as additional compounds are tested. The number of drugs tested varies with each assay, and the substances tested are chosen for a variety of reasons:

- Frequency of use and structural similarities to the analyte
- Use with common "street forms" of the abused drug
- Requests by experts and customers

The cross-reactivity is calculated from the following equation: [8]

$$\% \text{ Cross-reactivity} = 100 \times \frac{\text{(measured concentration of analyte)}}{\text{(actual concentration of the analyte)}}$$

C. ADJUSTABLE THRESHOLD

The threshold establishes the concentration of the drug or metabolite that must be present before a specimen is considered positive.[8] If the specimen does not demonstrate results at or above the threshold level, then it is considered negative. The selection of the threshold should relate to the purpose of the test and may not reflect the inherent sensitivity of the analytical system.

Through user-defined software edits, the operator may choose and store a threshold for each assay. The threshold may be defined beginning at the sensitivity limit of the assay continuing over the dynamic range of the calibration curve. The threshold value should be consistent with the confirmation technology. The correct selection of threshold is a major factor in determining the efficiency of the screening and confirmation assays.[13] Adjustable threshold allows the demands of the various testing systems, regulating agencies, and abused drug testing market to be considered. For example, the threshold that is desirable in a drug rehabilitation center, which chooses not to confirm screening positives, may not be appropriate for a private laboratory using GC/MS for confirmation on all screened positives.

IV. DIVERSITY IN TESTING SYSTEMS

In response to an ever-growing and diverse abused drug testing market, Abbott developed both assay systems and analytical instrument to solve the needs of a variety of testing environments. Hospitals, emergency rooms, sporting organizations, rehabilitation centers, industry, penal institutions, and government and military facilities all perform abused drug testing for different purposes. To meet the needs of these groups, a variety of testing systems is required.

Amphetamine testing is a good example of the flexibility built into Abbott FPIA Abused Drug Assay Systems. The original amphetamine assay was a specific assay designed to detect amphetamine and methamphetamine along with some of the amphetamine analogs or designer amines, such as MDMA (ecstasy), MDE, etc. This reagent system offered the single most specific assay on the market for the detection of amphetamine/methamphetamine. The specificity of the X SYSTEMS™ Amphetamine/Methamphetamine Assay was further improved and released as the X SYSTEMS™ Amphetamine/Methamphetamine II. The new reagent system has improved specificities for the d-isomer of amphetamine and methamphetamine.

To meet the needs of emergency rooms and sports testing, a broad specificity assay was required. Abbott developed the FPIA Amphetamine Class reagent system which detects central nervous system stimulants as well as over-the-counter medications in the sympathomimetic amine class.

A. INSTRUMENTATION OVERVIEW

In addition to assay systems, the instrumentation needed to process samples in diverse environments was addressed. Batch, stat panel, and high volume systems have been developed.

1. The TDx® System

In 1981, the TDx® Clinical Analyzer was introduced as a batch therapeutic drug analyzer. The TDx® System now provides analysis of more than 60 assays and is in use in 90% of the hospitals in the United States. Currently, the TDx® System offers assays for the most requested abused drugs as well as toxicology reagent systems. These include

- Amphetamine/Methamphetamine II
- Amphetamine Class
- Benzodiazepines (urine and serum)
- Barbiturates (urine and serum)
- Cocaine
- Cannabinoids
- Delta-9 Calibrators and Controls
- Methadone
- Opiates
- Phencyclidine
- Ethanol (whole blood, plasma, and urine)
- Acetaminophen
- Salicylate
- Tricyclic Antidepressants

2. The ADx® System

The ADx® System offers the capability of specific paneling and can operate in the batch, combination, and panel mode as follows:

- Batch — one assay performed on multiple samples
- Combination — varied combinations of assays performed on multiple samples
- Panel — specific series of assays performed on multiple samples

The TDx® System software and the ADx® System software provide for identification and documentation of the sample and operator and maintains a controlled testing environment to ensure result integrity.

3. The MTDxç System

The MTDx™ FPIA Abused Drug System addresses medium volume requirements by interfacing four TDx analyzers to an IBM® Personal System 2/Model 50 computer. ABBOTT DATATRAC™ System, a data management software, collates patient reports and provides quality control tracking.

4. The HTDx™ System

The HTDx™ FPIA Abused Drug System is designed to handle high volume testing. Multiple TDx analyzers operate in an accelerated mode using HTDx instrument software. The combination of the TDx analyzer and the HTDx software produces the HTDx analyzer. The HTDx™ System includes the HTDx analyzer and a Digital Equipment Corporation MicroVax computer with VMS operating system software. The HTDx™ System provides full capability to accession and analyze samples, acquire, collate and report results while assuring that the specimen integrity is documented. A full spectrum of supervisor management reports and control functions are also provided.

V. SUMMARY

The inherent characteristics of the Abbott FPIA technology offered solutions to problems associated with drug analysis. To solve the problems related to the abused drug testing, the Abbott FPIA reagents systems incorporated the following features:

1. Six-point calibration curves
2. Improved antibody specificity
3. A stable fluorescent tracer
4. Inverse relationship of concentration to polarization to improve sensitivity and specificity
5. Use of small sample volume
6. Correction for background interference
7. Comprehensive evaluation of selective reactivity and interfering substance
8. Use of FPIA instrumentation to improve the integrity of the sample and results.

Recognizing the need for both specific and drug class analysis, amphetamine/methamphetamine and amphetamine class reagent systems offer a broader approach to abused drug testing, depending on the requirements of the testing protocol. The TDx® System continues to offer a broad menu of therapeutic and abused drug and toxicology assays for batch mode analysis. The ADx® System is adapted to both classic and nontraditional, small-volume testing environments. The need for medium volume abused drug testing lead to the development of the MTDx™ System, while the HTDx™ System provides an option for high-volume testing needs.

As a result, Abbott FPIA technology offers solutions for many abused drug testing requirements. Those requirements include the need for (1) accuracy, specificity, and sensitivity; (2) numerical results and adjustable thresholds; and (3) reliable, flexible assay systems and instrumentation.

ACKNOWLEDGMENTS

We wish to thank Sandra H. Kinchen, Senior Technical Writer at Abbott Diagnostics Division, Irving, TX.

REFERENCES

1. **Dandliker, W. B., Schapiro, M. C., Meduski, J. W., and Alonso, R., et al.,** Application of fluorescence polarization to the antigen-antibody reaction, *Immunochemistry*, 1, 165–191, 1961.
2. **Dandliker, W. B. and Saussure, V. A.,** Review article: fluorescence polarization immunoassay in immunochemistry, *Immunochemistry*, 7, 799–828, 1970.
3. **Dandliker, W. B., Kelly, R. J., and Dandliker, J.,** Fluorescence polarization immunoassay: theory and experimental method, *Immunochemistry*, 10, 219–27, 1973.
4. **Jolley, M. E.,** Fluorescence polarization immunoassay for the determination of therapeutic drug levels in human plasma, *J. Anal. Toxicol.*, 5, 236–240, 1981.
5. **Weber, G.,** Rotation Brownian motion and polarization of the fluorescence of solutions, *Adv. Protein Chem.*, 8, 425–459, 1953.
6. **Blecka, L. J.,** Fluorescence polarization immunoassay: a review of methodology and applications, *Therapeutic Drug Monitoring, Continuing Education and Control Program*, American Association for Clinical Chemistry, March 1983, 1–6.

7. **Popelka, S. R., Miller, D. M., Holen, J. T., and Kelso, D. M.,** Fluorescence polarization immunoassay II. Analyzer for rapid, precise measurement of fluorescence polarization with use of disposable cuvettes, *Clin. Chem.*, 27(7), 1198–1201, 1981.

8. **Abbott Diagnostics Division,** *TDx System Assay Manual*, Rev. 110, Abbott Laboratories, Abbott Park, IL, 1990.

9. **Baselt, R. C., Ed.,** Urine drug screening by immunoassay: interpretation of results, *Adv. Anal. Toxicol.*, 81, 1984.

10. **Jolley, M. E., Stroupe, S. D., Wang, C. J., et al.,** Fluorescence polarization immunoassay I. Monitoring aminoglycoside antibiotics in serum and plasma, *Clin. Chem.*, 27, 1190–1197, 1981.

11. **Jolley, M. E., Stroupe, S. D., Wang, C. J., et al.,** Fluorescence polarization immunoassay III. An automated system polarization immunoassay for therapeutic drug determination, *Clin Chem.*, 27, 1575–1579, 1981.

12. **Lu-Steffes, M., Pittluck, G. W., Jolley, M. E., Panas, H. N., et al.,** Fluorescence polarization immunoassay IV. Determination of phenytoin and phenobarbital in human serum and plasma, *Clin. Chem.*, 28, 2278–2282, 1982.

13. **Walters, R.,** An abused drug assay system, *Am. Clin. Prod. Rev.*, March 1987.

Chapter 20

RADIOIMMUNOASSAY AND DRUG MEASUREMENTS: THE ART OF THE POSSIBLE

R. A. Moore, C. W. Hand, D. Carroll, and H. J. McQuay

TABLE OF CONTENTS

I.	Introduction	122
II.	Aspects of the Method	122
III.	Morphine and Glucuronide Metabolites	122
IV.	Differentiating Codeine From Heroin or Morphine Use by Radioimmunoassay	124
	A. Samples	125
	B. Analysis	125
	C. Results	125
V.	Pharmacogenetics of Codeine Demethylation	126
VI.	Conclusions	127
	Acknowledgments	127
	References	127

I. INTRODUCTION

In clinical chemistry and endocrinology, RIA has long been the method of choice for the analysis of low concentrations of protein, steroid, and thyroid hormones in biological fluids. Indeed, the explosive growth in understanding of the pathophysiology of endocrine disorders began, and continues, because of the use of RIA as an analytical tool. Careful and detailed investigations by the Association of Clinical Biochemists in the U.K. have led to certain radioimmunoassay methods being promoted for the provision of routine biochemistry service for some hormones.[1-3]

Immunological methods have thus been demonstrated over many years and in circumstances of great complexity have sufficient accuracy, precision, simplicity, and analytical robustness for routine use. It is difficult to square this appreciation of immunoassays with how they are often described in drug abuse analysis; here immunoassays come close to being contemptuously dismissed as inaccurate, insensitive, and imprecise.

The reasons in part stem from the growth (particularly in the United States) of abused-drug analysis from forensic science; many of the doubts arise from legal rather than scientific problems. Again, the growth in abused-drug testing has been explosive, with perhaps too little opportunity for the scientific community (and the customers) to ask (or answer) some basic questions regarding exactly what their analytical goals are. Drawing again from the example of endocrinology, it happens that products can often fit rapidly changing criteria rather than the other way around.

Because RIA is a technique that has been described definitively in many publications, this essay will not attempt a detailed description of the method. Rather it will point to ways in which RIA can be used as a subtle analytical tool, hopefully to stimulate discussion on the future goals of immunological methods.

II. ASPECTS OF THE METHOD

In order to discuss how RIA may be used confidently in drug analysis, it is first necessary to dispel some doubts concerning the method. For precision, the measurement of plasma cortisol in the U.K. External Quality Assessment Scheme has demonstrated that a wide variety of RIA techniques in use in routine laboratories give concordant results over long periods of time.[2] These results also demonstrate accuracy, in that laboratories using these methods report values identical to those found by GC/MS. RIA methods for drugs can also give identical values to GC/MS, and PCP is a good example.[4]

Another criticism of RIA methods is that they are slow to reach equilibrium. Again, this need not necessarily be so, as antibodies can be selected for speed of equilibrium, as well as for cross-reaction. As an example, in a double-antibody method for morphine, antibodies can achieve equilibrium within 5 min (Figure 1).

One of the most appealing properties of RIA is its sensitivity. By using high specific-activity tracers and appropriate antisera, analytical sensitivities of the order of 100 pg/ml are easily achieved. While this degree of sensitivity is unnecessary for most currently abused drugs, the emergence of highly potent "designer drugs" may make this important in the future. An example of this was the finding that 62% of patients attending a drug addiction clinic in Dublin, Ireland in 1987 were using the highly potent opiate buprenorphine.[5] Racing horses are already being doped with agents like fentanyl and etorphine because of the increased locomotor activity induced by subtherapeutic opiate doses in horses. A 500 kg horse may be given as little as 2 mg of fentanyl, but for etorphine effective doses are as low as 30 μg. With etorphine RIA, however, the drug can still be detected in equine urine 24 hours after a dose as low as 5 μg (Figure 2).

III. MORPHINE AND GLUCURONIDE METABOLITES

Morphine is extensively metabolized in man, and in recent years the importance of morphine-6-glucuronide (M6G) as an active metabolite has increasingly been recognized.[6] M6G is not only active, but may be 20 to 40 times more potent than morphine in the central nervous system.

The use of antibodies with different cross-reactions to morphine, M6G, and morphine-3-glucuronide (M3G) (Table 1) has allowed the development of differential radioimmunoassays which can produce analytical resolution between morphine and the two glucuronidated metabolites in human serum (Figure 3).[7] Concentrations of morphine and metabolites found in serum after intravenous or oral administration of morphine are similar whether measured by differential RIA or HPLC.[6-8] The use of antibodies to morphine with different specificities has also been used, for instance, in the investigation of endogenous opiate alkaloids.[9]

Morphine-6-glucuronide crosses the blood-brain barrier and may be responsible for a significant proportion of the pharmacological effects of morphine.[10] Moreover, the

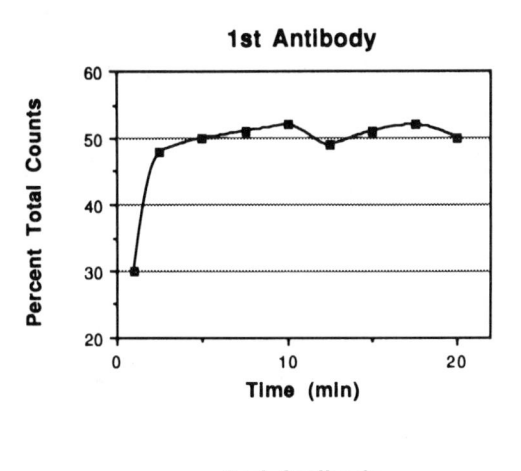

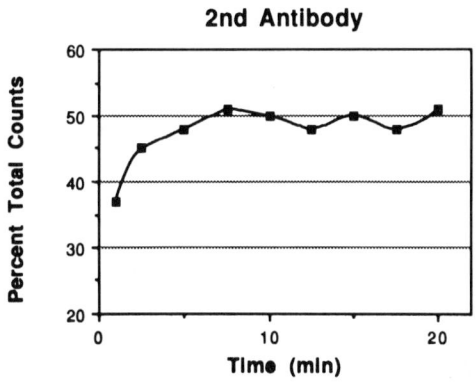

FIGURE 1. Time to reach equilibrium for first and second antibodies in a double-antibody assay for morphine.

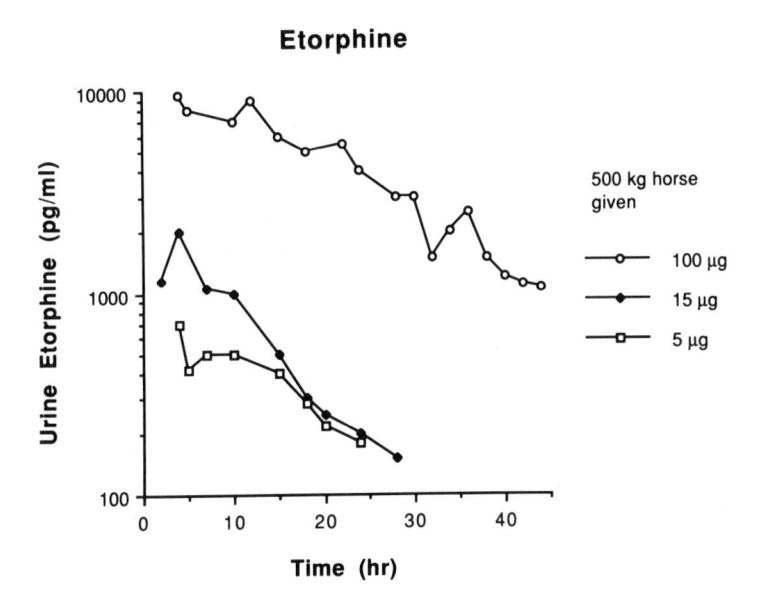

FIGURE 2. Urine etorphine values for a 500 kg horse given doses of 100, 15, and 5 µg intramuscular etorphine on three occasions separated by at least 1 week.

TABLE 1
Cross-Reaction Data with Three Different Antimorphine Sera

Percentage Relative to Morphine

	Antiserum A	Antiserum B	Antiserum C
Morphine	100	100	100
M-3-G	<0.1	100	1.1
M-6-G	<0.1	<0.1	300

All curves are parallel

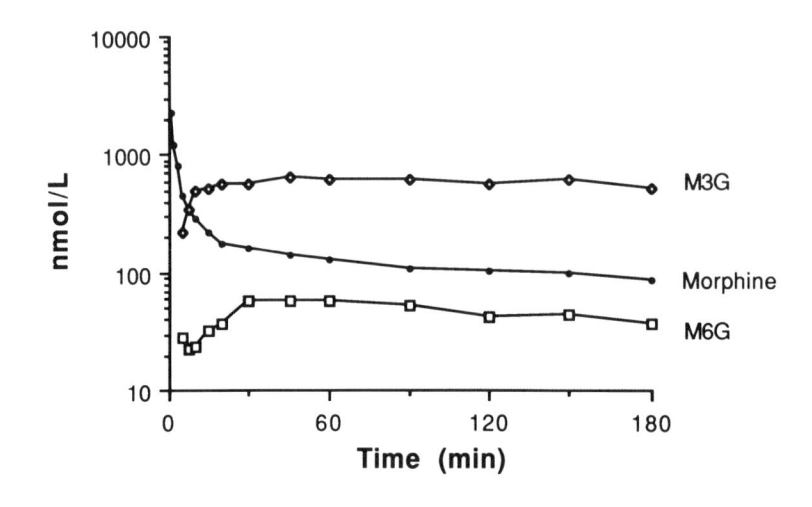

FIGURE 3. Mean plasma concentrations of morphine, M3G, and M6G following in 14 anaesthetized subjects given a bolus of 10 mg morphine (as sulfate).

accumulation and persistence of the glucuronides in any slight degree of renal dysfunction has been recognized as being clinically important.[6,11] This use of differential RIA can also be used for much more potent drugs like buprenorphine, where (inactive) metabolites also accumulate in the serum of patients with renal failure during chronic dosing.[12]

IV. DIFFERENTIATING CODEINE FROM HEROIN OR MORPHINE USE BY RADIOIMMUNOASSAY

Biotransformations of codeine include loss of the 3-O-methyl group and production of morphine. In rats, a substantial part of a codeine dose is converted in this way,[13] but in man the proportion is much lower.[14] Moreover, the demethylation enzymes in man may be subject to genetic polymorphism, as some patients produce much smaller amounts of morphine.[15] Codeine and morphine are then further metabolized, mainly by glucuronidation.[16]

Heroin shares some of these metabolic pathways; it does not itself bind to opiate receptors,[17] but works through conversion to its active metabolites 6-acetylmorphine, morphine, and morphine-6-glucuronide.[18,19] Heroin deacetylation to morphine occurs rapidly, and urinary excretion is mainly as morphine and its metabolites.

These metabolic interconversions can give rise to problems of interpretation in screening urine samples for abuse of heroin or morphine. A particular problem is that many hours after a dose of codeine, the amount of total morphine (free plus hydrolyzed) may be much greater than the amount of total codeine.[20] In addition, combination analgesic preparations containing codeine are freely available as nonprescription medicines in many parts of the world.

Attempts have been made to discriminate between use of codeine and heroin or morphine by a number of techniques. Gas chromatography for morphine and codeine in urine after hydrolysis of glucuronide conjugates and the use of a codeine/morphine ratio failed to separate use of the drugs,[21] but was more successful in post-mortem studies of death due to codeine overdose.[22] The ratio of specific to nonspecific morphine radioimmunoassays provided an almost complete separation of heroin and morphine use from that of codeine or dihydrocodeine.[23]

A. SAMPLES

Urine samples were obtained from patients or volunteers known to be using a particular drug (or drugs), in which the presence of the drug had been confirmed by at least one of a number of techniques including immunological analyses, TLC, and GC/MS.

Heroin	Fifty-five samples from known heroin abusers
Codeine/ dihydrocodeine	Thirteen samples from known abusers of codeine or dihydrocodeine but not heroin or morphine
Mixed users	Six samples from abusers of both heroin and codeine or dihydrocodeine
Morphine patients	Thirteen samples from patients receiving oral morphine for the relief of chronic pain of malignant origin
Codeine volunteers	Thirty samples from human volunteers taking 30 or 60 mg codeine daily

B. ANALYSIS

Analysis for morphine was with Morphine Coat-A-Count (DPC, Los Angeles, CA). Samples with values greater than 100 ng/ml were diluted 1:100 with drug-free human urine and re-assayed to provide a quantitative value for morphine in urine.

Samples were also measured for morphine plus codeine using an antibody (491) which cross-reacted to both morphine, codeine (129%), dihydrocodeine (78%), and ethylmorphine (76%), but not the glucuronide metabolites. The antibody was coated onto polypropylene test tubes; calibrators were morphine (1 to 250 ng/ml, as base) in human urine, and the radioactive tracer was 2-iodomorphine. Values greater than 250 ng/ml were diluted 1:100 or 1:1000 with human urine and re-assayed to provide a quantitative value for codeine plus morphine. The results of assay for morphine (M) and morphine plus codeine (C) were expressed as the ratio C/M.

C. RESULTS

The concentration range found in the samples was very wide, over three orders of magnitude for results obtained with both assays (5 to 100,000 ng/ml for urine morphine and 30 to 200,000 ng/ml for urine morphine plus codeine). Despite this, there was a clear differentiation between those patients taking morphine or heroin who had C/M ratios below 3.5, and patients or volunteers taking codeine who had C/M ratios above 7.5 (Figure 4).

Individuals taking a mixture of heroin and codeine or dihydrocodeine had intermediate C/M ratios between 3.8 and 15.6. Using the C/M ratio, heroin users also taking codeine were not distinguished from volunteers taking codeine alone. However, volunteers taking codeine had urine morphine concentrations of 552 ng/ml or below (median 33 ng/ml), while the heroin users who also took codeine had urine morphine concentrations of 3900 ng/ml and above (median 5000 ng/ml).

Codeine is a commonly prescribed analgesic and in many parts of the world is available as a nonprescription co-analgesic in combination with nonopiate drugs such as aspirin, acetaminophen, and ibuprofen. Analytical problems arise because both codeine and heroin share a major route of metabolism through morphine, and morphine and its glucuronides are found in the urine of both codeine and heroin users.[24] The situation is complicated because, many hours after a dose of codeine, urinary levels of total morphine may exceed those of total codeine.

The strategy used here was to compare not the ratio of total codeine to total morphine, but rather the ratio of unconjugated codeine plus morphine to unconjugated morphine in urine. Two separate radioimmunoassay procedures were used which differed only in the specificity of the antisera used; neither cross-reacted to morphine glucuronides or normorphine, but one cross-reacted to codeine and dihydrocodeine as well as morphine. The assays had excellent interassay precision and recovery.

Urine samples were diluted to provide quantitative estimates of the concentrations of morphine and morphine plus codeine, and this allowed the generation of a ratio between the tests. Given the low cross-reaction with morphine metabolites, the theoretical C/M ratio in users of heroin or patients on morphine should have been ap-

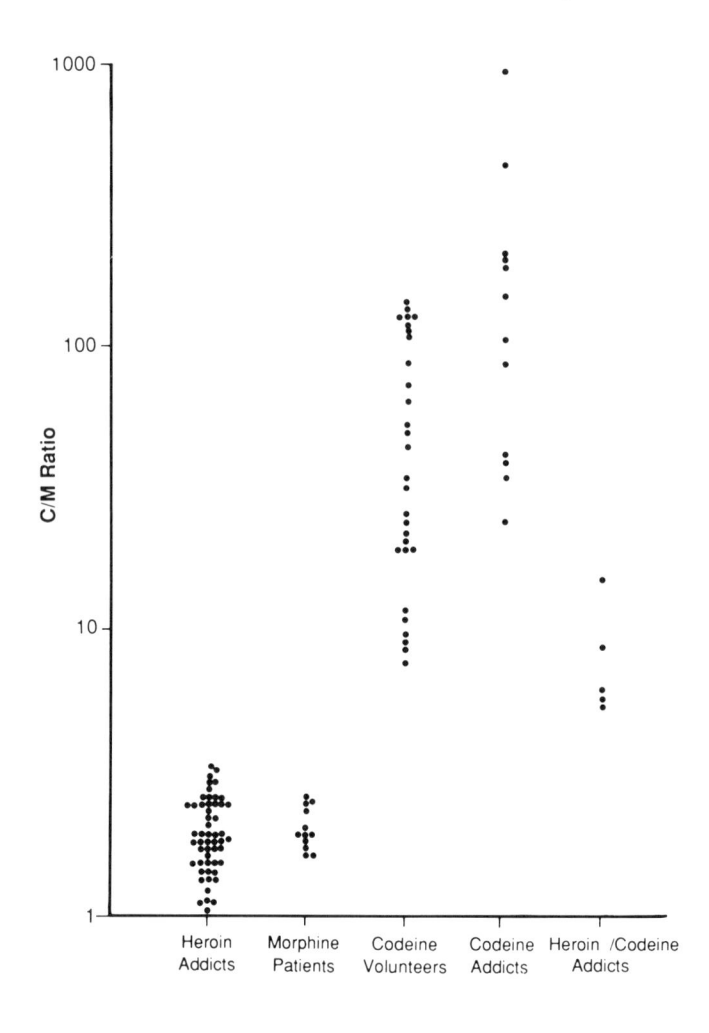

FIGURE 4. Urine codeine/morphine (C/M) ratios in different patient groups.

proximately unity. The actual range found was between 0.94 and 3.3 (Figure 4).

There was complete separation between use of heroin or morphine from use of codeine. Where codeine was used by volunteers or abusers, the range of the ratios was 7.9 to more than 100 (Figure 4). This degree of separation was significantly better than that achieved by Cassani et al.[23] using the ratio of a nonspecific assay cross-reacting to morphine, codeine and their glucuronide metabolites, and the same specific morphine assay as used here. That study did not demonstrate complete separation.

The use of the C/M ratio alone did not differentiate between codeine volunteers and those who abused both heroin and codeine together (Figure 4). However, the latter group all had measured urinary morphine concentrations of above 3900 ng/ml, whereas volunteers taking codeine had urine morphine levels below 650 ng/ml (Figure 3). Since generation of a quantitative value for urine morphine was essential for producing the C/M ratio, it is unlikely that heroin abusers would be able to mask their heroin intake by simultaneous ingestion of codeine.

V. PHARMACOGENETICS OF CODEINE DEMETHYLATION

Work by Findlay and colleagues in the early 1980s had suggested that some individuals metabolize codeine to morphine only very slowly,[15] with the suggestion that the analgesic activity of codeine depends on its biotransformation to morphine. It was likely that codeine O-demethylation was achieved by the microsomal cytochrome P-450 system, and it is known that a genetic polymorphism exists for this enzyme system. About 7% of humans have a deficient system using the drug debrisoquine as a probe.[25]

Some elegant work by a Swiss group has linked deficient codeine demethylation in man to debrisoquine-like cytochrome P-450 deficiency in a few patients.[26] Our previous observations showing wide variation in the

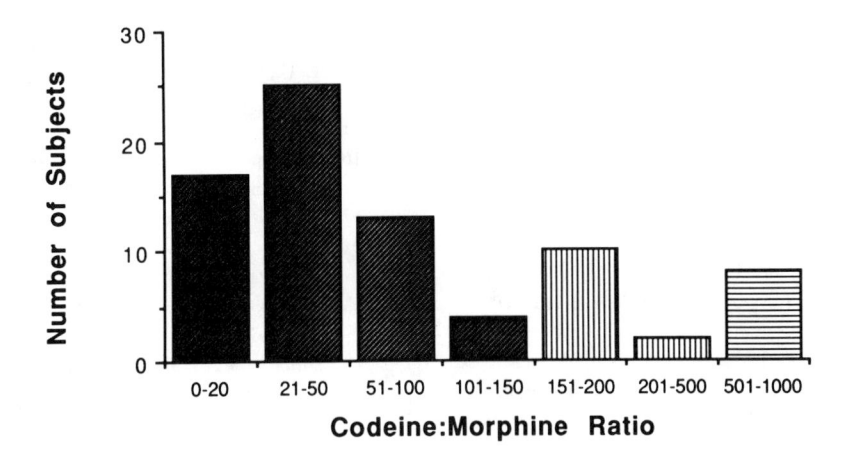

FIGURE 5. Urine codeine/morphine (C/M) ratios found in 8-hour urine collection from 76 subjects given 8 mg oral codeine phosphate.

amount of morphine formed from a standard codeine dose led us to investigate the use of C/M ratios as a probe for codeine demethylation in man.

Seventy-six adult men and women were given a capsule of codeine phosphate (8 mg) between 6:00 and 10:00 a.m., and all urine passed during the succeeding 8 hours was collected. None of the subjects was taking any medication or drugs. Urines were analyzed for the ratio of codeine plus morphine to morphine (C/M ratio) as described above.

Three groups of individuals were identified by this analysis (Figure 5). Fifty-seven subjects (75%) had considerable urine morphine concentrations (median 64 nmol/l) and C/M ratios below 200. A further 12 subjects (16%) had low concentrations of urine morphine (median 14 nmol/l) and C/M ratios between 201 and 1000. Seven subjects (9%) had negligible morphine in their urine (median 2 nmol/l), and C/M ratios were all above 1000.

This last group could not metabolize codeine to morphine, and the proportion of the population studied (9%) was very close to that commonly found for debrisoquine hydroxylation deficiency (8%). The population was probably too small to establish definitively whether a true heterozygous intermediate group was distinguished.

VI. CONCLUSIONS

Radioimmunoassay can be used as a powerful method for investigating many different aspects of clinical pharmacology. The use of a radioactive tracer is not an absolute requirement, and other nonisotopic tracers may also be used with similar benefits. The key is the flexibility of immunological methods to analytical variables, despite their use in situations of complex metabolic interactions.

There is no *a priori* reason why the power of immunological methods should not also be applied with benefit to drug-abuse screening, and such methods may well be able to accommodate the different analytical requirements obtained in different parts of the world.

ACKNOWLEDGMENTS

We wish to thank the staff of the Oxford Regional Pain Relief Unit, Abingdon, Oxfordshire, Dr. Tony Tetlow, Dr. Naresh Jain, and Mr. Brian Smith for providing human samples; and Mr. Laurie Jackson of the Horse Racing Forensic Science Laboratories in Newmarket for equine urine samples. We are grateful to Dr. M. Cassani for stimulating our interest in differentiating between heroin and codeine administration.

REFERENCES

1. **Wood, P., Groom, G., Moore, R. A., Ratcliffe, W., and Selby, C.,** Progesterone assays: guidelines for the provision of a clinical biochemistry service, *Ann. Clin. Biochem.*, 22, 1–24, 1985.
2. **Moore, R. A., Aitken, R., Burke, C. W., Gaskell, S., Groom, G., Holder, G., Selby, C., and Wood, P.,** Cortisol assays: guidelines for the provision of a clinical biochemistry service, *Ann. Clin. Biochem.*, 22, 435–454, 1985.
3. **Ratcliffe, W. A., Carter, G. D., Dowsett, M., Hillier, S. G., Middle, J. G., and Reed, M. J.,** Oestradiol assays: applications and guidelines for the provision of a clinical biochemistry service, *Ann. Clin. Biochem.*, 25, 466–483, 1988.
4. **Jain, N. C. and Sneath, T. C.,** An evaluation of a simple and rapid RIA procedure for cocaine and phencyclidine using Coat-A-Count, *Proc. TIAFT*, Banff, Alberta, Canada, 1987.

5. Hand, C. W., Ryan, K. E., Dutt, S. J., Moore, R. A., O'Connor, J., Talbot, D., and McQuay, H. J., Radioimmunoassay of buprenorphine in urine: studies in patients and in a drug clinic, *J. Anal. Toxicol.*, 13, 100–104, 1989.
6. Moore, R. A., Hand, C. W., and McQuay, H. J., Opiate metabolism and excretion, *Bailliere's Clin. Anaesthesiol.*, 1, 829–858, 1987.
7. Hand, C. W., Moore, R. A., McQuay, H. J., Allen, M. C., and Sear, J. W., Analysis of morphine and its major metabolites by differential radioimmunoassay, *Ann. Clin. Biochem.*, 24, 153–160, 1987.
8. Osborne, R. J., Joel, S. P., Trew, D., and Slevin, M. L., Morphine and metabolite behavior after different routes of morphine administration: demonstration of importance of the active metabolite morphine-6-glucuronide, *Clin. Pharm. Therap.*, 47, 12–19, 1990.
9. Goldstein, A., Barrett, R. W., James, I. F., Lowney, L. I., Weitz, C. J., Knipmeyer, L. L., and Rapoport, H., Morphine and other opiates from beef brain and adrenal, *Proc. Natl. Acad. Sci.*, 82, 5203–5207, 1985.
10. Hand, C. W., Blunnie, W. P., Claffey, L. P., McShane, A. J., McQuay, H. J., and Moore, R. A., Potential analgesic contribution from morphine-6-glucuronide in CSF, *Lancet*, 2, 1207–1208, 1987.
11. Osborne, R. J., Joel, S. P., Trew, D., and Slevin, M. L., The analgesic activity of morphine-6-glucuronide, *Lancet*, 1, 828, 1988.
12. Hand, C. W., Sear, J. W., Uppington, J., Ball, M. J., McQuay, J. H., and Moore, R. A., Buprenorphine disposition in patients with renal impairment: single and continuous dosing, with special reference to metabolites, *Br. J. Anaesthesiol.*, 64, 276–282, 1990.
13. Yeh, S. Y. and Woods, L. A., Physiologic disposition of N-C14-methyl-codeine in the rat, *J. Pharm. Pharmacol.*, 166, 86–95, 1969.
14. Quiding, H., Anderson, P., Bondesson, U., Boreus, L. O., and Hynning, P. A., Plasma concentrations of codeine and its metabolite, morphine, after single and repeated oral administration, *Eur. J. Clin. Pharmacol.*, 30, 673–677, 1980.
15. Rogers, J. F., Findlay, J. W. A., Hull, J. H., Butz, R. F., Jones, E. C., Bustrack, J. A., and Welch, R. M., Codeine disposition in smokers and nonsmokers, *Clin. Pharmacol. Ther.*, 32, 218–227, 1982.
16. Boerner, U., Abbott, S., and Roe, R. L., The metabolism of morphine and heroin in man, *Drug Metab. Rev.*, 4, 39–73, 1975.
17. Inturrisi, C. E., Schultz, M., Shin, S., Umans, J. G., Angel, L., and Simon, E. J., Evidence from opiate binding studies that heroin acts through its metabolites, *Life Sci.*, 33, 773–776, 1983.
18. Inturrisi, C. E., Heroin pharmacokinetics, *Adv. Pain Res. Ther.*, 8, 117–127, 1986.
19. Inturrisi, C. E., Max, M. B., Foley, K. M., Schultz, S. U., and Houde, R. W., The pharmacokinetics of heroin in patients with chronic pain, *N. Engl. J. Med.*, 310, 1213–1217, 1984.
20. Posey, B. L. and Kimble, S. N., High-performance liquid chromatographic study of codeine, norcodeine and morphine as indicators of codeine ingestion, *J. Anal. Toxicol.*, 8, 68–74, 1984.
21. Dutt, M. C., Lo, D. S., Doris, L. K., Woo, Ng, and Woo, Soo-on, Gas chromatographic study of the urinary codeine-to-morphine ratios in controlled codeine consumption and in mass screening for opiate drugs, *J. Chromatogr.*, 267, 117–124, 1983.
22. Nakamura, G. R., Greisemer, E. C., and Noguchi, T. T., Antemortem conversion of codeine to morphine in man, *J. Forens. Sci.*, 21, 518–524, 1976.
23. Cassani, M., Vanzetti, G., Villa, A., Clerici, M. C., and Valente, D., La discriminazione della sostanza oppiacea assunta: un approccio immunologico, *Giorn. It. Chim. Clin.*, 9, 27–37, 1984.
24. Cone, E. J., Darwin, W. D., and Gorodetzky, C. W., Comparative metabolism of codeine in man, rat, dog, guinea-pig and rabbit: identification of four new metabolites, *J. Pharm. Pharmacol.*, 31, 314–317, 1979.
25. Steiner, E., Bertilsson, L., Sawe, J., Bertling, I., and Sjoqvist, F., Polymorphic debrisoquine hydroxylation in 757 Swedish subjects, *Clin. Pharmacol. Ther.*, 44, 431–435, 1988.
26. Dayer, P., Desmueles, J., Leeman, T., and Striberni, R., Bioactivation of the narcotic drug codeine in human liver is mediated by the polymorphic monooxygenase catalysing debrisoquine 4-hydroxylation, *Biochem. Biophys. Res. Comm.*, 152, 411–416, 1988.

Chapter 21

GAS CHROMATOGRAPHY AND LIQUID CHROMATOGRAPHY COUPLED TO MASS SPECTROMETRY

Carles Barcelo

TABLE OF CONTENTS

I. Drug Analysis Using GC/MS 130

II. Drug Analysis Using PB LC/MS 131

III. Drug Analysis Using GC/FT-IRD/MSD 132

I. DRUG ANALYSIS USING GC/MS

The analysis of drugs of abuse in body fluids is usually performed in a two-step process: an initial screen followed by a second test using a different technique for confirmation of samples which test positive by the screen. A positive screen can have potentially serious consequences, so it is important that the confirmation method of choice be unambiguous. An HP5970/5890 GC/MS with an HP7673 autosampler provides an excellent solution for confirmation of drugs of abuse. The 59970C MS Chemstation software can be used manually or in an automated fashion for customized drug analysis.

How does GC/MS work? In GC/MS, a complex sample is separated into its components by the gas chromatograph, and then the components are ionized and identified by the characteristic spectra produced by the mass spectrometer.

There are several steps in GC/MS analysis.

1. The compound of interest is separated from the mixture by the gas chromatograph.
2. The compound is ionized in the mass spectrometer source.
3. The fragment ions are separated by the mass filter.
4. The filtered ions strike the surface of the detector.
5. The work station processes each mass signal to produce one unique mass spectra. This mass spectra is like a "fingerprint" of the compound and can be used to identify the drugs.

We have four steps to ionization as follows:

1. Electrons bombard the neutral molecule
2. Which becomes energized and loses an electron
3. The unstable molecule breaks apart into reproducible fragments
4. And the process is repeated

IONIZATION:

$$ABC + e^- \rightarrow ABC^{\ddagger} + 2e^-$$
Neutral molecule, Excited molecular ion

FRAGMENTATION:

$$ABC^{\ddagger} \rightarrow AB^+ + C^{\bullet}$$
$$A^+ + BC^{\bullet}$$
$$AB^+ + C \text{ (loss of neutral)}$$
$$AC^+ + B \text{ (rearrangement)}$$
etc.

But, how do we know that our mass spectrum is accurate? We know by running autotune. Autotune sets instrument parameters for proper detection of the following:

- Correct masses
- Ion abundances
- Resolution

All is operator independent.

And how do we analyze our data? By pressing a softkey "spectrum" and another softkey "library search", our drug is identified. We have six steps in drug analysis by GC/MS.

1. Prepare samples and add internal standard
2. Run autotune
3. Specify method (qualitative or quantitative)
4. Inject sample (manual or automatic)
5. Analyze data
6. Print final report

The steps from 3 to 6 can be automated.

The operator needs to prepare and inject the sample, to specify methods for data acquisition and data analysis, and to review the results (this last point should be done by a qualified expert).

Once the methods are established, it is possible to automate injection, acquisition, and analysis. The work station does the following steps: tunes the instrument, controls GC/MS and ALS in data acquisition, displays data in real time, analyzes data, generates reports, stores data and does file management, and other functions.

For drug confirmation quantitation, selected ion monitoring (SIM) is necessary; qualitative analysis (scanning) is not enough. The reason is that in scan mode we scan samples each 0.1 amu while in SIM we scan only selected discrete masses. In this way, we can increase the selectivity and the sensitivity because we are monitoring a few ions instead of many.

A calibration table is used to identify and quantitate drugs in an unknown mixture. The calibration table is prepared by measuring ion abundances for known quantities of drug standards according to

$$\frac{\text{AMOUNT}_{\text{drug std.}}}{\text{AREA}_{\text{drug std.}}} = \frac{\text{AMOUNT}_{\text{drug unknown}}}{\text{AREA}_{\text{drug unknown}}}$$

An internal standard (ISTD) is used for accurate quantitation. The internal standard is a compound chemically similar to the drug being analyzed, and a known amount is added to the sample and all calibration standards. Ion ratios of drug are compared to those of the internal standard.

The final report gives us the identity and amount of drug found in sample. A drug must meet the following criteria to be reported present in the sample:

- Proper retention time
- Proper ions
- Proper ion ratios

The internal standard must also meet the above criteria. Then the concentration of the drug is reported, and the report also states when the drug is not found.

It is also important to describe the GC/MS requirements for drug analysis. These are as follows:

- Capillary chromatography
- Classical electron impact (EI) spectra
- Reproducible data (retention time, spectra, peak areas, and ion ratios)
- Sensitivity
- Wide dynamic range and digital instrument control
- Reproducible tuning
- Automation
- Library search and drug libraries
- Easy to use
- Reliable
- One vendor solution with full service and training

But, a word of caution: using a GC/MS for drug analysis does not guarantee the correct answer! While GC/MS provides the most conclusive technique for confirmation of drugs of abuse, the reliability of the analysis is dependent on many noninstrumental factors — primarily the extraction techniques used as well as the skill and experience of the GC/MS operator.

We cannot overemphasize the importance of proper training and methodologies, written standard operating procedures, and good quality control. Also, it is essential to have a qualified person, who is experienced in drug analysis, reviewing the results.

II. DRUG ANALYSIS USING PB LC/MS

The HP Particle Beam (PB) LC/MS interface design is derivated from the original magic LC/MS interface created at the Georgia Institute of Technology from whom Hewlett-Packard has obtained the exclusive rights to develop and market this product. In simple terms, the PB interface is a sample transport device, very similar to a two-stage jet separator, where the solvent vapor is pumped away and the analyte particles are concentrated in a beam. The beam of particles then enters the MS source where they are first vaporized and then ionized. It is the simplicity of the particle beam design which provides ideal interface performance, providing rich spectral information without major hardware or data system changes in a user's existing MS system.

The most significant advantage of PB LC/MS is the production of classical EI spectra. Previous LC/MS techniques such as Direct Liquid Introduction (DLI), early designs of thermospray, and fast atom bombardment (FAB) yielded only molecular weight information or chemical ionization (CI) spectra. However, none of these techniques yield classical EI spectra. Qualitative work is expedited with higher confidence levels when classical EI spectra are available.

In many lab applications, the customer has to deal with large volumes of complex matrices such as water, blood, and urine. Sample cleanup and concentration for these types of samples often takes hours and represents a significant factor in determining productivity and profitability of a lab. The combined use of column switching and precolumn concentration can be used in PB LC/MS to save hours of sample preparation time. LSD in urine was analyzed by injecting a sample of raw urine spiked with LSD into a PB LC/MS system. Through the use of column switching and a precolumn concentration process, the detection limit of LSD was determined to be less than 4 ppb! Typical analysis of LSD requires length sample workup and derivatization for negative chemical ionization (NCI)/MS analysis to achieve comparable levels of detection.

The use of precolumn concentration techniques allows large volumes (200 ml) of sample to be injected under noneluting conditions and collects the analyte on the head of the column. The retained sample is then eluted by gradient elution and analyzed on the PB LC/MS system without adverse effects. Where sample response is low or column overloading appears, larger capacity columns may be substituted to eliminate the problem.

HP PB LC/MS requires very little modification of either LC methodology or MS operation. Typical flow rates range from 0.1 to 1.0 ml/min and a wide range of solvents can be used. The primary restriction is the mandatory use of volatile buffers when buffering is needed. Additionally, the PB technique may be useful for most compounds having sufficient volatility to be run by Direct Insertion Probe (DIP) or Desorption Chemical Ionization (DCI). On the other hand, compounds such as proteins, peptides, and azo dyes which have very limited volatility are not well suited to PB and can be more successfully run by either thermospray or FAB as alternative techniques.

In conclusion, PB LC/MS offers an exciting new approach to interfacing LC and MS. PB can generate EI, CI, and NCI spectra. It can provide very good quantitative performance for drug confirmation and has ease-of-use features.

III. DRUG ANALYSIS USING GC/FT-IRD/MSD

The current federal guidelines for drug testing programs call for a screening technique followed by independent GC/MS confirmation of samples which screen positive. Now it is also possible to combine the HP5965A infrared detector (IRD) and the HP5970B mass selective detector (MSD) to provide results which can meet the sensitivity requirements of the federal guidelines. Because of the two completely independent principles of detection, the IRD/MSD system provides the highest level of confidence currently available for drug identification.

This capability will be of most value to those laboratories doing a broader range of drug testing, such as the analogs and isomers of the amphetamine family where mass spectrometry alone may not always provide unequivocal identification. Although the IRD contribution to the combined system would be mainly qualitative information, a good quantitation is also possible.

The configuration used for drug mixture consist of two columns installed in one injection port. A 0.1 mm i.d. column was directed to the MS while the IRD had a 0.32 mm i.d. column installed. The two-column configuration was found to be superior to the serial configuration due to the apparent reactivity of some compounds (like monoacetyl-morphine) to the 300°C light pipe.

The IRD/MSD combination has a combined library search reporting capability unequivocal identification by the two completely independent dimensions of IR and MS data greatly enhances the chances for successful prosecution of illicit drug cases. In addition, the simplicity and convenience of a single injection can add greatly to the fast turnaround time often required in forensic labs.

Chapter 22

CORRELATIVE INFORMATION BY GC/MS IN DOPING ANALYSIS

D. Fraisse, M. Becchi, and M.J. Bobenrieth

TABLE OF CONTENTS

I.	Objective of Mass Spectrometry	134
II.	Gas Chromatography Information	134
III.	Derivatization	136
IV.	Chemical Ionization (CI)	138
V.	Negative Chemical Ionization (NCI)	138
VI.	Conclusions	140
	References	144

In the environment of doping control in sports, analyses are currently performed on the urine. The complexity of that biological matrice requires a sample preparation more or less dedicated to the different classes of compounds forbidden by the International Olympic Committee (IOC), i.e., stimulants, β-blockers, narcotics, corticosteroids, anabolic steroids, and diuretics. These undesirable substances are first detected by enzyme immunnoassay or radioimmunoassay and chromatographic techniques. In the latter case, the technique requires sample preparation which can include one or several of the following steps: hydrolysis of the conjugates, extraction and cleanup, and derivatization.[1] Immunoassay techniques are fast, inexpensive, and easily automated, but as chromatographic techniques, they are not specific and the positive results must be confirmed by reliable and undisputable techniques. In this paper, we will expose the capabilities of gas chromatography/mass spectrometry to confirm the absence or presence of a substance, the identity of a substance, and to identify the unknowns.

I. OBJECTIVE OF MASS SPECTROMETRY

The objective of mass spectrometry is to provide a mass spectrum which is the "fingerprint" of the substance under investigation. Figure 1 shows the mass spectrum of a stimulant, mefenorex, recorded with 70 eV electron energy. It is clear that the mass molecular of the molecule is not obtained straightforward in this case; nevertheless, all the information needed to identify the molecule can be deduced from the major fragment ions. The mass spectrum shows a base peak at m/z 216 which can be associated to m/z 218; the intensities ratio of the two peaks shows the presence of one chlorine atom. These two ions are formed by cleavage in α-position of the nitrogen atom. Another typical feature is the presence of m/z 91 ion formed by benzilic cleavage initiated by the aromatic ring. The molecular weight of the molecule is then calculated from these two complementary ions. The m/z 216 ion further fragments by loosing C_3H_5Cl which gives a relatively intense fragment ion at m/z 140.

For qualitative analysis in doping control, repetitive scanning of the analyzer provides several complete full scan mass spectra which identifies the compound under investigation. When the amount of sample is not large enough to acquire a full scan spectrum whatever the injection mode, a dedicated mass spectrum is obtained. This second way of monitoring a limited number of representative ions instead of getting a full scan spectrum is more sensitive because, for the entire time of scanning, only the selected ions are recorded. In other words selected ion monitoring is capable to provide a dedicated mass spectrum of a substance with a few hundreds of picograms where tens of nanograms are required for a full scan spectrum.

These two possibilities are currently utilized in dope analysis for confirmation.

The quantitation of a substance is often performed by monitoring the most specific ions together with the ions of a reference compound called internal standard. A chemically similar compound will be preferentially chosen as internal standard.

II. GAS CHROMATOGRAPHY INFORMATION

The first parameter provided by gas chromatographic separation is the retention time (RT) which is the elapsed time between the injection and the emergence of the peak of the sample. This parameter is a characteristic property of each compound under the current operating conditions. However in practice we rely on the relative retention times (RRT) calculated relatively to a convenient selected internal standard. The values are applied effectively as indicators of the presence of drugs. The calculation of RRT is illustrated in Figure 2 for methoxyphenamine with diphenylamine as internal standard.

In 1966, Kovats[2] introduced the retention index system which was designed to normalize instrument variables. The retention indices are used in dope analysis for identification. In practice, a substance is identified by its retention index relative to the retention indices of a suitable mixture. Because of the nature of the banned substances, a mixture of diisopropyl alkylamines, developed by Donike et al.,[1] is preferred to the traditional mixture of normal paraffins. To the normal hydrocarbon chain of each diisopropyl amine of the mixture is assigned an indice equal to its carbon atom number × 100. As illustrated in Figure 3, methoxyphenamine is identified by its calculated retention index. Therefore, the question of the confirmation of a substance by its retention index using homemade compilations could be an interesting approach. This is more valuable if the identification of a substance is sustained by more than one metabolite. Also, the preparation of different derivatives should permit to reduce the probability of interfering compounds.

To summarize, gas chromatography does provide highly definitive information through correlation established with reference compounds.

MEFENOREX

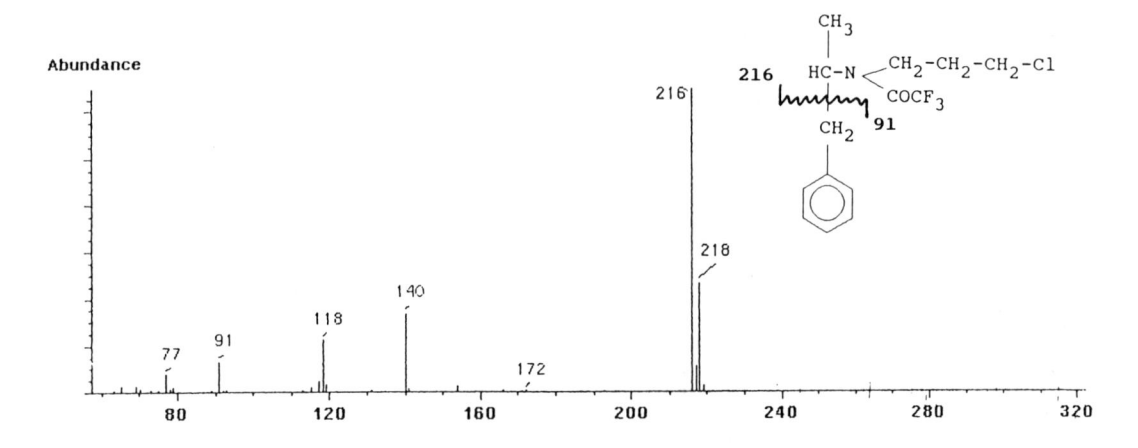

FIGURE 1. EI mass spectrum of mefenorex.

RELATIVE RETENTION TIME DETERMINATION

$$RRT = \frac{\text{RETENTION TIME OF THE COMPOUND}}{\text{RETENTION TIME OF DIPHENYLAMINE}}$$

a25 = Methoxyphenamine

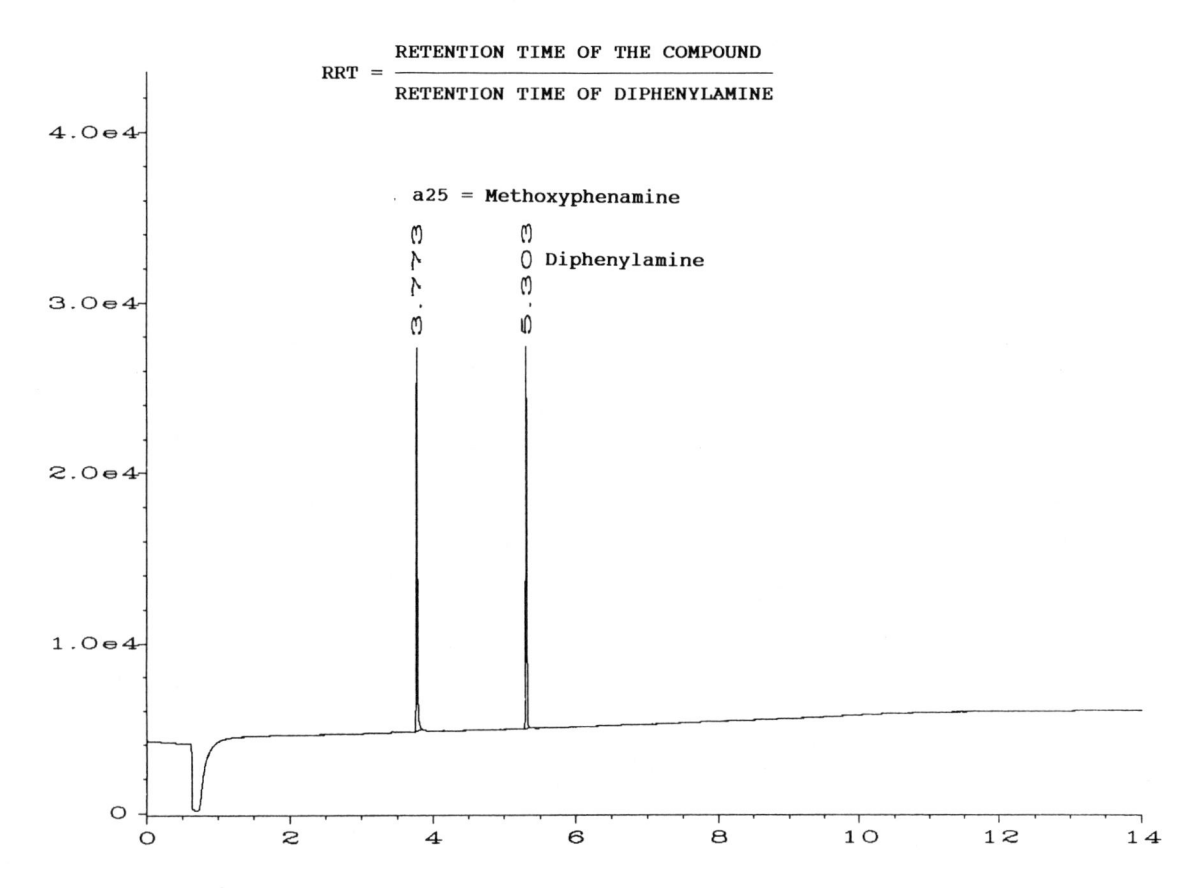

Diphenylamine

FIGURE 2. Relative retention time determination in GC.

RETENTION INDEX CALCULATION

$$RI = RI_n + (RI_n - RI_{n+1})\left(\frac{RT_i - RT_n}{RT_{n+1} - RT_n}\right) \text{ with } RT_n < RI_n < RI_n$$

a25 = methoxyphenamine

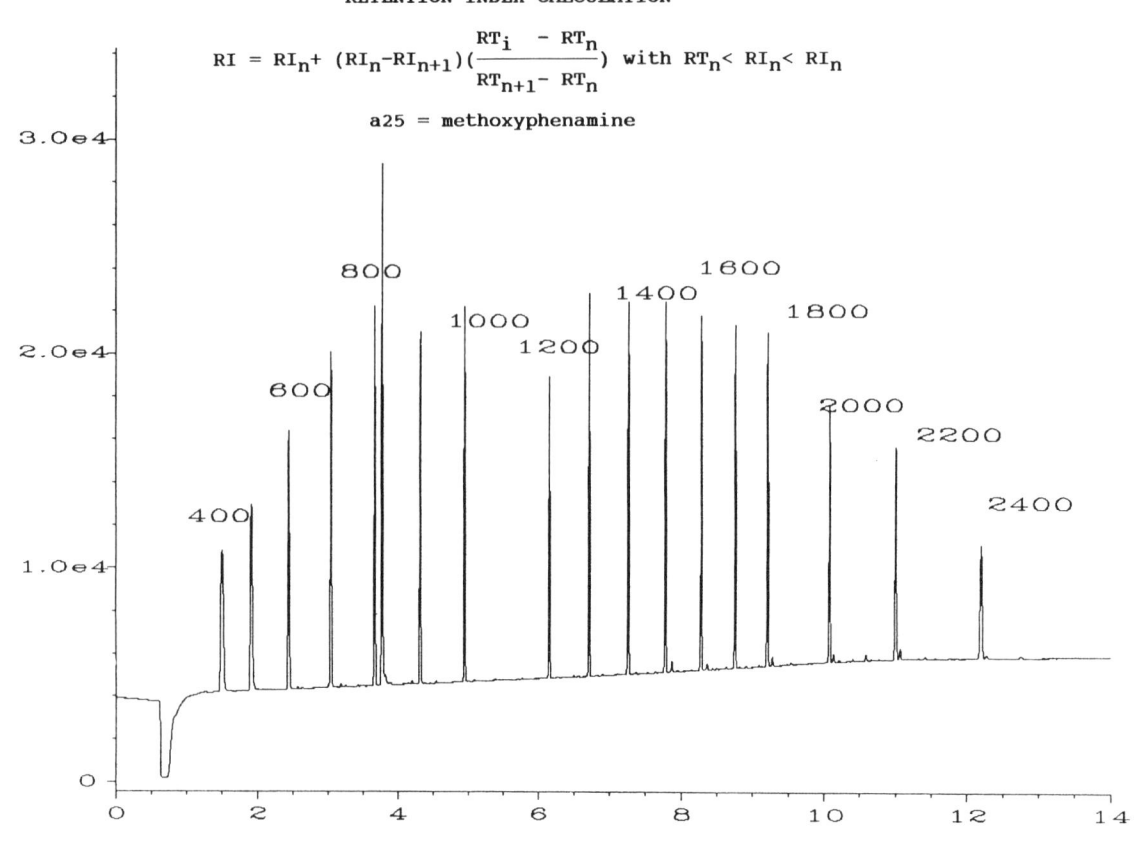

FIGURE 3. Identification of methoxyphenamine by its Retention Index calculation.

III. DERIVATIZATION

In analysis by GC and GC/MS, volatility and thermal stability of the compounds under investigation are required. Therefore, the preparation of derivatives is compulsory for polar and thermolabile doping agents to make them amenable to analysis. Besides the protective function of the derivatization, the preparation of a derivative will be performed when the mass spectrum of the underivatized molecule is poor as shown in Figure 4. In such a case, the derivative can introduce changes that facilitate interpretation and thus identification. Figure 5 shows the electron impact mass spectrum of the derivatized phenylpropanolamine (pseudoephedrine). The trifluoroacetyl (TFA) derivative has been prepared to improve the thermal stability of the molecule and to shift the masses of the fragment ions. Therefore, the replacement of the two exchangeable hydrogens by TFA groups increases the reliability of the mass spectrum. The molecular weight of the compound can be proposed on the base of the fragment m/z 230 ion formed by loss of the radical $CF_3\text{-}COO^\bullet$ specific to the TFA-derivatives. It is worthwhile to keep in mind that derivatization changes the retention time of the molecules by changing their polarity and thus increasing confidence in the identification.

Additional molecular indication of molecular weight are also available by preparing more than one derivative. The mass spectrum of the N-TFA, O-TMS (trimethylsilyl) derivative of phenylpropanolamine (Figure 6) provides an $(M-CH_3)^+$ ion characteristic of TMS-derivatives. An interesting feature of the O-TMS derivative spectrum is the presence of an intense fragment ion at m/z 179 which is observed for the whole ephedrines family. Therefore, that ion will be monitored to charaterize these drugs. This feature defines the strategy utilized in dope analysis.

Figure 7 illustrates the utility of preparing several derivatives for confirmation of 3'-hydroxy stanozolol, a metabolite of stanozolol. Another feature of derivatives that the analyst has to keep in mind, is their stability with time. For example, the N-acylated derivatives are very stable, but their EI spectra are less informative than those of N-TMS derivatives which are unfortunately less stable. In other words, the program temperature of the chroma-

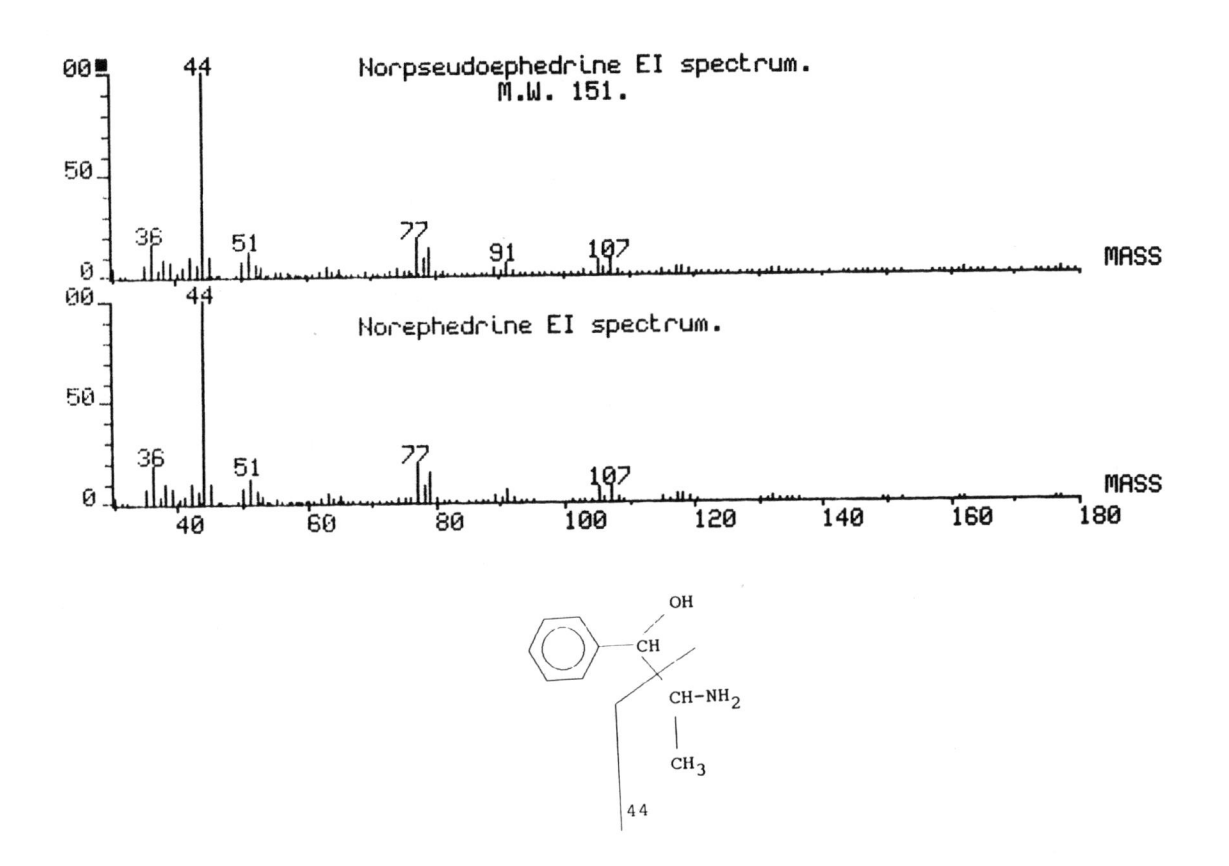

FIGURE 4. Underivatized EI mass spectrum.

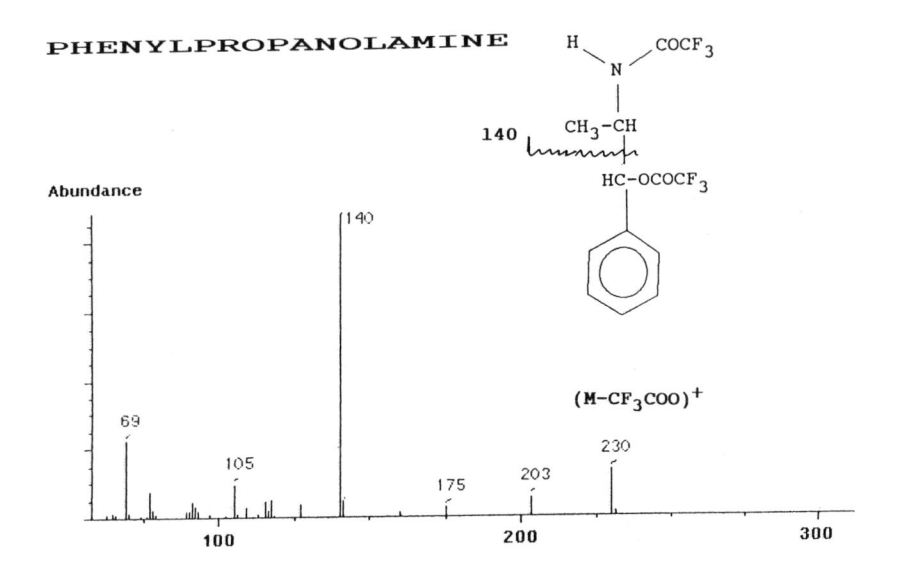

FIGURE 5. Mass spectrum of the TFA derivative of phenylpropanolamine.

tographic analysis will be set relative to the derivative stability. A discerning choice of derivatizing reagents and derivatization operating conditions produces different degrees of derivatives. The derivatization of the β-blocker, hydroxymetoprolol, leads to the formation of the bis- and tri-TMS derivatives (Figure 8A and 8B).

As stressed by Donike et al.,[1] derivatization is a powerful analytical tool that must be used by experienced

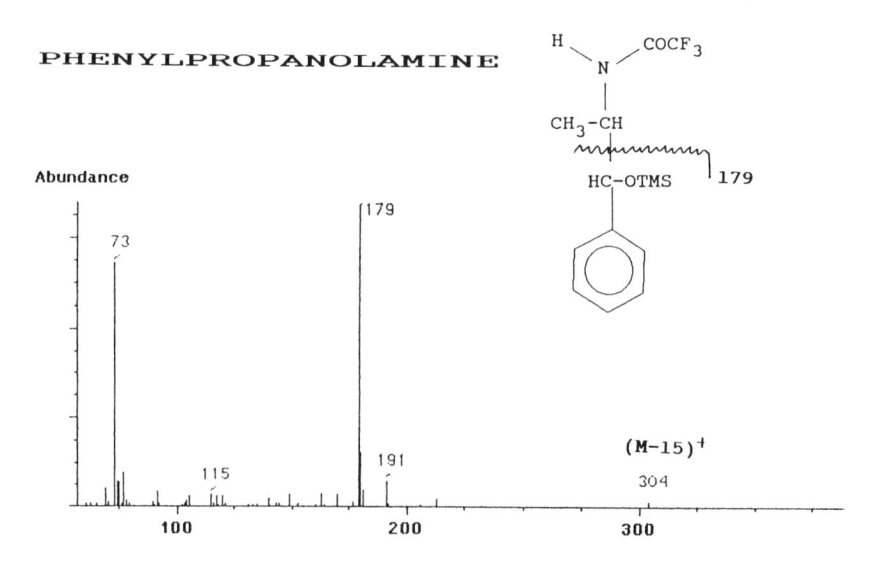

FIGURE 6. Mass spectrum of the N-TFA, O-TMS derivative of phenylpropanolamine.

people. Even though side effects can occur frequently in the derivatization reactions, they can be of interest if they are properly understood. Figures 9 and 10 illustrate the incomplete methylation of bumetanide, a diuretic used in doping, which ends up with a mixture of mono-, di-, and trimethyl derivatives. Again, an experienced analyst will utilize this side effect to confirm the presence of bumetanide.

To summarize, the establishment of correlative data between retention data, derivatives, and mass spectra can provide strong evidence of the presence or absence of a drug.

IV. CHEMICAL IONIZATION (CI)

Electron impact (EI), the commonest method of ionization used in dope analysis is somewhat rather nonspecific and because of the large amount of energy involved in the ionization process molecular ion information is not straightforward available. Chemical ionization,[3] in which the ionization is produced by ion-molecule reactions, is widely used to confirm the molecular weight of a suspected compound. As the energy involved in the ionization process does not exceed 5 eV, the stability of the protonated molecular ion MH$^+$, formed by ion-molecule reaction between M and the protonating reactant ions, is greater than that of M$^{+\theta}$ (EI). As shown in Figure 11, the electron impact ionization of nylidrin fails to give a molecular ion, whereas CI with isobutane as reagent gas shows an intense protonated molecular ion MH$^+$ at m/z 300. Electrophilic addition of cations produced by isobutane provides an adduct ion (M+C$_3$H$_7$)$^+$ which confirms the molecular weight of the compound.

As it was emphasized, fragile compounds such as ephedrines and amphetamines give very poor electron impact spectra. Definitive molecular weight information are provided in chemical ionization as shown in Figure 12. Cocaine, a very powerful stimulant, is rapidly metabolized by de-esterification by liver enzymes into benzoylecgonine, the predominant metabolite. The acidic function of benzoylecgonine has to be derivatized before analysis. Figure 13 shows the CI (isobutane) spectrum of the TMS-derivative of benzoylecgonine in an extract of urine. Notable is the rather clean GC/MS total ion current of the urine extract which shows the specificity of CI.

V. NEGATIVE CHEMICAL IONIZATION (NCI)

During the electron impact ionization process, negative as well as positive ions are formed. Nevertheless, in the conventional EI process, the formation of negative ions is inefficient relative to that of positive ions. By increasing the population of thermal electrons with a moderator gas in a tight source, Hunt et al.[4] introduced an alternative soft ionization technique to positive chemical ionization. There are two mechanisms involved in negative ions formation: electron capture and ion-molecule reaction. Electronegative compounds easily capture an extra electron to form negative ions which eventually

3′-HYDROXY-STANOZOLOL

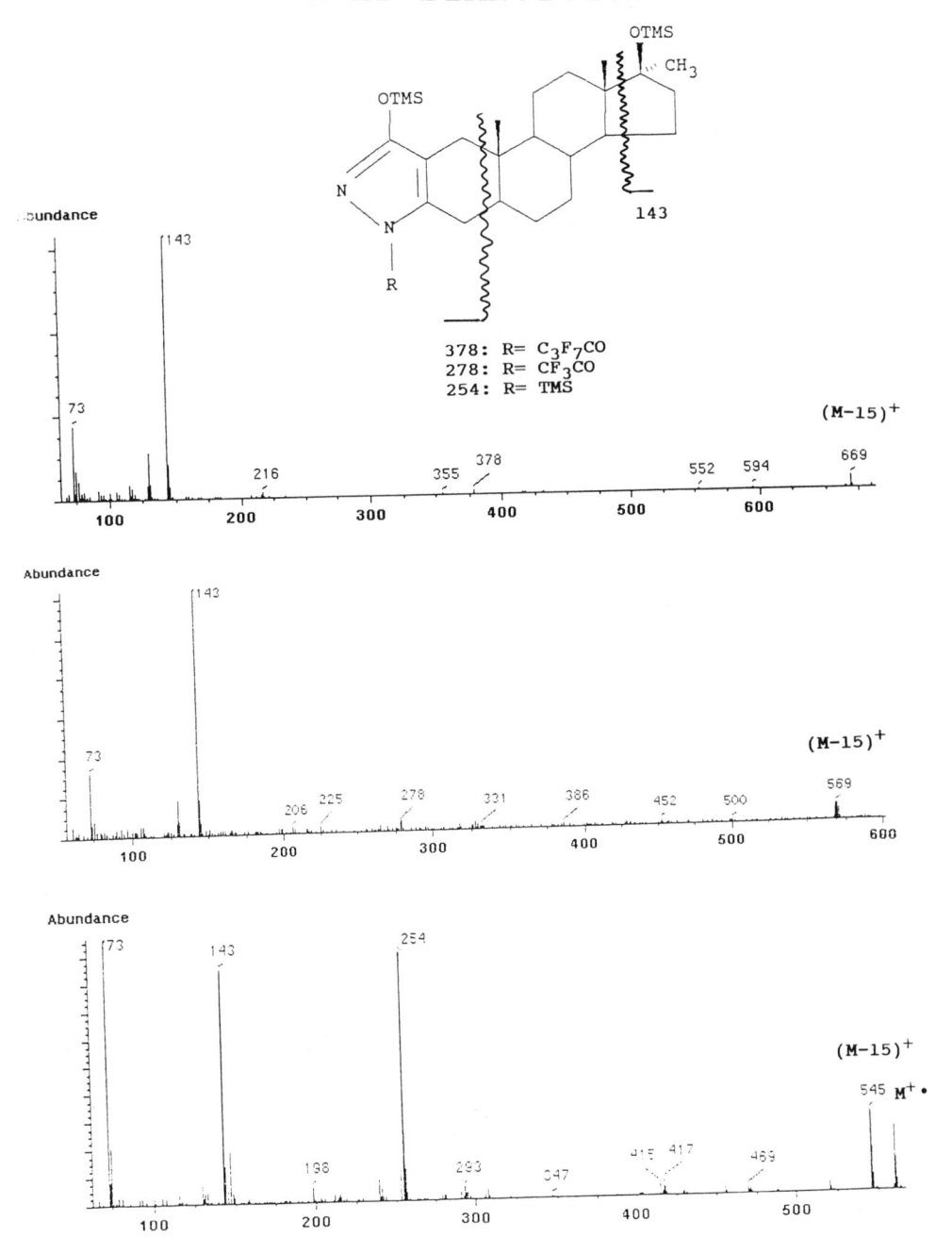

378: R= C$_3$F$_7$CO
278: R= CF$_3$CO
254: R= TMS

FIGURE 7. Example of complementary information by multiple derivatives of 3′-hydroxy-stanozolol.

fragment. True negative chemical ionization involves an ion-molecule reaction with a reactant ion such as O⁻· or OH⁻. The predominant reaction is then a proton abstraction leading to the formation of a deprotonated molecular ion (M-H)⁻ which is very stable as most of the exothermicity of the reaction is carried away by the reactant ion.

Figure 14 displays the NCI spectra of the two isomers of methyl ephedrines. In contrast to the EI spectra, the OH⁻ negative spectrum affords an intense (M-H)⁻ ion which is the base peak. In addition, the fragmentation profiles of the two spectra allow the differentiation of the two ephedrine isomers.

HYDROXY–METOPROLOL BIS–TMS

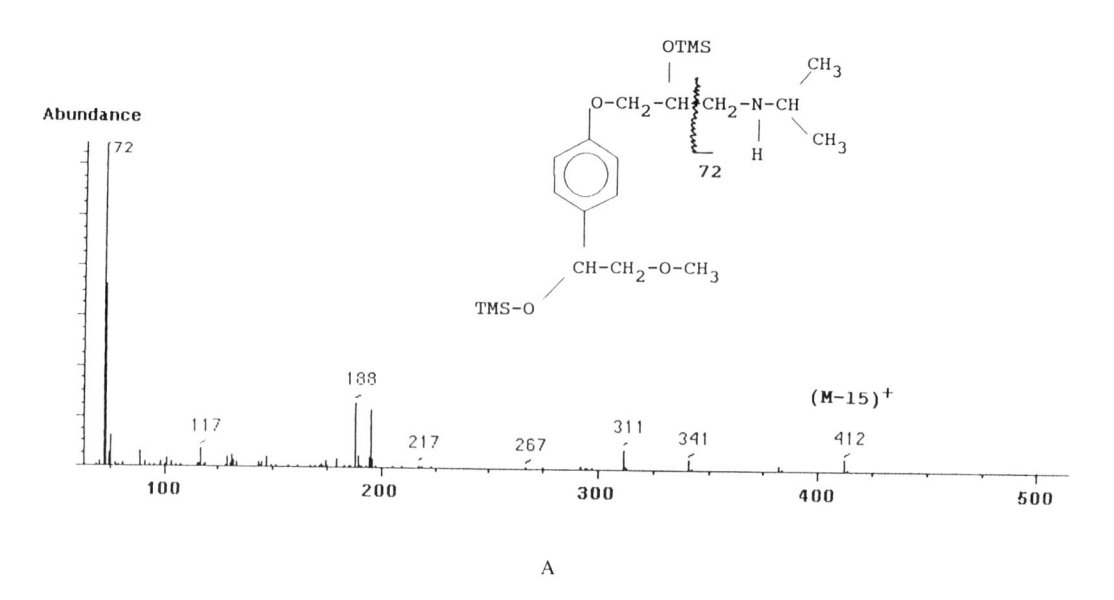

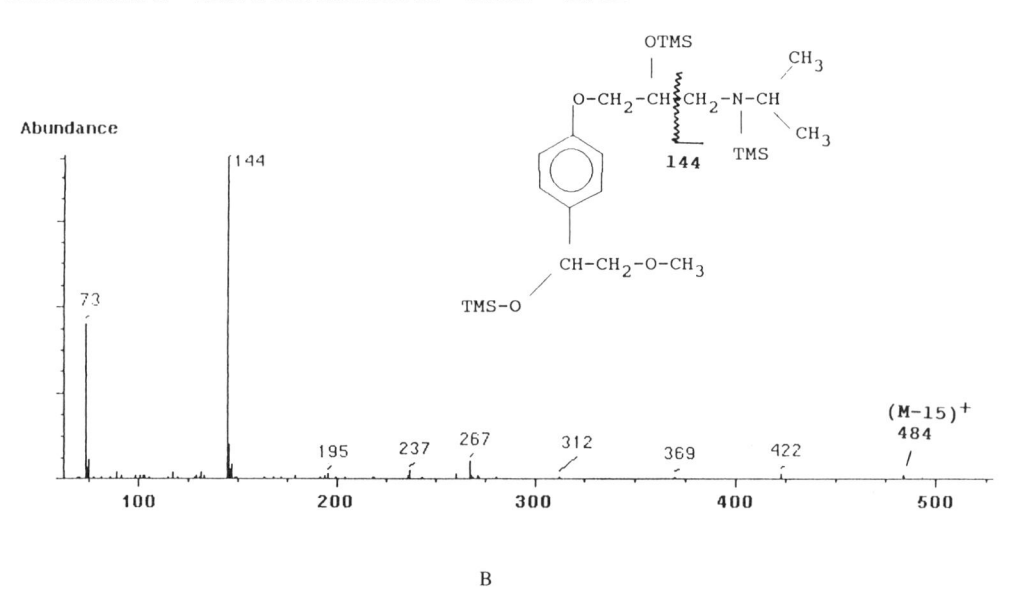

FIGURE 8. Example of the complexity of derivatization process. (A) EI mass spectrum of bis-TMS hydroxy-metoprolol. (B) EI mass spectrum of tri-TMS hydroxy-metoprolol.

VI. CONCLUSIONS

The reading of this paper might induce a half-false opinion about confirmation in dope analysis. The accomplishment of an undisputable mass spectrum of a suspected drug is very dependent upon the sample extract preparation. This important part of an analysis protocol includes several steps such as hydrolysis, cleanup, and derivatization. The formation of different derivatives is of great interest for structural confirmation and to eliminate potential interferences. At this time, GC/MS is definetely the method of choice to confirm the presence of banned drugs in urine. Correlative data provided by gas chromatography and mass spectrometry allow laboratories to reach a reasonable certainty which should satisfy the analyst and the lawyer.

TRI-METHYL BUMETANIDE

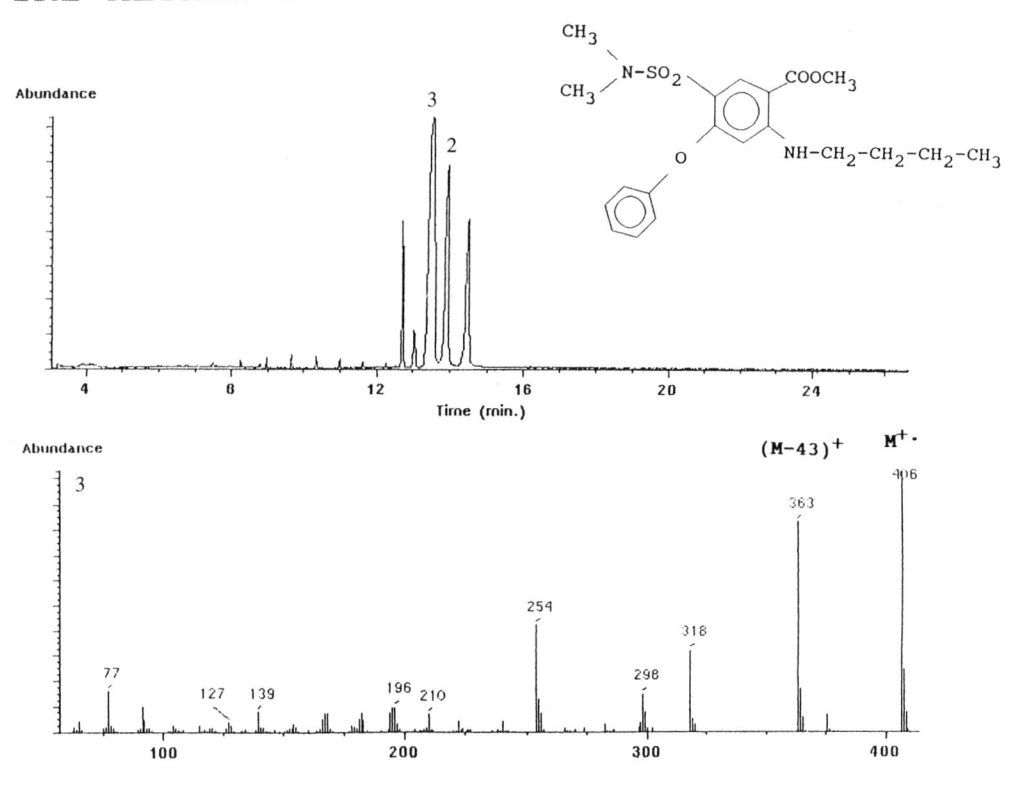

FIGURE 9. Side effect of bumetamide methylation.

MONO and DI-METHYL BUMETAMIDE

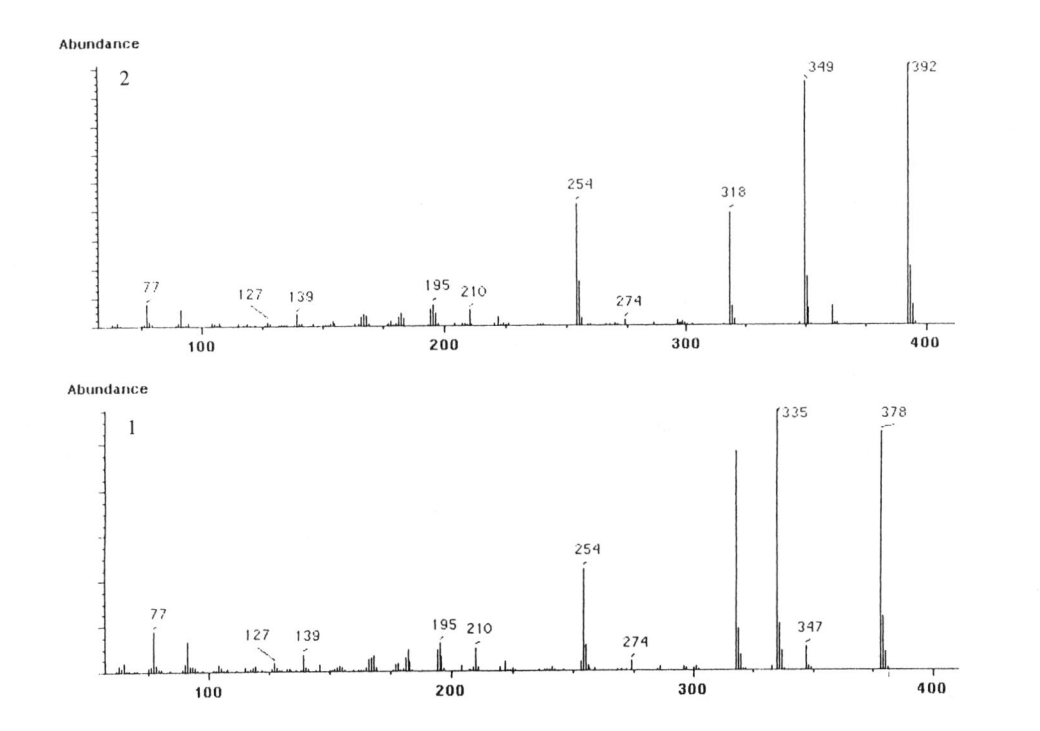

FIGURE 10. Side effect of bumetamide methylation.

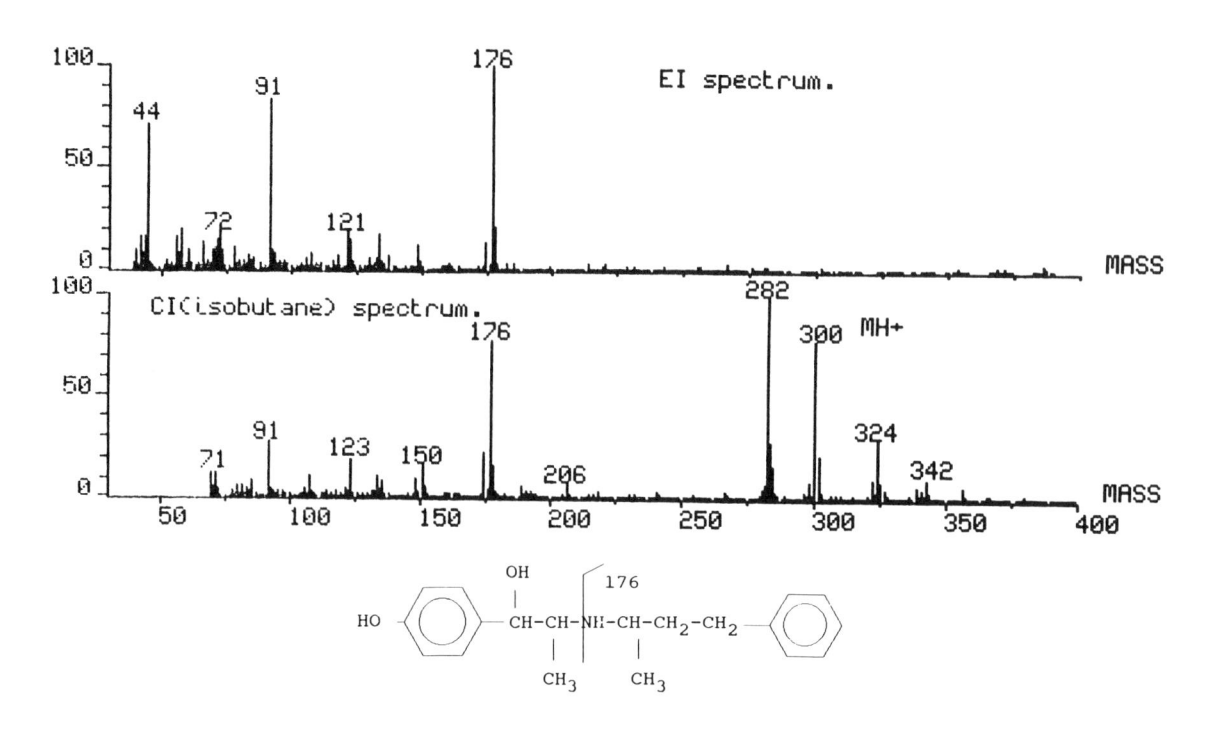

FIGURE 11. EI and CI (isobutane) mass spectrum of nylidrin.

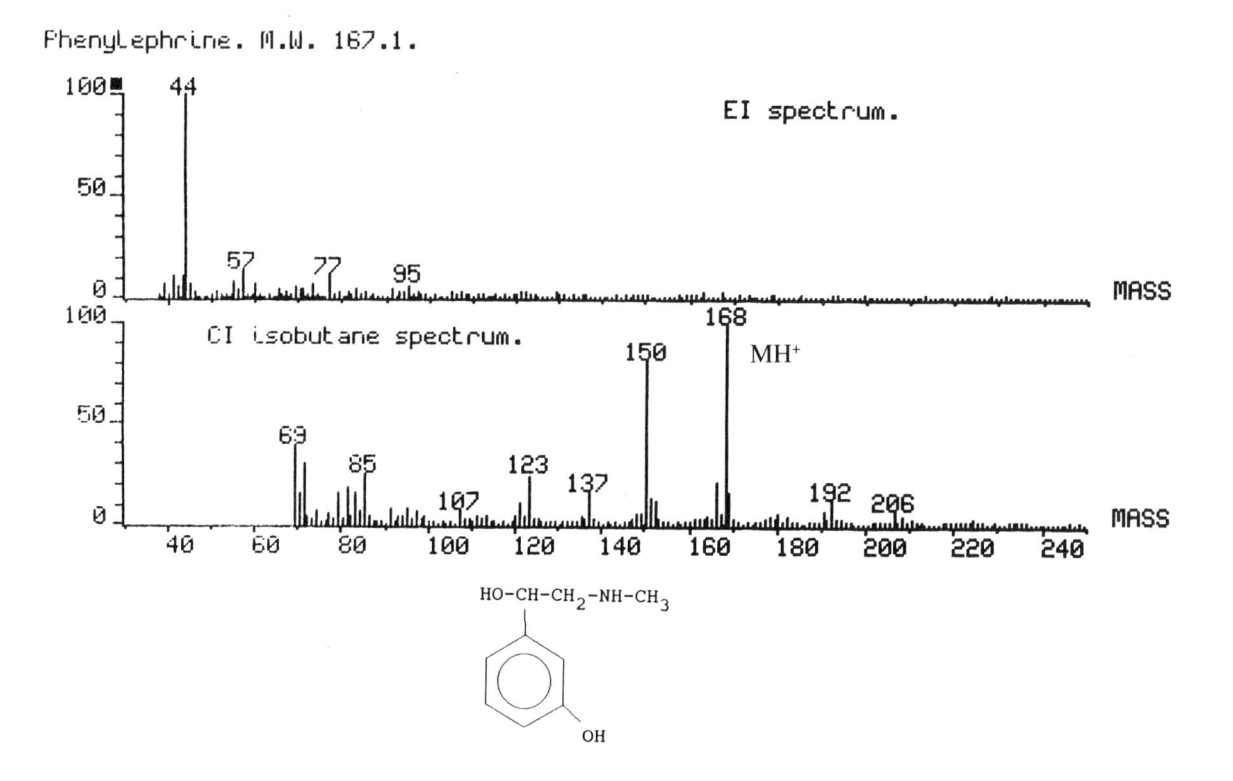

FIGURE 12. Confirmation of molecular weight of phenylephrine in CI (isobutane).

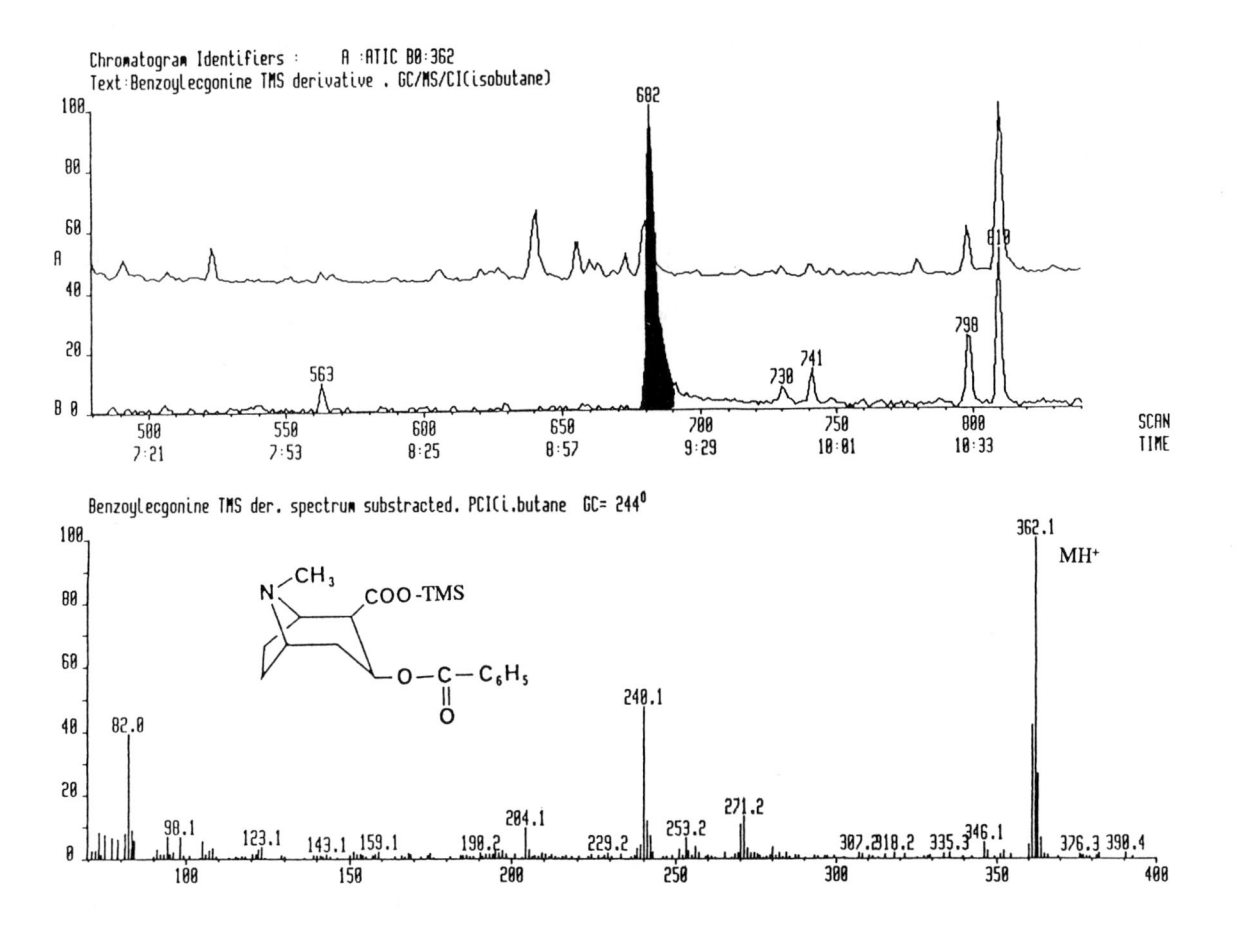

FIGURE 13. TMS derivative CI mass spectrum of benzoylecgonine.

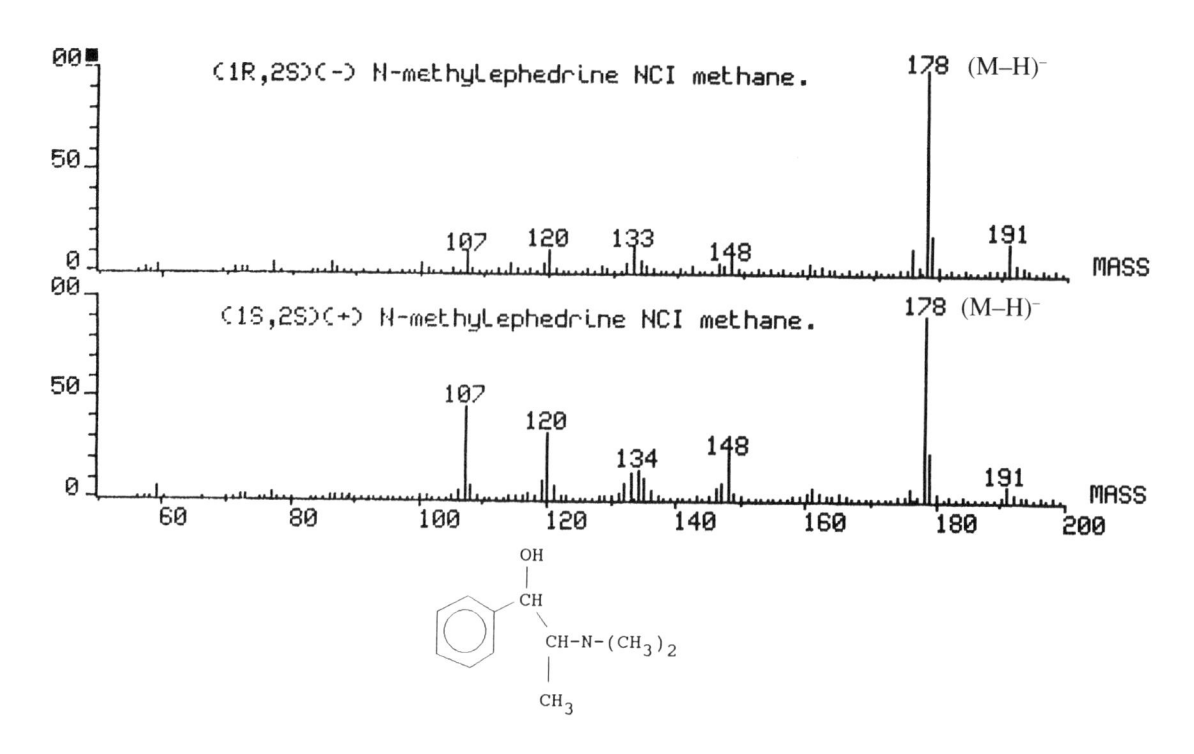

FIGURE 14. NCI (methane) mass spectra of N-methylephedrine isomers.

REFERENCES

1. **Donike, M., Geyer, H., Gotzmann, A., Kraft, M., Mandel, F., Nolteernsting, E., Opfermann, G., Sigmund, G., Schanzer, W., and Zimmermann, J.,** International Athletic Foundation World Symposium on Doping in Sport, Florence, May 1990.
2. **Kovats, E.,** *Advances in Chromatography*, Giddings, J.C. and Keller, R.A., Eds., Marcel Dekker, New York, 1, 1966, 229–247.
3. **Munson, M. S. B. and Fields, F. H.,** *JACS*, 88, 2621–2630, 1966.
4. **Hunt, D. F., Stafford, J. C., Jr., Crow, F. W., and Russell, J.W.,** *Anal. Chem.*, 48, 2098, 1976.

Chapter 23

DISCUSSION ON ANALYTICAL METHODOLOGY

Gelpí: I think we have attended to an interesting session which will undoubtedly generate different kinds of questions. A point, however, that is probably lacking in this session is the point of view of the user. When listening to these marvelous techniques, it appears that we should sell our mass spectrometers and begin to perform EMIT or FPI or any other system. I don't know how accurate is this thinking, but it is something that I am offering to the audience. However, in order not to monopolize the session, we will open the time for questions.

Minty (Charing Cross Hospital, London, U.K.): GC/MS is the gold standard for confirmation. Do you consider any combination of other techniques to be a suitable alternative?

Cook: I think the question was would any other combination of techniques be equal to GC/MS. This is certainly an area for debate, and I am sure there are many opinions here, so I will give my own. I think in terms on the amount of information obtainable in GC/MS, the total amount of information is more than in any other combination technique. So, I still think I will favor that procedure, particularly in view of the consequences of a positive result.

Gelpí: May I add here that we should make a distinction between the use of GC/MS with an internal standard that is analog or analyte related. When we are talking about validation by GC/MS we should talk about isotope dilution mass spectrometry using the same labeled analyte. I would like to remind people that these are the so-called definitive methods in the literature. But only when you are working with your compound isotopically labeled.

Rincon (Forensic Institute, Valencia, Spain): We have an experience when analyzing cadavers' blood from autopsies. The problem is that usually there is not urine available for an EMIT analysis and the available blood is usually hemolyzed which generate analytical inconveniences. Do you have an alternative for that problem?

Kelly: Yes, I think if you will talk with Dr. Christophersen, there are methods by extraction with methanol and the use of EMIT assays in the methanol extracts which I can guarantee that will get around the problem because we at Syva really have not done these studies, but there is some evidence to suggest that methanol extracts will work.

Segura: Sometimes it has been raised that a possible confirmation technique for an unspecific immunological method could be the use of another immunological methodology with monoclonal antibodies. What is the experts's opinion about that possibility?

Kelly: Certainly, the monoclonal antibodies are not necessarily more specific; They are certainly more consistent. You may run into the same problem with monoclonal antibodies if you attempted to make it more specific. There is always the potential of cross-reacting with some compound that you do not understand or have not seen before. So the use of an alternative antibody will surely enhance the surety that you have with the result, but it will not totally eliminate the possibility of a molecule cross-reacting that you will not suspect.

Moore: Can I just add that I don't think it makes any difference really whether there is a monoclonal antibody or a polyclonal antibody. Some antibodies are good and some are bad. I think however good your antibody is I would never for a moment suggest that you should use one immunoassay to confirm another immunoassay. We will point towards GC/MS or whatever technique that is based in a totally different chemical principle. I think this is an absolute. We have a lot of thanks to the people in the United States who developed that sort of basic philosophy for us.

Unidentified Speaker: What about mass spectrometry-mass spectrometry coupling? Is it really useful from the practical point of view? What about HPLC with the supercritical fluid and microcapillary electrophoresis in the drug abuse analysis field?

Barceló: GC/MS coupling is at present a practical method which works without problem as a routine method. Although HPLC/MS coupling may have some further difficulties, this is not the case for GC/MS.

Cook: I think that one point I had in my talk is that there are a multitude of analytical techniques. The one you mentioned or some of the newer ones which obviously will be applied in the future to drugs of abuse as well as other areas should be assessed under the same principles as we do when we look to the immunoassays or gas chromatography or GC/MS. The best method is dependent on the purpose for which you are doing, the procedure and the skill of the people, and so forth. I don't think we can make generalizations about this one technique that may be the best in the future.

Gelpí: There is also one point in regards to costs. In our experience, the mass spectrometer is expensive when bought, but, depending on the number of samples, may become less expensive than radioimmunoassay, especially when antibodies are not available and kits should be bought.

Vereby: It seems that the Du Pont system is a different version of the EMIT or probably is the same system. Could you comment on the advantages because it seems to be that each kit is for one analysis and this could be tremendously expensive. How do you compare it with the EMIT system?

Lehane: What is the same in both systems of course is the chemistry; specificity and the performance are almost identical. And I think what separates the Syva system, the Abbot system, and the Du Pont system is the target audience for which is intended. The Syva system is really ideal in large volume situations where you have large batches. The Abbot system is somewhat in between: smaller batches and hospital situations. The Du Pont system is really more suited for hospitals and clinics where you have a small number of tests, but a very urgent need to do those in a short time, with relatively untrained people, and a need to have high quality, reliability, and ease of use into the hospitals. There is, in the United States, a problem getting qualified people. So, while (it) is in a cost base apparently somewhat more expensive to do single unit dose test, if you look at the situation where the test is being done, then the cost is cut away as a factor.

Vereby: What is the shelf-life of this unit; lets say if you want to keep it on hand for emergency purposes.

Lehane: All of the chemistry packs have a 12-month shelf-life at 4°C so they are quite well suited to that need.

Sunshine: In the Du Pont system, I didn't quite get whether you imply that you could do blood analysis for the drugs of abuse or just urines. Would you distinguish that for us please?

Lehane: Most of my presentation was on urine drugs of abuse. One slide referenced a number of similar methods that were for use in serum. They are screens, in some cases, for benzodiazepines, tricyclic antidepressants, and barbiturates. The other slide was for quantitative analysis in serum: alcohol, salicilates, and acetaminophen.

Gelpí: I would like to reconcile in my mind some statements I heard from Dr. Kelly and Dr. Stewart. Dr. Kelly seemed in favor of no quantitation, while Dr. Stewart mentioned that FPI is the only company supplying semiquantitative reports. The question here is to quantitate or not to quantitate (... to be or not to be).

Stewart: As I was trying to demonstrate in the slide presentation in my discussion, we have recognized that there is a need to have versatility in our abuse drug testing systems. Because of that, we wanted to allow our customers the option of having qualitative analysis if they have decided that numerical or semiquantitative results do not fit they needs or they have problems with the numbers. However, there are other customers who are interested in numerically assessing the reliability of their system by having numerical QC values to look at precision or accuracy. Also, the question that has come up is how can you asses or determine the recency of use issue if you don't have a numerical result. This is not to say that we do agree or we don't agree with that. We are trying to provide many options for the individuals that are performing drug testing.

Gelpí: Yes, but how you can really talk about precision or accuracy with semiquantitative data?

Stewart: This is done through the assessment of your quality control material. With each of the calibration curves we offer various controls with known concentrations, and those concentrations of the controls can be reviewed with the ranges of the targeted values. You can determine from that if your calibration curve is stable; therefore, you can feel more comfortable if you are looking at any trend in your control values. This gives you more confidence in what your instrument or reagent is actually doing.

Kelly: Again, as far as quantitation goes, as I said earlier in my presentation, we do not believe that the ability to quantitate in a random urine sample when you are screening for potential drug abuse really adds anything to the fact that all the assays are really telling you is that the individual has been exposed to the drug. As far as the need to have numbers in order to do quality control, obviously this is not correct. Laboratories regularly do quality control on positive and negative samples and also they actually use delta absorbance units on their instruments to do quality control in that way. So, it isn't necessary to have numbers in order to do quality control assessment.

Gelpí: One observation about the comment by Dr. Moore on the specificity or unspecificity of radioimmunoassay. In my experience, there are two separate worlds as is the assay of exogenous compounds as compared to endogenous compounds and the potentiality of radioimmunoassay may differ according to the objective.

Moore: Looking back over the last 15 or 20 years, I have been involved with radioimmunoassay for hormones or drugs or a variety of other compounds. I get the sense that when one comes to the immunoassay in drug abuse testing, it is like where immunoassay for endocrine testing was may be 10 years ago. And that the customers are not coming along to us, the producers, and telling us exactly what is what they want; there is a huge wait particularly coming out from the United States because of the trust of drug abuse testing there and the NIDA Guidelines. The most important thing is to say what specificity you want. I give an example on serum progesterone. The reason why serum progesterone is specific is not because it is specific on its own, but because the customers in the laboratories and the doctors that were using the tests demanded to the companies that were making the kits that the degree of specificity and at the end, they got it. And I think that if the customers here demand that degree of specificity in their assays, I think, within limits always, they will get it.

Gelpí: That brings me to the point one of the conclusions I had from all this. It is that when we consider analytical methods we should also consider the sample, the user, and the analytical method. This is an interrelated kind of triangle that sometimes you cannot separate one from the other. I mean the analytical method may be wonderful, but the quality of the sample may be too bad to get something out of the method, or the method is good, the sample is excellent, but the user is totally unqualified; or the user is highly qualified and the sample is a total lost. I mean you cannot get anything out of it and the method is wonderful or the method is bad; you can do as many permutations as you want.

Sunshine: The thing that bothers me with the immunoassays is that many times we are comparing apples to oranges to pears. A hundred on amphetamine in EMIT system is not a hundred in a FPIA system and is not a hundred in the RIA system. All too frequently, someone says that cutoff is one hundred and we assume automatically that each of these assays have the same hundred, and they do not. There is part of the problem of what you consider a presumptive positive test in your initial program because the hundreds are not the same, and which one will go on to confirmation will vary with the procedure you are using. We should say a hundred plus or minus, particular minus, a certain amount because they will all vary and we should have the final judgement on the quantitative assessment by whatever the confirmation technique is.

Gelpí: Thank you. That was the last point I wanted to raise: the definition of cutoff points.

Moore: A recent work has been done taking GC/MS as a gold standard and working out what is the best cutoff for any particular assay for any particular circumstance. If you want to have a value of a hundred and to have a hundred, as you say, what you must do is not to say it is a hundred, but a hundred what. You have to define specificity of that technique.

Unidentified Speaker: I think that part of the difficulty is obvious. It is important to strive to have every assay that says it is a hundred of amphetamine or a hundred of cannabinoid be the same assay by assay. The difficulty is that for many assays there are class drugs of assays, for example, opiates, I am not sure what a hundred means. Even for drug assays that are not for a class, again we are not sure what a hundred means (THC metabolite/s). Certainly, we should try to get a screening test as close as possible when we all say a hundred is a hundred. We should not forget, however, that the role of the screening tests is not to make everyone's hundred exactly the same; the role of the screening tests is to eliminate those people who are negative for drugs in their urine. In other words, we get back to the fact that the screening test is supposed to be simply a way from detecting potential positives and along the hundreds are close enough to one another in GC/MS or some other confirmation technique resolves that problem then is not all that bad that they are not exactly the same.

Gelpí: I will come back with my first question and a couple of comments. I have been astonished by the statement by Dr. Kelly: 59,000 blank samples, not a single false positive result in 8 years. Then we are speaking in

EMIT of a 100% reliability, not statistics to apply to: 100% absolute. I would like to know the opinion, in addition to that of Dr. Kelly, of people that are using EMIT. If it is so excellent, what are we doing with other techniques?

Kelly: What the study and many studies show is not so much the reliability and accuracy of EMIT, but the reliability and accuracy of the drug testing process. The EMIT screen and the confirmatory method are, as far as we know, currently close to a 100% accurate. For almost all of the screening done in the U.S., drug screening is a two test process. No matter how good EMIT is, how good FPIA is, or how good RIA is, you must have a confirmation by an alternative chemical method. That is really the key to drug testing.

Gelpí: But still, you had in 8 years no false positive from 59,000 samples. That means that going back to the comment of Dr. Vereby this morning, he mentioned the need for well-qualified personnel. Congratulations to the personnel in your facility.

Kelly: The laboratory that did that is the oldest and largest drug testing laboratory in the world. And that is the one I was talking about. All they do is drug testing. They run 100,000 samples a month.

Gelpí: As a last comment, it is obvious that the methods with immunological grounds dominate the analysis of abusable drugs. Mass spectrometry appears in the second line for the confirmation of all that needs to be confirmed and validated. Other low technology methods exist, but they have not generated extensive comments. Finally, it also appears that all systems, when in qualified hands, may become excellent.

Section III
Interpretation of Results

Chapter 24

INTERPRETATION OF RESULTS: AN INTRODUCTION

Jordi Camí

The massive increase in the use of urine analysis testing to detect drugs of abuse forces the need to define the terms of the relationship which exists between the testing laboratory and the person being tested. A very precise procedure must be established so that neither party is left indefensible. It must be recognized that laboratory proficiency testing has improved greatly in recent years. In addition, the current regulations for the chain of custody assure the security of the test samples. In contrast, the legitimate rights of the persons being tested have not received the same in-depth consideration. This is difficult because the importance of a given test analysis is not the same when it is done as part of clinical treatment, as an accident investigation, or as a means of selection or control in the work place or military situation.

The correct interpretation of the urine analysis test is not exempt of difficulties. In a wide sense, a positive test result for a given drug indicates that the person being tested has consumed or currently is consuming that particular drug. A negative result indicates that the person being tested has not consumed that drug. In a strict sense, it may be exactly the opposite. A negative result does not exclude the possibility that the person being tested consumes drugs, and a positive result not only can be obtained from a person who does not use drugs, but also it does not exclude that their performance may be impaired by other factors. The possibilities that one must keep in mind in order to adequately interpret a negative analysis result are diverse. The most probable possibility is that the person being tested is not a drug consumer. Another possibility is that the person being tested is not using drugs detectable by the test. It is also possible that the person being tested is consuming one of the drugs detectable by the test but that he or she is not taking sufficient quantities to be detected. Or that the subject is not using them with enough frequency to be detected. Or that the urine sample may have been diluted or otherwise tampered with or switched with another sample by the subject. The final other possibility is that the person being tested is taking the drug, but that the analysis used may not be sensitive enough to detect the drug in the urine. In any case, urine sample testing for drugs must never be the only analytical testing used when the situation deals with a test taken after an accident. The reason for this is that these urine sample tests still cannot adequately determine the amount of alcohol ingested, which is the drug involved in approximately 50% of fatal accidents.

In general, the main pharmacological factors which determine if a test is positive or negative are the dosage, the frequency of usage, and the time which lapses between the consumption of the drug and the collection of the urine sample. Thus, the presentations that follow, concerning metabolism and pharmacokinetics of abused drugs, will demonstrate the relevance of those factors with the most characteristic examples. The recent advances in the field of pharmacogenetics constitutes also a case of special interest, because they demonstrated the basis of interindividual variability of the metabolism of some drugs.

For an adequate interpretation of a positive analysis result, it is also necessary to look at diverse possibilities. A positive result indicates that a certain drug is present in the urine of an individual. But it does not mean that the person being tested was under the influence of the drug when the specimen was taken. One of the main challenges today is to advance in the knowledge about the relationship between the amount of drug present in the organism and the performance-impairment induced by the drug. It is known that according to the learning or the presence of cellular or metabolic tolerance, subjects under the influence of Cannabis present less impairment than naive subjects. This also occurs with a heavy drinker of alcohol in comparison to a social drinker. It has recently been demonstrated that women present a greater sensitivity on alcohol than men due to metabolic reasons. Another obstacle in the interpretation of a positive result is constituted by the special case of subjects under passive exposure to a drug. In the case of Cannabis, the possibility to falsely label a person being tested as a consumer exists.

In conclusion, today we can know with sufficient precision if a person consumes or has consumed drugs, but we cannot infer the degree of impairment that the drugs may be causing or may have caused. A confidential interview must be combined with repeated analysis at regular intervals to determine if the subject has taken the drug under medical supervision, if he or she is using the drug intermittently or chronically, or if the subject is an addict. The problem of the interpretation of drug analysis results is one more example of the limitations of testing and shows why the urinalysis cannot be undertaken indiscriminantly if there are no guarantees that the results will not be used in a correct form and without endangering the rights of the person being tested.

Chapter 25

METABOLISM OF DRUG ABUSE

Randall C. Baselt

TABLE OF CONTENTS

I. Introduction 154

II. Methamphetamine 154
    A. Case 1 154
    B. Case 2 155
    C. Case 3 155

III. Cocaine 155
    A. Case 4 155
    B. Case 5 155

IV. Opiates 156
    A. Case 6 156
    B. Case 7 156

References 157

I. INTRODUCTION

Persons who perform urine drug testing are often required to interpret analytical results, either via a verbal communication, a written report, or testimony at an adversarial proceeding. In our role as a reference laboratory, we are frequently requested to re-analyze specimens previously tested by the primary laboratory and to offer interpretation of the findings in controversial situations.

Most of us are probably familiar with, and capable of, answering the typical questions that arise after we have reported a positive urine drug test result, such as

- How long does the urine remain positive after drug use?
- Is the individual a light, moderate, or heavy user?
- Was the individual impaired at the time of the test?

But there are other, more difficult questions for which information is not generally available and which are often answered incorrectly, including

- Does the result indicate the donor definitely abused drugs?
- What route of drug administration was employed?
- Could the result be due to inadvertent, accidental, or unknowing exposure?
- Could the result be due to contamination of the specimen?

Many laboratories in the United States operate without specific standards regarding performance of their drug tests. Some laboratories may report a positive result using only a nonspecific presumptive test. Other laboratories may employ a confirmation test, but do not necessarily quantitate the result. Even when a laboratory's operation falls under governmental control, the analytical scheme may be directed to only a single metabolite or the parent drug. Currently, there are no established standards regarding metabolic patterns of abused drugs or reference ranges for parent/metabolite ratios.

A working knowledge on the part of the laboratory director of normal pathways of metabolism of abused drugs, common or uncommon routes of administration, and concentration relationships of the drugs and their metabolites in urine would help laboratories to minimize misunderstandings in such situations.

It is not the objective of this presentation to discuss all details of the metabolic patterns for the known drugs of abuse, but rather to present examples of actual cases from our laboratory to illustrate some important principles. These may be rare and unusual situations, but the fact that they have occurred should make us all cautious when providing answers to drug testing questions, especially when punitive measures await the unfortunate test subject.

II. METHAMPHETAMINE

d-Methamphetamine is the most frequently abused of the phenylisopropylamine class of drugs and is usually administered by nasal insufflation or intravenous injection. It can also be taken orally and, more recently, may be smoked in the form of "ice", a crystalline form of methamphetamine hydrochloride. Street grades of the drug have been found to average 40 to 50% in purity and often contain trace amounts (<0.5%) of amphetamine. Approximately 43% of a single dose is excreted in the 24-hour urine as methamphetamine and about 5 to 6% as amphetamine, but these figures may vary significantly due to the extensive pH-dependence of the elimination rate.[1]

Therapeutic administration of the drug usually produces urine methamphetamine concentrations of 1000 to 10,000 ng/ml, while methamphetamine abuse may result in levels of 20,000 to 400,000 ng/ml or higher (Table 1). Of course, if abuse has ceased, then over a period of several days the urine levels will fall first into the therapeutic range, and then eventually below that. In our experience, methamphetamine in the urine is always accompanied by the presence of amphetamine in a level of 5 to 30% of the methamphetamine concentration (i.e., at a urine methamphetamine concentration of 1000 ng/ml, one would expect to see amphetamine within a range of 50 to 300 ng/ml).

A. CASE 1

A urine specimen collected on demand from a state probationer was found presumptively to be positive for amphetamines; on the basis of this, the individual was returned to prison. On request of the defense attorney, the specimen was tested quantitatively by an independent laboratory and found to contain 60,000 ng/ml methamphetamine and 28 ng/ml amphetamine. The defense and prosecuting attorneys were informed of the physiological improbability of this result and further investigation followed, the outcome being that the probation officer was placed under suspicion of tampering with the specimen in this case and in several other similar cases.

TABLE 1
Methamphetamine

	Daily dose (mg)	Urine concentrations (ng/ml) Methamphetamine	Amphetamine
Normal use	5–15	1,000–10,000	50–3000
Abuse	20–800	20,000–400,000	1,000–120,000
Vicks Inhaler	1–10	200–6000	10–500
Benzphetamine	25–150	1,000–6000	50–1,000

B. CASE 2

Urine from a federal prisoner was found positive for amphetamines, and the subject offered up as a possible explanation a list of nonprescription drugs that included Vicks Inhaler containing l-desoxyephedrine (l-methamphetamine). Stereoisomeric analysis showed the presence of 728 ng/ml of l-methamphetamine, 35 ng/ml of d-amphetamine, and 47 ng/ml of l-amphetamine. We considered this to be consistent with, and recent reports have confirmed,[2] the normal use of a Vicks Inhaler for nasal decongestant purposes. Apparently, isomerization of l-amphetamine takes place to a certain degree during the biotransformation process.

C. CASE 3

Urine from a state government employee obtained in a random testing program was found positive for methamphetamine. At the employee's request, the specimen was referred for independent testing and found to contain 3200 ng/ml methamphetamine and 200 ng/ml amphetamine. After discussions with the employee's attorney, it was disclosed that the employee had been taking an appetite suppressant provided by a close relative. Further analysis of the specimen using a more appropriate analytical technique showed the presence of benzphetamine. The case was resolved as the ill-advised and unknowing, but probably not illegal, use of a prescription drug.

III. COCAINE

Cocaine is frequently abused for its stimulant properties by nasal insufflation or smoking and occasionally by intravenous injection. Street grades of the drug are generally of 40 to 80% purity. The drug degrades spontaneously to benzoylecgonine in aqueous solution, especially in an alkaline environment.[1] The presence of cocaine in microgram quantities has been demonstrated on approximately one half of all United States paper currency tested. Cocaine is present in milligram quantities in "deco-cainized" coca leaf tea imported from Peru (such importation is now banned in the United States).[3] One published report describes a young child who demonstrated benzoylecgonine in urine, apparently due to passive exposure to cocaine vapor following abuse of the drug by her parents[4] (see Table 2).

A. CASE 4

Two professional athletes provided urine specimens during an unannounced annual testing that were found positive for benzoylecgonine at levels of 16,000 and 26,000 ng/ml. They were placed on suspension and required to provide urine specimens 2 to 3 times per week upon demand until proven to be drug free for a 1-month period. During the next 4 months, urine specimens from these individuals were found to sporadically contain benzoylecgonine at concentrations by GC/MS of 25 to 65 ng/ml. The program director wanted to discharge these individuals for continued cocaine abuse, but we argued that this situation was not representative of abuse, rather, it was more consistent with unknowing or passive exposure to pharmacologically insignificant amounts of the drug. Recent experiments in our laboratory have demonstrated that urine benzoylecgonine concentrations of this magnitude are produced over a 4-day period after single dermal application of 5 mg cocaine base to the intact forearm surface.[5]

B. CASE 5

Urine was collected from a person suspected by the police of driving under the influence of alcohol or drugs, and the specimen tested presumptively positive for cocaine. Our retesting showed the presence of 18,000 ng/ml cocaine, 1500 ng/ml benzoylecgonine, and no detectable methylecgonine. We explained the physiological improbability of these results to the attorneys involved and the charges against the defendant were eventually dropped. The possibility of accidental or intentional contamination of the specimen was raised, but no satisfactory explanation for the situation was ever received.

TABLE 2
Cocaine

	Daily dose	Urine Concentrations (ng/ml)		
		Cocaine	Benzoylecgonine	Methylecgonine
Normal use	50–200 mg	0–10,000	500–50,000	100–40,000
Abuse	50–1,000 mg	0–50,000	1,000–400,000	500–250,000
Coca-leaf tea	2–20 mg	0–300	100–15,000	—
Dermal exposure	2–5	0	0–200	—

TABLE 3
Heroin

	Daily dose	Total Urine Concentrations (ng/ml)		
		Morphine	Codeine	6-Acetylmorphine
Abuse	20–200 mg	2,000–150,000	50–10,000	0–10,000
Codeine use	60–240 mg	1,000–10,000	5,000–50,000	0
Poppy seeds	1–10 mg	100–18,000	0–2000	0

IV. OPIATES

When heroin is used intravenously by addicts in amounts of 20 to 200 mg daily, it leads to total urine morphine concentrations (Table 3) of 2000 to 150,000 ng/ml, with codeine present as an impurity in amounts representing 2 to 10% of the morphine value. The determination of urinary 6-acetylmorphine has been suggested as a means of substantiating heroin usage, but that substance is present in only 60 to 70% of all specimens from known heroin users even when the urine is tested within a short time after collection.[1]

When codeine is taken orally in daily doses of 60 to 240 mg, total urine codeine and morphine concentrations are generally in the range of 5000 to 50,000 ng/ml and 1000 to 10,000 ng/ml, respectively; however, the amount of morphine in the urine usually exceeds that of codeine within 24 to 30 hours after the last codeine dose, and the urinary excretion pattern can resemble that of a heroin user during the 24 to 72 hour post-codeine period.[1]

The oral ingestion of poppy seed foods is capable of providing a morphine dose of 1 to 10 mg and has been shown to result in total urine morphine concentrations of 100 to 18,000 ng/ml within the first 24 hours of consumption, with 2 to 47% of those levels being present as codeine. Again, these urinary excretion patterns may resemble those of heroin users depending on the recentness and extent of exposure to poppy seeds.[6-8]

A. CASE 6

Urine from a federal probationer was found to contain 270 ng/ml morphine and 31 ng/ml codeine; on the basis of these results, his probation officer recommended revocation of his parole and return to prison. After discussions with the concerned parties, it was determined that the individual had consumed several poppy seed rolls on the day prior to supplying the urine specimen. The probation officer was initially very resistant to accepting this explanation, especially since the primary testing laboratory had denied its plausibility, and it was necessary for us to supply articles from the literature as well as to furnish names of other reliable experts who could support this explanation prior to successful resolution of this matter.

B. CASE 7

Urine from a private sector employee was tested as part of his application for promotion and found to contain 730 ng/ml morphine and 256 ng/ml codeine. When confronted with these results, the employee furnished a prescription for codeine; however, the company's medical officer gave the opinion that the finding indicated abuse of either morphine or heroin. Interestingly, the medical officer was willing to accept poppy seed ingestion as an explanation, but the employee denied this! It was necessary for us to appear at an arbitration hearing and to present scientific data supporting the codeine prescription theory in order to resolve this situation.

In conclusion, it is apparent that while the science of urine drug testing has made great technological strides during the past decade toward achieving a very high degree of accuracy, the interpretation of these results in terms of what substance was used, how and when it was used, whether it was used knowingly, and whether it ever impaired performance is still largely an art. Certainly this art will improve as our understanding of metabolic pathways and patterns evolves, but we must always employ a certain degree of conservatism in expressing our opinions in order to allow for that unforeseen possibility that could exonerate the urine donor as an abuser of drugs.[9]

REFERENCES

1. **Baselt, R. C. and Cravey, R. H.,** *Disposition of Toxic Drugs and Chemicals in Man*, 3rd ed., Year Book Medical Publishers, Chicago, IL, 1989.
2. **Fitzgerald, R. L., Ramos, J. M., Bogema, S. C., and Poklis, A.,** Resolution of methamphetamine stereoisomers in urine drug testing: urinary excretion of R(–)-methamphetamine following use of nasal inhalers, *J. Anal. Toxicol.*, 12, 255–259, 1988.
3. **Elsohly, M. A., Stanford, D. F., and Elsohly, H. N.,** Coca tea and urinalysis for cocaine metabolites, *J. Anal. Toxicol.*, 10, 256, 1986.
4. **Bateman, D. A. and Heagarty, M. C.,** Passive freebase cocaine ("crack") inhalation by infants and toddlers, *Am. J. Dis. Child.*, 143, 25–27, 1989.
5. **Baselt, R. C., Chang, J. Y., and Yoshikawa, D. M.,** On the dermal absorption of cocaine, *J. Anal. Toxicol.*, in press.
6. **Hayes, L. W., Krasselt, W. G., and Mueggler, P. A.,** Concentrations of morphine and codeine in serum and urine after ingestion of poppy seeds, *Clin. Chem.*, 33, 806–808, 1987.
7. **Streumpler, R. E.,** Excretion of codeine and morphine following ingestion of poppy seed, *J. Anal. Toxicol.*, 11, 97–99, 1987.
8. **Zebelman, A. M., Troyer, B. L., Randall, G. L., and Batjer, J. D.,** Detection of morphine and codeine following consumption of poppy seeds, *J. Anal. Toxicol.*, 11, 131–132, 1987.
9. **Cone, E. J. and Huestis, M. A.,** Urinary excretion of commonly abused drugs following unconventional means of administration, *Forensic Sci. Rev.*, 1, 121–136, 1989.

Chapter 26

THE RELATIONSHIP BETWEEN PHARMACOKINETICS AND PHARMACODYNAMICS

Gene Barnett

TABLE OF CONTENTS

I.	Introduction	160
II.	Pharmacokinetics	160
III.	Pharmacodynamics	162
IV.	On the Nature of the Relationship between Pharmacokinetics and Pharmacodynamics	163
	A. Marijuana	163
	B. Diphenhydramine	166
V.	Conclusions	168
	Acknowledgments	169
	References	170

I. INTRODUCTION

Efforts to understand the nature of the interactions of exogenous chemical agents with the human body, and their use in treatment of human disease, eventually resulted in the formation, almost a century ago, of the American Society of Clinical Pharmacology and Therapeutics.[1] Medical and research interests focused on the nature of the drug effect relationship and eventually a basic part of medical education came to rely on such books as the treatise *The Pharmacological Basis of Therapeutics*, now in its seventh edition.[2] Research studies of this type attempted to determine a measured degree of physiologic response, usually related to a maximal effect, due to a measured amount of chemical agent administered, the drug dose, and thereby construct a quantitative correlation between drug effect and drug dose. This is shown as the drug-effect curve in Figure 1. Such studies successfully focused classical pharmacology indetermining the nature of human response to drug consumption/exposure for many classes of chemical agents. In some cases, these studies also lead to the establishment of the relationship between drug effect and the concentration of the drug in a measurable body fluid thus establishing, for example, the therapeutic window of plasma/blood levels vs. efficacy/toxicity. There is clearly a great amount of information that is not available from the dose-response curve such as in Figure 1. For each dose, there is the variation of drug concentrations in the body which occurs over the course of a period of time that may range from minutes to days. Likewise, the maximal effect shown on such a curve is only one value selected from the range of values that vary over a similar extended time period.

The aspect of dose-effect studies that was not pursued in great detail in early work was the time dependence of such relationships, even though it was clear that after ingestion of a drug the resulting biological response varied over time. The classical studies frequently attempted to determine the maximal drug effect which required following the observation of drug response during the time course of observability. This concept of observation and measurement of drug effect over the time course of response is given the name pharmacodynamics; the formally expressed relationship of the time dependence of drug response, which can often be expressed in quantitative terms. It was realized very early that the administered chemical entity was often excreted from the body in an altered form due to transformations that occurred within the body. The formal study of the nature of the time course of drug transport throughout the body, as well as the nature of any transformation that occur, is given the name pharmacokinetics; also, a formally developed area of study that can usually be expressed in quantitative terms.

The study of relationships between the pharmacokinetics and pharmacodynamics of a drug, the kinetic/dynamic relationship, is one of the most active areas of research in clinical pharmacology at the present time. To understand the relationship allows a greater insight into the mechanism(s) of drug action and can provide the means to more quantitative control of drug plasma levels and the corresponding drug response, thus providing safer and more effective drug therapy.

II. PHARMACOKINETICS

The study of the fate and time course of a drug in the body was described in terms of differential equations by Teorell about a half a century ago and has since become an area of incredible activity with a large rate of scientific publications. Quantitative parameters can be defined which allow description of the rate of drug entry into the body, the extent of distribution throughout the various tissues and organs, the extent and rate of biotransformation within the body, the rate of disappearance from measurable body fluids, and the nature of excretion of drug from the body in its unchanged and biotransformed molecular structures. This discipline of biomedical science is now supported by many textbooks of which we mention two outstanding ones: Gibaldi and Perrier[3] and Rowland and Tozer.[4]

Drug pharmacokinetics can often be expressed in terms of models, but there are many examples where no definitive model has yet been established. One underlying reason that it is often difficult to establish a pharmacokinetic model lies in the complexity of nature. For all drugs, it is usually assumed that there is a dose range for which the plasma concentration vs. time relationship is superimposable due to linearity of the processes which govern drug transport within the biological system. It is equally likely that this linear range is a subdomain within the dose range, however, and at doses sufficiently large, it is reasonable to expect nonlinearities to occur due to saturable processes for binding, transformation, transport, etc. At doses sufficiently small, on the other hand, the laws of mass action upon which kinetic theory is based will no longer be valid. In the history of pharmacokinetics, it has frequently been necessary to await technological advances in applied analytical chemistry in order to be able to perform measurement of molecules in biological fluids. Such advances have always lead to a greater understanding of the fate of a drug in the body.

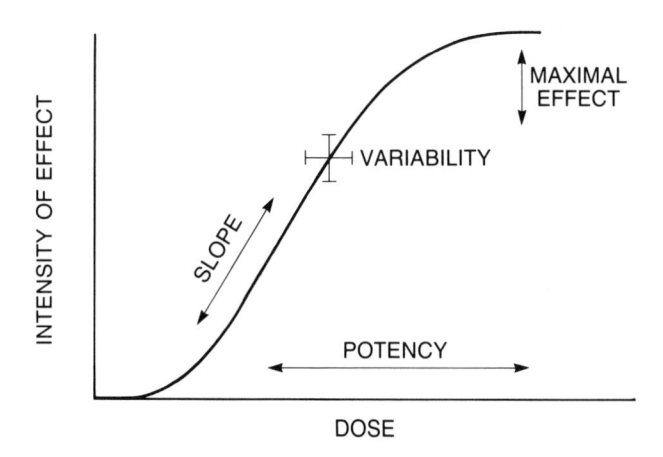

FIGURE 1. Classical dose-response relationship. (From Gilman, A.G., Goodman, L.S., Rall, T.W., and Murad, F., *The Pharmacological Basis of Therapeutics*, 7th ed., Macmillan, New York, 1985, 44. With permission.)

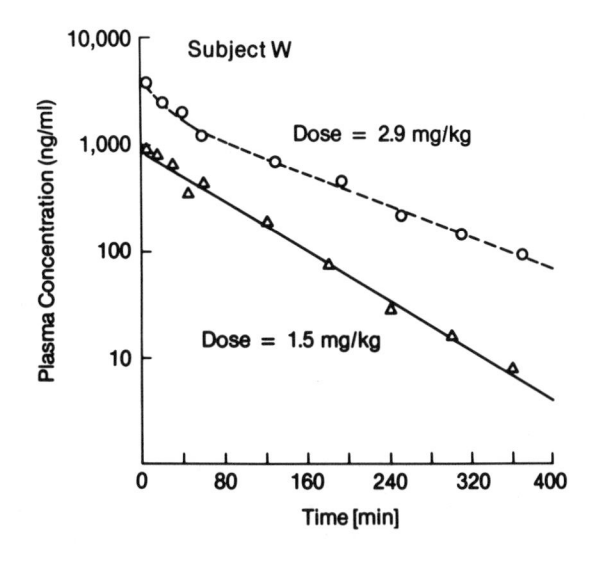

FIGURE 2. Pharmacokinetic curve: comparison of log plasma concentration vs. time curves for two doses of cocaine. (From Barnett, G., Hawks, R., and Resnick, R., *J. Ethnopharmacol.*, 3, 353–366, 1981. With permission.)

The pharmacokinetic graph shown in Figure 2 provides an example of apparent simplicity that is in fact considerably more complex. The figure, the log-linear plot of the plasma concentration of cocaine in man after intravenous administration, shows a simple kinetic relationship for the small dose and the model for the drug can be described by a one-compartment open model.[5] For the larger dose, the graph appears slightly more complex due to the biphasic plasma curve, which might be described as a simple two-compartment model of the drug. However, it was pointed out that the differences in the curves for the two doses might also be due to nonlinear kinetic processes related to the elimination of cocaine via metabolic pathways for the larger dose. The numerical simulation study of kinetic models for nonlinear elimination via metabolic transformation with competitive product inhibition[6] were proposed to provide a basis for understanding the complexities of Figure 2. The characteristic of this type of elimination mechanism results in larger doses demonstrating a curve with an apparent distribution phase

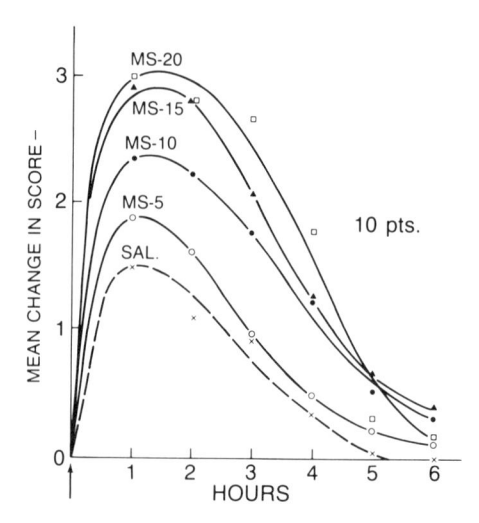

FIGURE 3. Pharmacodynamic curve: comparison of pain relief vs. time after administration of morphine sulphate or placebo. (From Houde, R.W., Wallenstein, S.L., and Rogers, A., *Clin. Pharmacol. Ther.*, 1, 163–174, 1960. With permission.)

and an elimination phase with a longer half-life. This observation of the nonlinearity of cocaine pharmacokinetics in humans has recently gained solid experimental support from the new reports of Ambre and colleagues,[7] where they also observed biphasic plasma curves with a longer terminal half-life at higher doses, and of Kumor et al.[8] This example serves as a reminder that although pharmacokinetics has evolved considerably more than pharmacodynamics as a discipline, it is still an area of biomedical research where challenging and exciting work remains to be done.

III. PHARMACODYNAMICS

The study of the nature and time course of biological response to drug consumption is not as well established as the area of pharmacokinetics. The physiological response to an administered drug is a complex manifold of actions and reactions that can occur via direct and indirect processes. Even when considerations are limited to the CNS class of compounds, the complexity of response is still a great challenge. Once a drug has entered the systemic circulation, the processes of distribution to the many organs and tissues, the possibilities of biotransformation, and the cascade of indirect mechanisms for various physiologic responses can all contribute to this complexity. The many variables encompassed within the descriptive term *biological variability* are not yet quantified, but one can expect this term to become more specific as the quantitative development of pharmacodynamics continues. While there are numerous textbooks on pharmacokinetics, the discipline of pharmacodynamics is still evolving, primarily within the research journals on clinical pharmacology.

The descriptive nature of reporting drug response can be put into more quantitative terms in some cases and can often be characterized in terms of the magnitude and duration of response, time of maximal or peak response, lag time to onset or first observation of response, some measure of decay or disappearance of response, and areas under the response vs. time curve. Some or all of this set of quantities can provide parametric descriptors for the pharmacodynamics of a drug. Because of the variability of response, from known or unknown sources, it is frequently difficult to analyze the time course of response on an individual patient basis as is usually possible for drug level vs. time measurements.

An early pharmacodynamic graph, published in the first volume of *Clinical Pharmacology and Therapeutics*,[9] and reproduced in Figure 3, shows the time course of pain relief due to administration of morphine sulfate for relief of pain due to cancer. A pain scale for patients to record their level of relief was applied before drug was administered and at hourly intervals for 6 hours after. In this study, with ten patients and a dose range of 5 to 20 mg, the time course shows a similar response for all doses with the maximum response proportional to the dose administered. This family of curves can be described in terms of magnitude and duration of effect, rate of onset and decay of effect, time and magnitude of peak effect, and area under the effect-time curve. However, it is both interesting and confounding to observe that when a saline solution is used in place of the drug, pain relief is still reported and the pharmacodynamic curve is not unlike the others in the figure. This type of drug response demonstrates the placebo effect, which plays a critical role in attempting to quantify drug response measures. The nature of the placebo effect and the need to consider it in the design of double-blind clinical studies has been a topic of investigation for over half a century.[10] To further complicate understanding of the placebo effect, the role of a patient's own state of anticipation of drug treatment, better called patient expectancy, confounds the nature of the placebo effect even further. To gain an improved understanding of drug response, the role of patient expectancy, a topic of current investigation,[11,12] and the nature of the feedback loops from drug effect to drug use are important parameters in need of further study both for understanding drug abuse and for improving drug therapy.

IV. ON THE NATURE OF THE RELATIONSHIP BETWEEN PHARMACOKINETICS AND PHARMACODYNAMICS

To study the kinetic/dynamic relationship of a drug, it is necessary to make a judicious choice as to the class of pharmacological agent. The tricyclic antidepressants and nonsteroidal anti-inflammatory drugs, for example, display a lengthy delay between achievement of steady state plasma levels and the onset of observable therapeutic response. Both indirect cascade mechanisms involved in drug action and lag times between the time-dependent kinetic and dynamic drug descriptors are critical parameters in determining the nature of such relationships. A number of studies which have focused on drugs of abuse provide a sufficient data base for discussion as they display a relatively rapid onset of effect and the pharmacokinetics is relatively well known. We will consider studies on marijuana and diphenhydramine as examples to present the principles involved in investigation of the nature of the relationships between controllable drug plasma levels and resulting drug response variables.

A. MARIJUANA

Pharmacokinetic studies have established that by smoking marijuana the cigarette delivers delta-9-tetrahydrocannabinol (THC) into the systemic circulation very rapidly and plasma levels increase to peak levels which may be reached even before the patient stops smoking the cigarette.[13] The pharmacodynamic response variables that can be considered include the objective measure of heart rate acceleration, a subjective measure of self-reported intoxication or psychological "high", and quantitative measures of complex task performance.

In the case of heart rate, quantitative analysis of the individual patient pharmacodynamic data demonstrate that heart rate response to smoking could be described by a biexponential function with a half-life of approximately 7 min for the rate increase and then a gradual return to the baseline rate with a half-life of approximately 17 min for the decrease.[13] In Figure 4, the relationship between THC plasma levels and heart rate, the kinetic/dynamic relationship, shows a linear relationship from 30 min (the post-distributive phase) to 120 min after smoking the cigarette, for data from six subjects that smoked three potencies of THC in a double-blind, cross-over, Latin square designed study.[14] The relationship spans the three potencies of cigarette (the actual dose ingested cannot be quantified). This is an example of a single-valued relationship between drug plasma levels and physiologic response to the drug. While the relationship appears to be independent of time, there is an implicit time dependence since the high THC concentrations occurred at the first response measures and the time course of the relationship reads from early time at the upper right side of each graph to late time at the lower left side. Such graphs have been referred to as phase plots.

The self-reported psychological "high" or intoxication pharmacodynamic response in the same study was found to lag behind the THC plasma levels, unlike the relation of heart rate response. Analysis for the "high" vs. plasma concentration of THC, shown in Figure 5 for mean data, demonstrates the lag of pharmacodynamic response relative to the pharmacokinetics of THC.[15] The relationship is a hysterisis loop where there is an obvious time dependence, with the time coordinate having a counter-clockwise direction. The highest plasma level occurs at 5 min after smoking and then decreases gradually, while the maximal drug response occurs at approximately 20 to 30 min and then decreases in an apparent linear fashion during 1 to 6 hours after smoking. The area enclosed within the loop appears to be proportional to the THC potency of the cigarette, which is assumed proportional to the dose. Since the kinetic/dynamic relationship is a loop, it is a double-valued relation where for a given plasma level there are two corresponding effect values occurring at different times. A similar looping relationship was

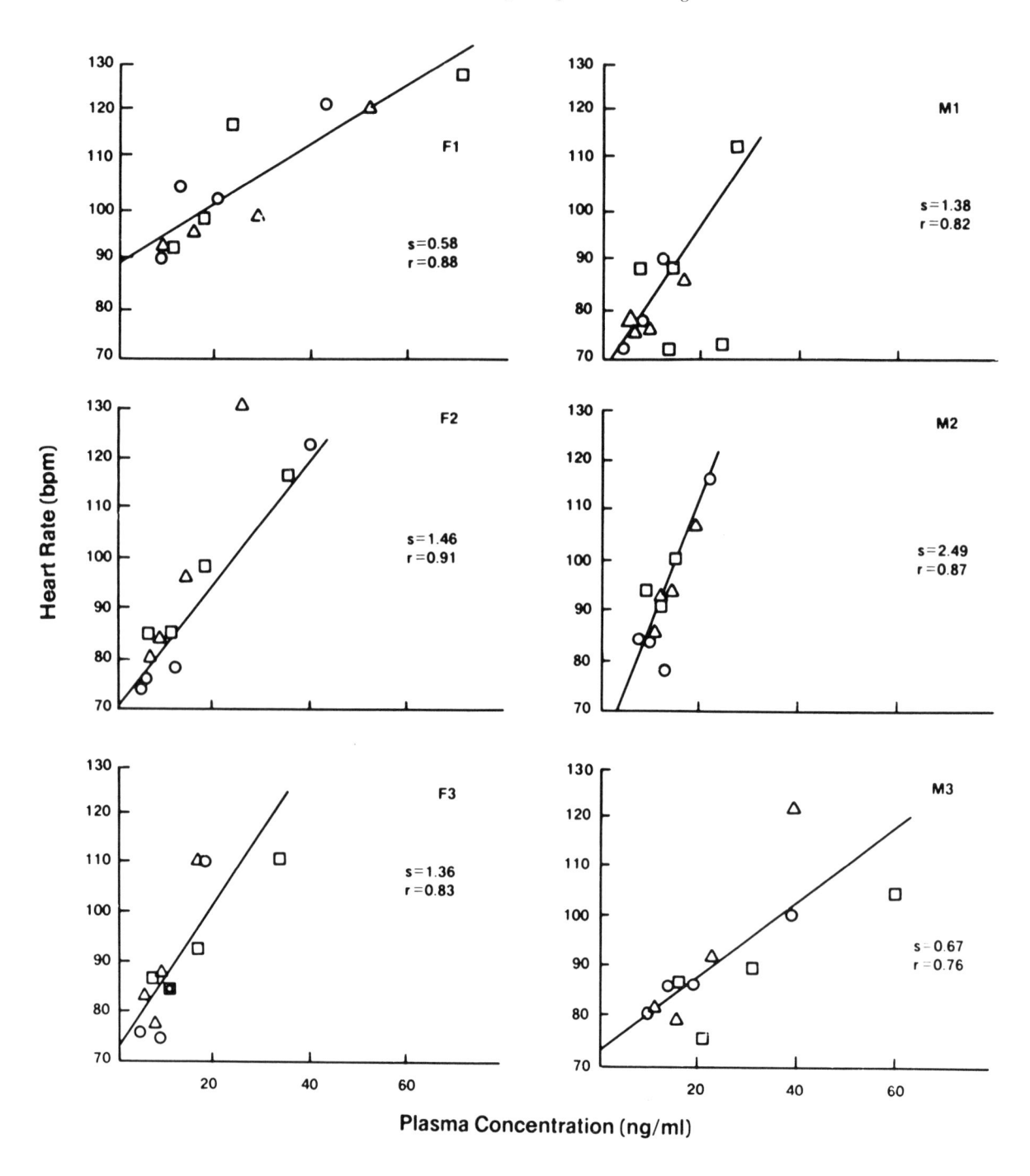

FIGURE 4. Relationship for individual subjects between heart rate and plasma concentration of THC from smoking marijuana. (From Chiang, C.N. and Barnett, G., *Cocaine, Marijuana, Designer Drugs: Chemistry, Pharmacology, and Behavior*, Redda, K., Walker, C., and Barnett, G., CRC Press, Boca Raton, FL, 1989, 13–25. With permission.)

in a comparison of kinetic/dynamic relations for THC from smoking, intravenous, and oral drug administration which demonstrated the effect of THC metabolism lowering THC plasma levels with a corresponding, but diminished, decrease in response. Again, the relationship is double-valued and a time coordinate must be assigned to the graphs. Consideration of variability and the statistically significance of the area enclosed within a loop is an area of needed research.

The relationships between pharmacodynamics of performance and the pharmacokinetics of THC from smoking were analyzed for several laboratory tasks related to

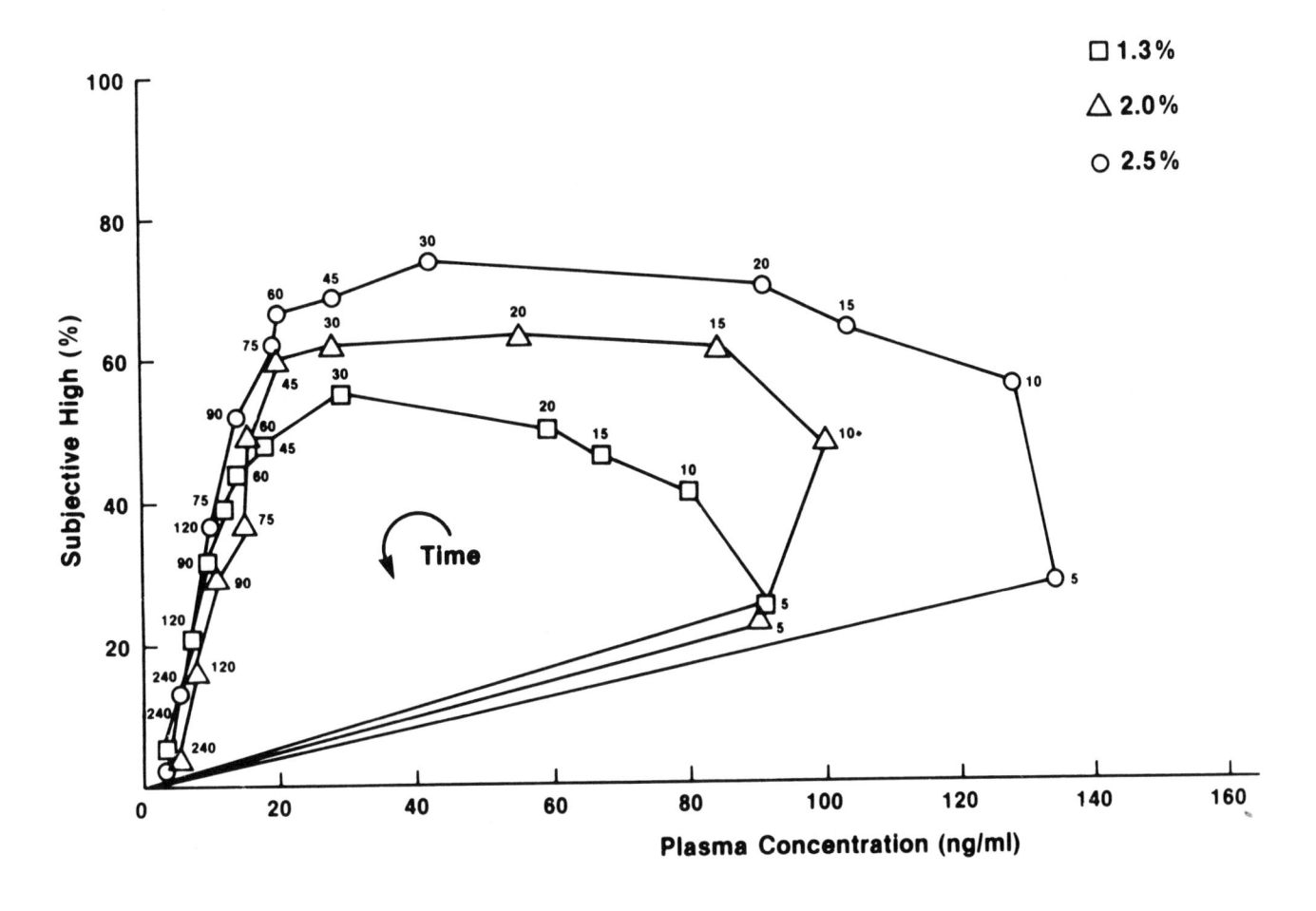

FIGURE 5. Relationship for average data of subjective "high" vs. plasma THC levels from smoking one marijuana cigarette. Numbers are time (minutes) after smoking when data were measured. (From Chiang, C. N. and Barnett, G., *Clin. Pharmacol. Ther.*, 36, 234–238, 1984. With permission.)

automobile driving.[16] The studies were designed in a placebo controlled double-blind fashion and the subjects performed laboratory tasks for tracking, divided attention, response time, and compensatory tracking. The performance or pharmacodynamic data was analyzed via quantitative methods and shown to decay in an exponential manner for all subjects on all tasks. That is, drug effects on performance were greatest immediately after smoking the cigarette and slowly decreased to drug-free levels of performance over a period of time. For the measure of response time required to search and identify a signal, the drug effect resulted in such variability that no clear kinetic/dynamic relation was found. The relationship between response and plasma levels of THC for two different measures of complex performance are shown in Figure 6. The measure of drug effect on tracking errors showed a strong dependence on plasma THC levels that was both linear and single-valued. The top curve of Figure 6 demonstrates that as THC levels increase the performance is more greatly impaired. For the more complex measure of critical tracking, which assays a mixture of reaction time and signal tracking, there is also a single-valued relation between drug effect and the log of THC plasma levels. In this case, the relationship is a sigmoidal curve that appears to saturate at plasma levels above 10 ng/ml. In both cases, the time course, which is implicit in the data, presents early time as the largest THC values and late time as the lower left side of each curve with the smallest THC levels. As pointed out by the authors, "the differential sensitivity revealed by the two behavioral measures may be due to different receptor systems and/or different components and/or metabolites of marijuana." These single-valued relationship allows a unique relationship between plasma levels and degree of drug effect or, in this case, drug impaired performance. There are, however, many questions in need of further research: what is the effect of multiple dosing? drug tolerance? subject learning abilities? and sensitivity and accuracy of the tasks?

The relationship between the pharmacodynamics of

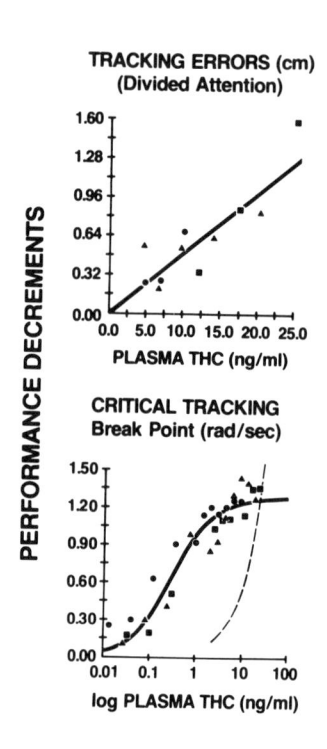

FIGURE 6. Correlation of decrement in performance with plasma levels of THC after smoking one marijuana cigarette. The upper curve is tracking errors under divided attention vs. plasma THC concentration. The lower curve is critical tracking break point vs. plasma THC concentration on a logarithm scale and the dashed line is tracking errors replotted from the upper curve. (From Barnett, G., Licko, V., and Thompson, T., *Psychopharmacology*, 85, 51–56, 1985. With permission.)

smoking marijuana and the pharmacokinetics of THC must be considered as a special case in the search for understanding the nature of such relationships. Smoking the marijuana cigarette is a very special dosage form of several reasons. As has been discussed,[14] it is not possible to establish the dose of drug (assumed to be THC) that enters the body and, in addition, the nature of the cigarette allows self titration of the dose, thus creating an interesting example of a response-dose feedback loop. Further, the rapid rise of THC plasma levels presents a significantly different pharmacokinetic profile than that encountered with oral drug administration. For this reason, we find it important to consider the different patterns and relationships in the following example.

B. DIPHENHYDRAMINE

Oral administration of commercially available doses of diphenhydramine produces plasma levels that gradually increase to maximum values at 1.5 to 2.5 hours and then decrease very slowly over the next 24 to 36 hours. As a result of this pharmacokinetic profile, the pharmacodynamic response profile is also much different than those discussed above for marijuana. Pharmacodynamic response profiles are shown in Figure 7 for drug effects on tracking errors and reaction time over a threefold range of doses. Since the drug effect curves are similar in shape to those of the drug plasma levels, there are several familiar quantitative parameters that can be used to describe the pharmacodynamics and its effect on these performance measures. There is a gradual increase in drug effects that reaches maximum values at 1 to 3 hours and then a gradually decrease over the next several hours. The shaded areas represent the span of variability which was found during placebo and pretreatment measurements. The solid curves are the best mathematical representation of the mean data points, and the dotted curves represent approximately one standard error of the mean values around the solid curve. The statistically significant onset of drug effect occurs when the lower dotted curve crosses above the baseline area. Thus, for reaction time, drug effect on performance starts at approximately 0.5 hours for the low and medium doses and at 1.2 hours for the high dose.

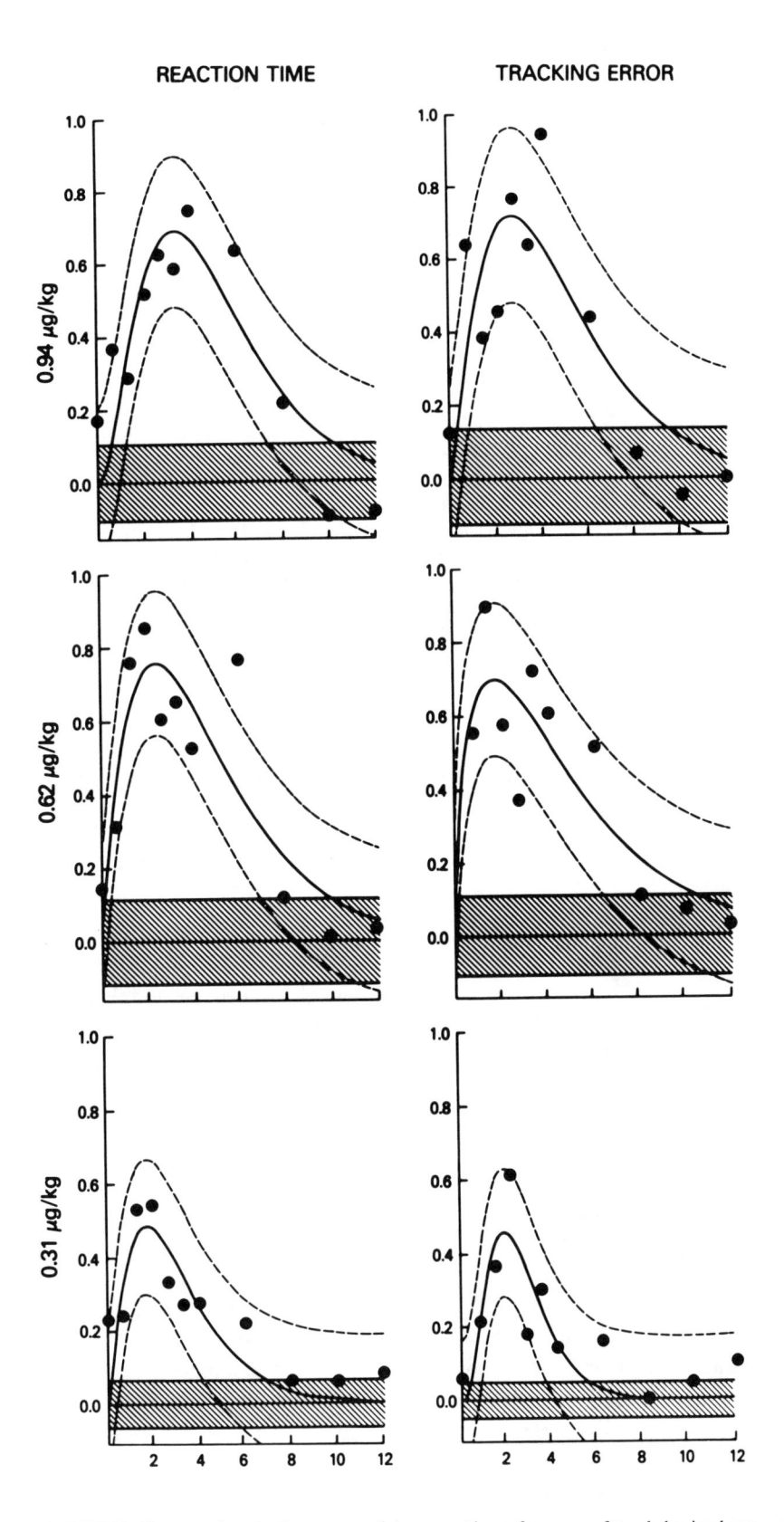

FIGURE 7. Pharmacodyamic time course of decrement in performance of two behavioral performance measures in response to one oral dose of diphenydramine. Experimental data points are shown as mean values and the solid curve is the computer fitted gamma distribution to the data. The dashed curves delimit upper and lower overall mean standard errors of the fitted curve. The shaded area represents the span of the standard error of the baseline. (From Licko, V., Thompson. T., and Barnett, G., *Pharmacol. Biochem. Behav.*, 25, 365–370, 1986. With permission.)

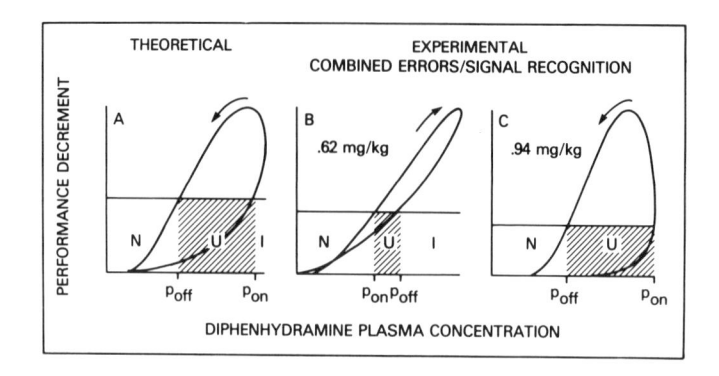

FIGURE 8. Illustration of the temporal relationships between plasma levels of diphenhydramine and drug effect on performance. The horizontal line indicates the threshold level of significant deviation of effect from baseline or unimpaired performance. The plots show the difference in the extent of three regions as a function of the degree of looping: N stands for the interval of plasma concentrations of no drug efect; U for the interval of uncertain effect due to the double-value relation; and I for the interval of certain impairment due to drug effect on performance. (From Licko, V., Thompson, T., and Barnett, G., *Pharmacol. Biochem. Behav.*, 25, 365–370, 1986. With permission.)

Significant effect ends when the same lower dotted curve crosses back down into the baseline, which occurs at approximately 4 hours for the low dose and 7 hours for the medium and high doses.

In this study, it was possible to determine several pharmacodynamic parameters.

1. Time of onset of effect
2. Duration of effect (the time interval from onset to offset)
3. Time of offset
4. Time of maximum effect
5. Area under the pharmacodynamic curve (which is the area within the duration of effect, above the baseline and below the lower dotted curve)

However, the dose dependence of the various parameters is confounded by the unusual pharmacokinetics of the drug as diphenhydramine tends to inhibit its own absorption. Therefore, even with all of this information, it was not always possible to determine a simple kinetic/dynamic relationship for a drug. Figure 8 presents this relationship for two doses on one measure of drug effect. In this case, there is no simple or single-valued relationship. The figure shows regions of the plasma concentration range within which it is not clear whether there is, or is not, a drug effect of significance, and it also shows a change in the direction of the time coordinate with respect to the hysteresis loops. This example emphasizes the importance of the time coordinate. Whether plasma levels are increasing or decreasing and whether drug response is increasing or decreasing present complexity in doing research to establish the kinetic/dynamic relationship.

V. CONCLUSIONS

We have seen that even in the case where the pharmacokinetic relationship is well characterized and, likewise, the pharmacodynamic relationship is well characterized in terms of quantitative parameters, the relationship between the two can still be complex. The complexity lies in the dissynchronous time evolution of the two relationships that generally exists. A theoretical example is shown in Figure 9[15] where the graphs show different perspectives of the relation between pharmacologic response (performance in this example) and pharmacokinetics (plasma drug levels) over time after oral administration of a drug. The pharmacodynamic profile is shown by the dotted curve and the pharmacokinetic curve is shown by the dashed curve. The critical kinetic/dynamic relation that we are searching for is that trajectory formed by the intersection of the pharmacokinetic and pharmacodynamic curves, which expresses the changing temporal relation between drug plasma level and pharmacologic response.

Understanding kinetic/dynamic relationships will provide insights into the processes involved in drug action. Such knowledge will also provide for more quantitative and thus safer, more effective drug therapy. While these

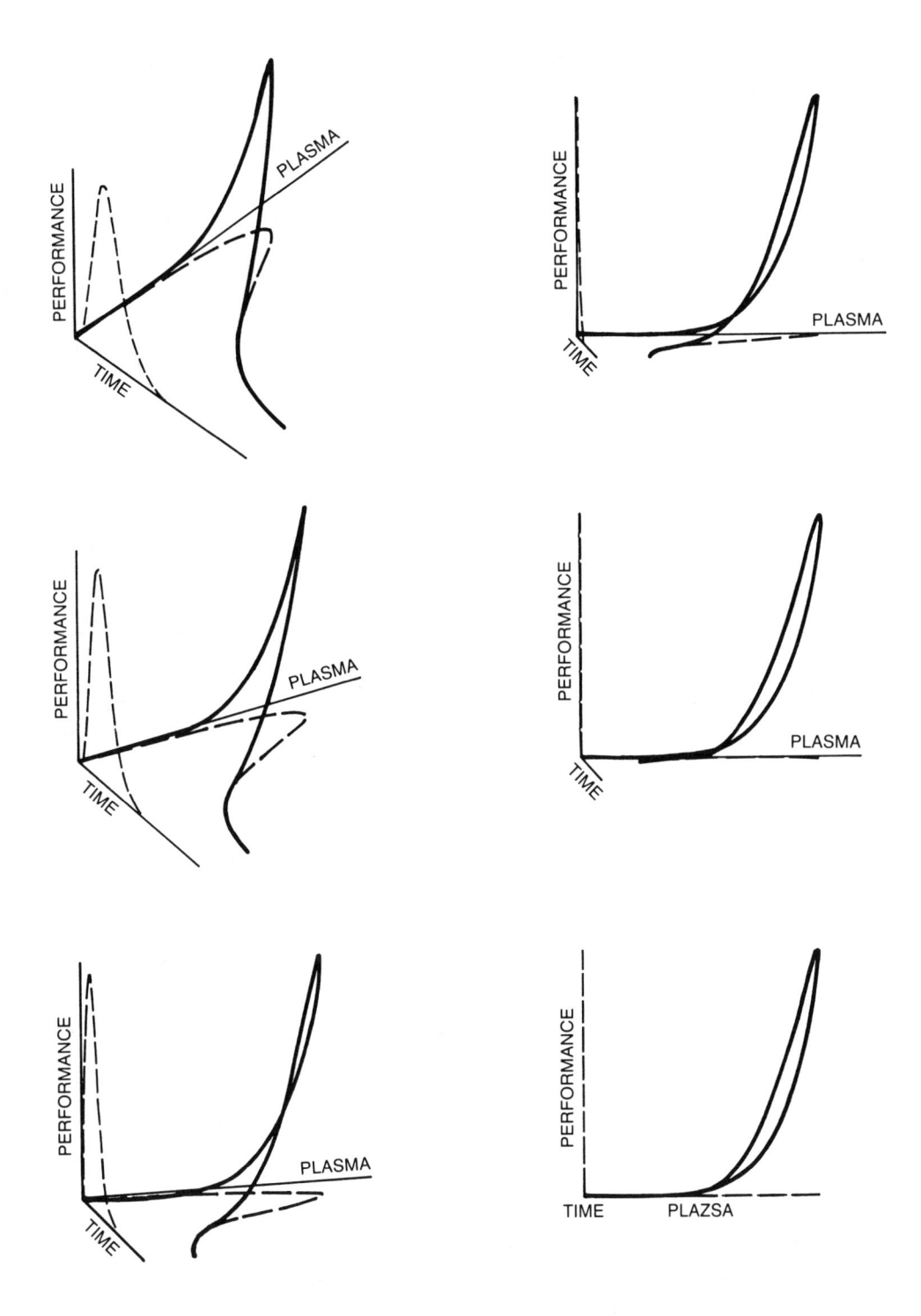

FIGURE 9. The general three-dimensional relationship between pharmacokinetics and pharmacodynamics with the time coordinate shown. (From Thompson, T., Licko, V., and Barnett, G., *Pharmacokinetics and Pharmacodynamics of Psychoactive Drugs*, Biomedical Publications, Foster City, CA, 1985. With permission.)

findings are also of forensic interest, caution is strongly recommended as many questions remain unanswered. This is obviously a field where considerable research is needed.

ACKNOWLEDGMENTS

It is a personal pleasure to acknowledge Nora Chiang, Vojtech Licko, and Travis Thompson, colleagues and friends with whom I collaborated on some of the work discussed in this chapter. They made the work exciting and enjoyable.

REFERENCES

1. **Aagaard, G. N.**, Ninety years of therapeutics — a history of the American Society for Clinical Pharmacology and Therapeutics — Preface, *Clin. Pharm. Ther.*, 47, 251, 1990.
2. **Gilman, A. G., Goodman, L. S., Rall, T. W., and Murad, F.**, *The Pharmacological Basis of Therapeutics*, 7th ed., Macmillan, London, 1985.
3. **Gibaldi, M. and Perrier, D.**, *Pharmacokinetics*, 2nd ed., Marcel Dekker, New York, 1982.
4. **Rowland, M. and Tozer, T.**, *Clinical Pharmacokinetics*, 2nd ed., Lea & Febiger, London,1989.
5. **Barnett, G., Hawks, R., and Resnick, R.**, Cocaine pharmacokinetics in humans, *J. Ethnopharmacol.*, 3, 353–366, 1981.
6. **Perrier, D., Ashley, J., and Levy, G.**, Effect of product inhibition on kinetics of drug elimination, *J. Pharmacokin. Biopharm.*, 1, 231–242, 1973.
7. **Connelly, T. J., Ambre, J. J., and Ruo, T. I.**, Kinetics of cocaine in humans, evidence for dose dependency, *Clin. Pharmacol. Ther.*, 47, 184, 1990.
8. **Kumor, K., Sherer, M., and Cascella, N.**, Cocaine use in man, subjective effects, physiologic responses, and toxicity, in *Cocaine, Marijuana, Designer Drugs, Chemistry, Pharmacology, and Behavior*, Redda, K., Walker, C., and Barnett, G., Eds., CRC Press, Basel, 1989, 83–96.
9. **Houde, R. W., Wallenstein, S. L., and Rogers, A.**, Clinical pharmacology of analgesics, *Clin. Pharmacol. Ther.*, 1, 163–174, 1960.
10. **Shapiro, A.**, The placebo effect, in *Principles of Psychopharmacology*, 2nd ed., Clark and del Giudice, Eds., Academic Press, London, 1978, 441–459.
11. **Camí, J.**, Analysis of the role of subject expectancy in the placebo effect, private communication, 1986.
12. **Cami, J., Guerra, D., Ugena, B., Segura, J., de la Torre, R., and Barnett, G.**, Effect of subject expectancy on disposition and response of THC from smoked hashish cigarettes, to be submitted, 1990.
13. **Barnett, G., Chiang, C. N., Perez-Reyes, M., and Owens, S.**, Kinetic study of smoking marijuana, *J. Pharmacokin. Biopharm.*, 10, 495–506, 1982.
14. **Chiang, C. N. and Barnett, G.**, Marijuana pharmacokinetics and pharmacodynamics, in *Cocaine, Marijuana, Designer Drugs, Chemistry, Pharmacology, and Behavior*, Redda, K., Walker, C., and Barnett, G., Eds., CRC Press, Boca Raton, FL, 1989, 113–125.
15. **Chiang, C. N. and Barnett, G.**, Marijuana effect and delta-9-tetrahydrocannabinol plasma level, *Clin. Pharmacol. Ther.*, 36, 234–238, 1984.
15. **Thompson, T., Licko, V., and Barnett, G.**, *Behavioral pharmacokinetics*, In *Pharmacokinetics and Pharmacodynamics of Psychoactive Drugs*, Barnett, G. and Chiang, C. N., Eds., Biomedical Publications, Foster City, CA, 1985, 247–263.
16. **Barnett, G., Licko, V., and Thompson, T.**, Behavioral pharmacokinetics of marijuana, *Psychopharmacology*, 85, 51–56, 1985.
17. **Licko, V., Thomson, T., and Barnett, G.**, Asynchronies of diphenhydramine plasma performance. Relationships, *Pharmacol. Biochem. Behav.*, 25, 365–370, 1986.
18. **Licko, V.**, Analysis of drug concentration-drug effect correlations, a theoretical model, in *Drugs, Driving, and Traffic Safety*, WHO Offset Publ. No. 78, World Health Organization, Geneva, 1983, 46–51.
19. **Barnett, G.**, Behavioral pharmacokinetics, in *Pharmacokinetics and Pharmacodynamics of Psychoactive Drugs*, Barnett, G. and Chiang, C. N., Eds., Biomedical Publications, Foster City, CA, 1985, 247–263.

Chapter 27

PHARMACOKINETIC APPROACHES ON DRUG TESTING

J. M. van Rossum, J. E. G. M. de Bie, and T. B. Vree

TABLE OF CONTENTS

I.	Introduction	172
II.	The Profile of the Body Transport Function	172
III.	Drug Input Profiles	173
IV.	The Absorption Process	174
V.	Drug Input by Inhalation	174
VI.	The Concentration Profile at the Observation Site	175
VII.	The Urine Profile of a Drug	175
VIII.	Observing Specific Drug Metabolites	177
IX.	Conclusions	179
References		181

I. INTRODUCTION

The drug concentration profile in the human body is dependent on three main entities[4] and the input:

1. The overall body transport function of the drug which in fact is a density function of residence times from a defined input site (vena cava) to a defined output site (aorta). So the drug concentration profile is only a direct reflection of the transport function when the drug is given as a bolus (pulse) in the vena cava and the blood sampling is done in the aorta.
2. The input profile (bolus, infusion, sustained release tablet, etc.).
3. The absorption process describing drug transport from application site (skin, GI-tract, etc.) to the vena cava.
4. The observation site being the arterial site where blood sampling is done (peripheral vena, urine) or where the action is supposed to occur (brain, heart, etc.).

Drugs of abuse are acting in some areas of the brain (cortex, N. accumbens, etc.), while they are used by oral route, intravenous injection, or inhalation. It will therefore depend on the purpose of drug testing, whether or not measurement of the drug or one of its characteristic metabolites in peripheral blood, saliva, or urine may provide relevant information.

If the aim is to detect the presence of a drug in the body, the terminal part of the transport function in relation to the analytical detection limit is important. If however the effect in relation to concentration is aimed at, rapid changes in the transport function may be most important. Such changes may be so fast that they can not be followed from measurements in the peripheral blood and certainly not from urine data.

II. THE PROFILE OF THE BODY TRANSPORT FUNCTION

Drug disposition kinetics is based on repetitive transits of drug molecules through the body, once they are introduced at the level of the vena cava until they are ultimately metabolized or excreted.

Essentially the pulmonary circulation and the systemic circulation are arranged in a positive feedback loop (see Figure 1). Defining the input at the vena cava and the output at the level of the aorta, an input pulse will be seen dispersed in the aorta, because of the transit time function of the pulmonary system (see Figure 2A). These molecules, at least the fraction that is not extracted, will be seen again after further dispersion in the systemic circulation and a second dispersion in the pulmonary circulation. Consequently, at each subsequent recirculation a further flattering occurs (see Figure 2A). Actually one observes the superposition of all recirculations, so that the disposition curve will be rapidly changing initially, but is mainly exponentially declining after some time (see Figure 2B).

The concentration profile after a pulse dose in the vena cava is

$$C(t) = \frac{D}{E \bullet CO} \bullet \psi(t) \qquad (1)$$

where $\psi(t)$ is the residence times distribution. The average number of recirculations and the slope of the terminal part of the curve depends directly on the extraction ratio.[2,4]

It must be noted that a fast transit curve in, e.g., the pulmonary circulation is lost by the slower dispersion thereafter in the systemic circulation. Since we are dealing with a zero order, positive feedback control system the steady state error is larger than one ($e_{ss} = 1/E$). Consequently, the mean time for the total body is e_{ss} times the mean time for a single transit:

$$MRT = \left[MTT_{\text{pulm}} + (1 + E) \bullet MTT_{\text{syst}} \right] / E \qquad (2)$$

So the mean residence time is a factor $1/E$ times the weighted mean body transit time. It must be emphasized that only the fraction $(1-E)$ of the molecules make a complete transit through the systemic circulation.

It may be noted that the terminal slope of the curves merely depends on the steady state error and therefore on the extraction ratio. This implies that if in the same individual the E may change in time or because due to the pharmacological action of the drug circulation may change and consequently the E may change. So it is likely that the nonlinear kinetics of cocaine at higher doses which has a strong cardiovascular effect may be due to a dose dependent change in extraction ratio.[1]

It is obvious that the transit time functions in the obese individual will be larger, and consequently, the dispersion during each recirculation is greater. Certainly then the mean residence time would be larger at the same extraction ratio, but the blood concentration profile is lower in the aorta and at any observation site, including the urine.

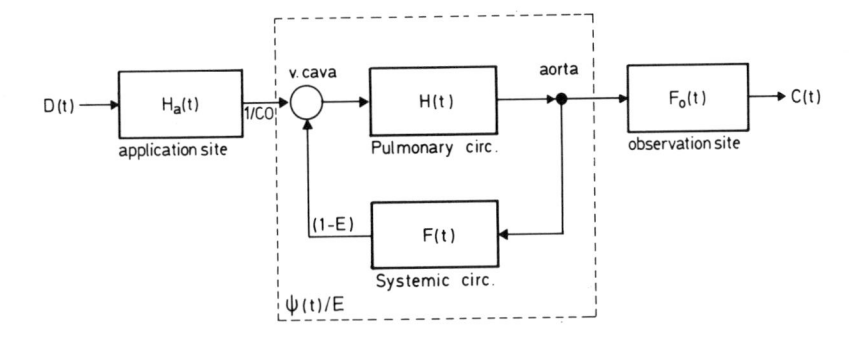

FIGURE 1. Block diagram of the positive feedback loop of the circulation. The body transport function ψ(t) is a density function of residence times based on repetitive transits through the pulmonary and systemic circulation. The drug input D(t) is at some application site. $H_a(t)$ is the absorption function. The concentration output is measured somewhere beyond the aorta, so $F_o(t)$ is the observation function. The input-output relationship depends on all three processes in succession.

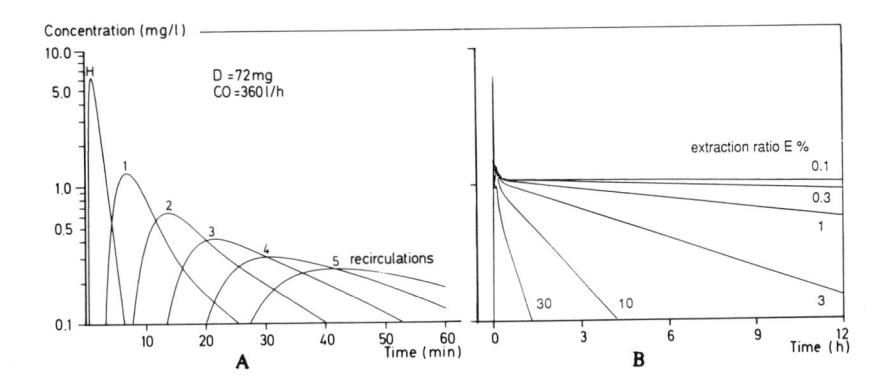

FIGURE 2. (A) The output concentration following a bolus injection simulated for molecules that for the first time pass the pulmonary circulation, those having made an additional complete passage through the entire body and so on. Note a progressive dispersion with every passage. (B) The superimposed curves for various extraction ratios. The feedback error (e_{ss} = 1/E) is larger for smaller extraction ratios and, consequently, the average number of recirculations is larger.

III. DRUG INPUT PROFILES

A bolus injection essentially is a momentary input of all molecules of the dose at the same time, $D \cdot \delta(t)$. The output curve then is directly proportional to the transport function located between input and output (see Equation 1).

A constant infusion of a dose D over a period T is a constant input rate D/T. It is in fact a step function (or block) over a period T. Then $D(t) = [U(t) - U(t-T)] \cdot D/T$. Other input profiles may occur if the drug is given as a sustained release tablet, applied on the skin as an ointment, or is inhaled in some way.

Unless the input profile is fast with respect to the transport function following it, the output is the convolution of both input and transport function. For any D(t):

$$C(t) = \frac{D(t)}{Cl} * \psi(t) \qquad (3)$$

Here "*" is the convolution operator, and the clearance (Cl) is E times the cardiac output (CO). It will be evident that if the time constant of the input curve is larger than the short time constant of the disposition curve, fast dynamics cannot be observed from the concentration output profile (see Figure 3).

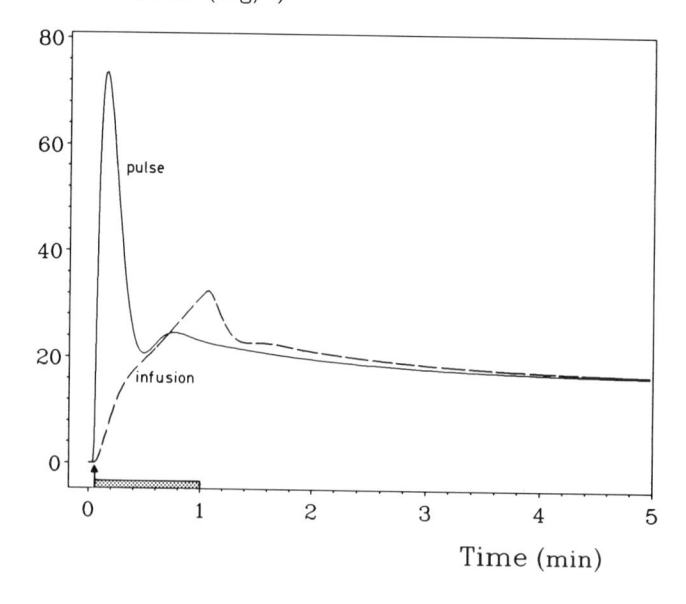

FIGURE 3. Output concentration curve over the first minutes following a bolus injection and following a short constant infusion. Fast processes are obscured by slow infusion.

IV. THE ABSORPTION PROCESS

The application site of drugs is not the vena cava, but either a peripheral vein in case of injection, the oral cavity, the GI tract, the skin, or otherwise. This implies that there is always a transit time function from application site to vena cava. Evidently, the mean transit time or mean absorption time (*MAT*) following an i.v. injection is much shorter than following oral intake.

Consequently, in the output concentration curve the fast changes disappear. After p.o. dosing the fast aspects of the transport function are certainly lost. The absorption curve can be simulated by a number of injections given after Δt delays (see Figure 4A). Each injection is reflected in the output by a dispersion governed by the transport function. Superposition of all curves gives the output curve (see Figure 4B). From this figure, it is evident that fast changes are lost. Following any input *D(t)* the output concentration in the aorta is the convolution of all functions involved.

$$C(t) = \frac{D(t)}{E \bullet CO} * H_a(t) * \psi(t) \qquad (4)$$

where $H_a(t)$ is the absorption function.

V. DRUG INPUT BY INHALATION

Abuse drugs are often given by inhalation. Absorption in the lungs occur for small particles and gases such that they bypass the vena cava and directly enter the vena pulmonalis. Consequently, the pulmonary transit time function will be faster so that dependent on the input profile — way and depth of inhalation — the drug may reach a higher peak in the aorta than after i.v. injection. The duration of a single short inhalation is about 1 s, but a deep inhalation may be several seconds. So if the short time constants of the transport function are larger than several seconds, the inhalation input may be regarded as a pulse of zero duration (see Figure 5).

Following inhalation, extremely high concentrations in the aorta may be encountered. Since the brain is highly vascularized, the high peak in the blood is little dispersed upon entering the brain. The influence of different input absorption curves in the aorta concentration are visualized in Figure 5. It is evident that at the site of blood sampling more dispersed concentration profiles are encountered.

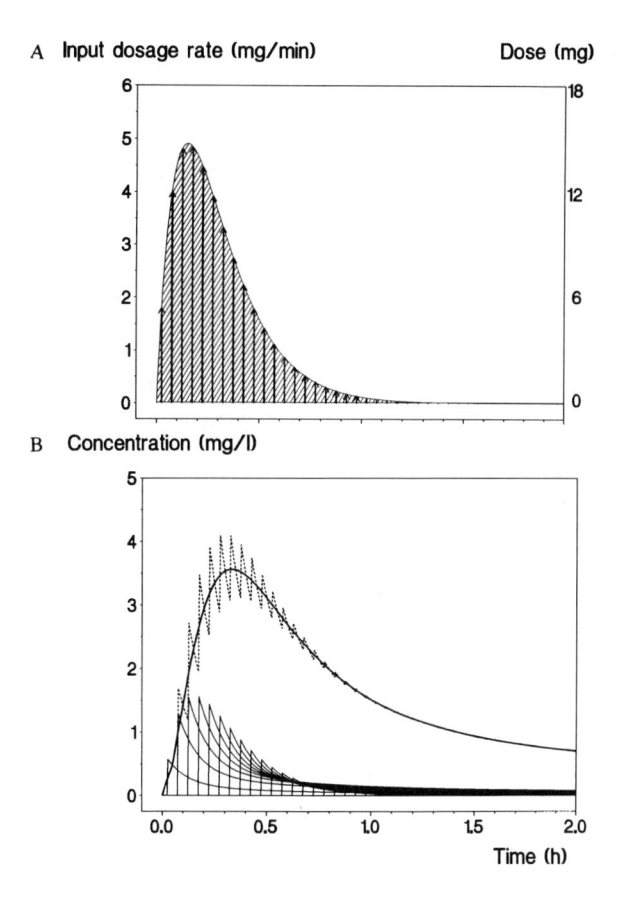

FIGURE 4. Demonstration of the convolution operator. The input ratio can be split up into a number of injections of different size, each of which causes an output concentration of different amplitude. The summation (convolution integral) of all the functions is the observed output. (Adapted from van Rossum and de Bie, 1989.)

VI. THE CONCENTRATION PROFILE AT THE OBSERVATION SITE

Often blood sampling is done in a peripheral vein. Consequently, a transport function $F_o(t)$ is included governing drug transport from aorta to observation site. The overall input/output relationship is then:

$$C(t) = \frac{D(t)}{E \cdot CO} * H_a(t) * \psi(t) * F_o(t) \qquad (5)$$

It is likely that fast changing concentrations in the aorta, due to inhalation, cannot be followed in the blood of a peripheral vein.

VII. THE URINE PROFILE OF A DRUG

The renal excretion rate (dQ_r/dt) is directly proportional with the blood concentration of arterial renal blood.

$$dQ_r/dT = Cl_r \cdot C(t) \qquad (6)$$

The renal clearance however may not be a constant but dependent on urine volume, urine pH, and the concomitant excretion of other drugs. The momentary renal excretion rate cannot be followed, since in the urine produced over a period Δt one can only calculate the average rate over that period as $\Delta Q_r/\Delta t$

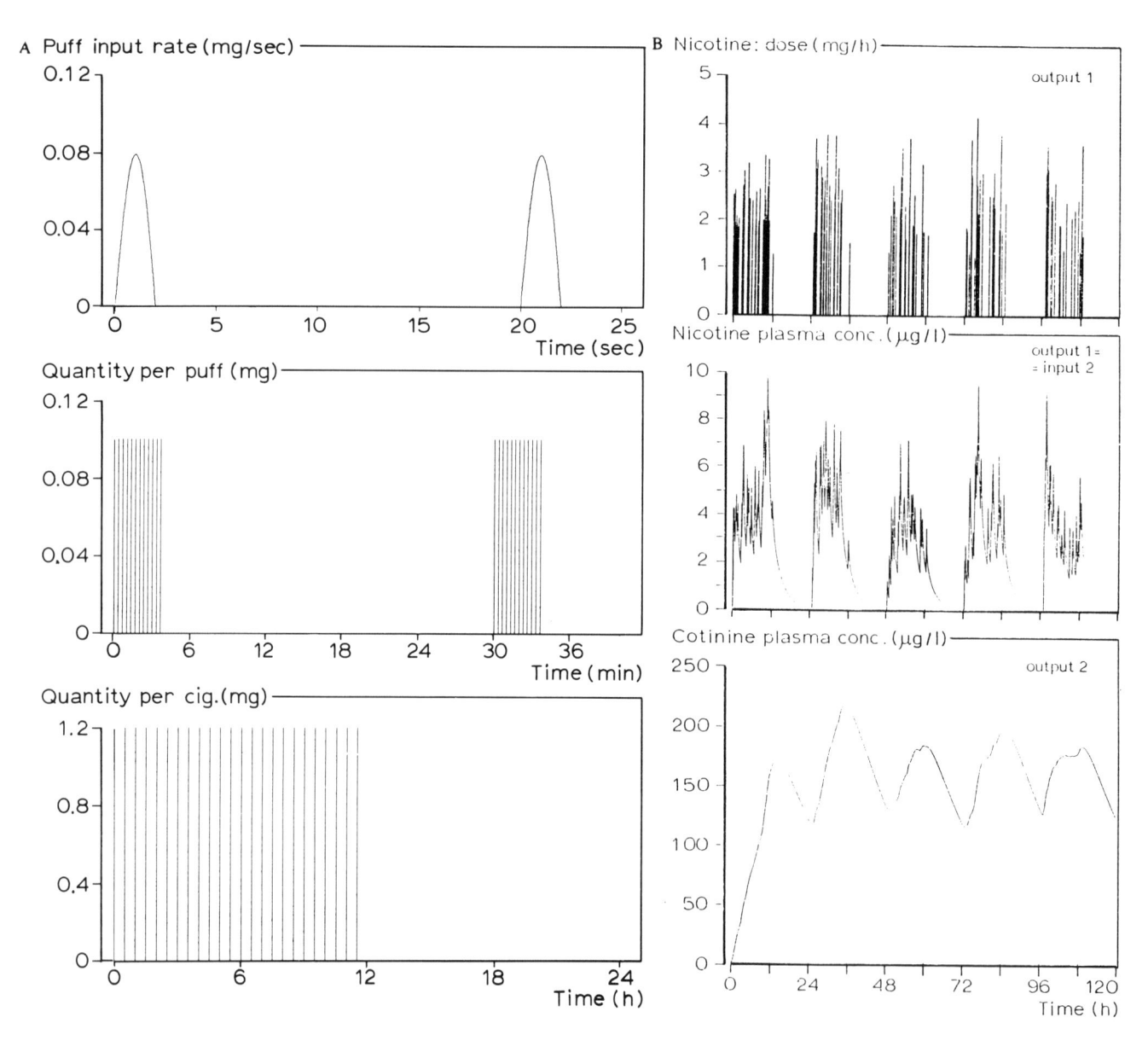

FIGURE 5. (A) Inputs of inhalation of, e.g., nicotine. These inputs are of short duration so that on a compressed time scale they resemble pulses, while the sum of such pulses resembles an infusion. (B) Variable inputs of cigarette smoking and the resultant nicotine output concentrations. Nicotine having a fast kinetics follows input variations, while its major metabolite cotinine, having a slow kinetics, averages the input variations.

$$\Delta Q_r = \overline{Cl_r} \bullet \int_t^{t+\Delta t} C(t)dt \qquad (7)$$

The clearance in that period is taken as the mean clearance over Δt. The average renal excretion rate reasonably follows the blood concentration when the urine flow and pH are constant. It is therefore a good custom to plot urine volume and pH together with the average renal excretion rate[8] (see Figure 6). Also, the cumulative excretion is plotted, which is the integral of the plasma concentration profile

$$Q_r(t) = \overline{Cl_r} \bullet \int_0^t C(t)dt \qquad (8)$$

The total ultimately amount excreted in the urine is

$$Q_r(tot) = \overline{Cl_r} \bullet AUC = D \bullet \overline{Cl_r} / Cl \qquad (9)$$

The fraction excreted unchanged may vary tremendously among various drugs in relation to the values of the renal clearance and the total clearance. See Figure 6 for a difference between amphetamine and phenylethylamine the latter which is rapidly metabolized.[8]

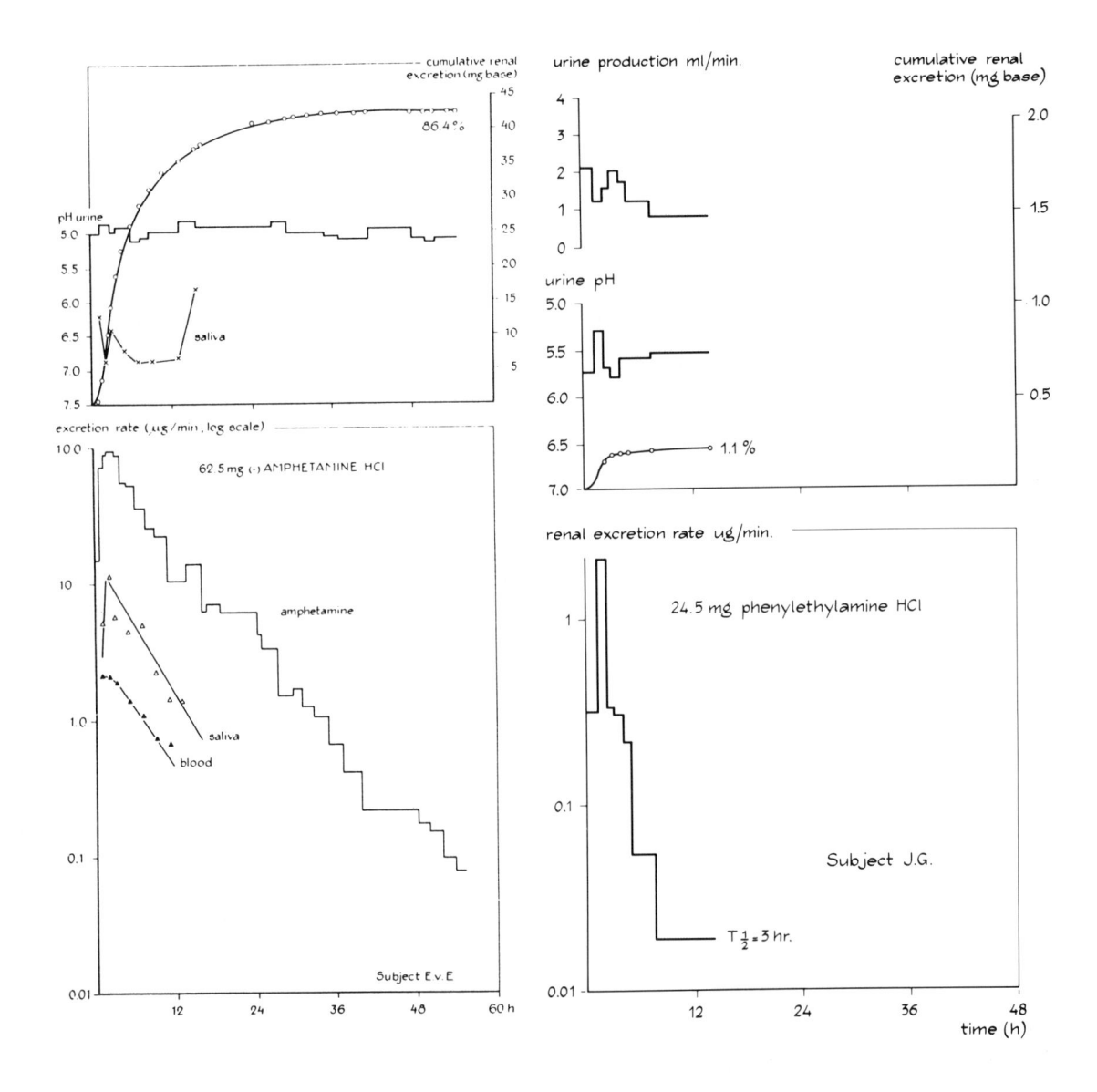

FIGURE 6. Renal excretion of amphetamine and its closely related homolog phenylethylamine. Amphetamine is excreted unchanged to a large extent, while its homolog is largely metabolized. (From Vree, 1974.)

Monitoring drugs of abuse in the urine focuses on the concentration in the urine. The urinary concentration may however vary much more as it depends again of the volume of urine produced.

Low water intake will lead to high concentrations and drinking of water to relatively low concentrations. An example is given in Figure 7 for ephedrine. Urine density and also urine pH has to be taken into account in interpreting cutoff limits for abuse drugs in the urine. The influence of the pH can be very large as is the case of fencamfamine, see Figure 8.[6]

VIII. OBSERVING SPECIFIC DRUG METABOLITES

During every recirculation of a drug in the body a certain fraction is either metabolized or excreted as such. So a fraction from of the extracted molecules are converted into a particular metabolite. The metabolite again is subject to recirculation and extraction. The metabolite profile therefore depends on the parent drug profile and the disposition profile of the metabolite:[4]

$$C_m(t) = \frac{D(t)}{Cl_m} * H_a(t) * \psi(t) * f_m S_F(t) * \psi_m * F_o(t) \qquad (10)$$

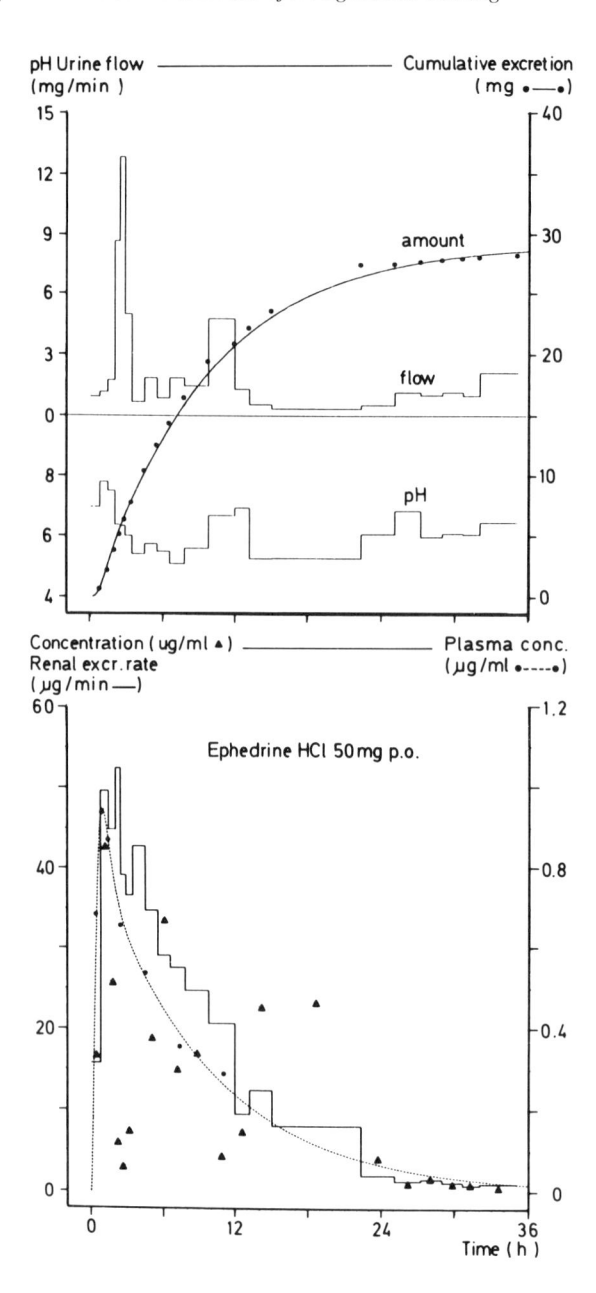

FIGURE 7. Renal excretion of ephedrine following an oral dose of 50 mg(HCL salt). The renal excretion rate $\Delta Q_r/\Delta t$ parallels the plasma concentration. Because of the large renal clearance of ephedrine, this compound can be followed in the urine much longer than in the blood. The urine concentration highly fluctuates due to variation in fluid excretion. Also the pH has some influence.

Here Cl_m is the total clearance of the metabolite, f_m is the fraction of parent drug converted into the particular metabolite, and $S_F(t)$ a survival function of parent drug from aorta to the moment of metabolic conversion; this process will be fast with regard to the two disposition profiles so that this function can be disregarded.[4]

Obviously, now more functions are involved and the concentration profile of the metabolite is further dispersed with regard to the profile of the parent drug (see Figure 9).[7] Also, from the urinary excretion rate curves, it may be seen that the metabolite curves are more dispersed than the curve of the parent drug. The total amount of metabolite

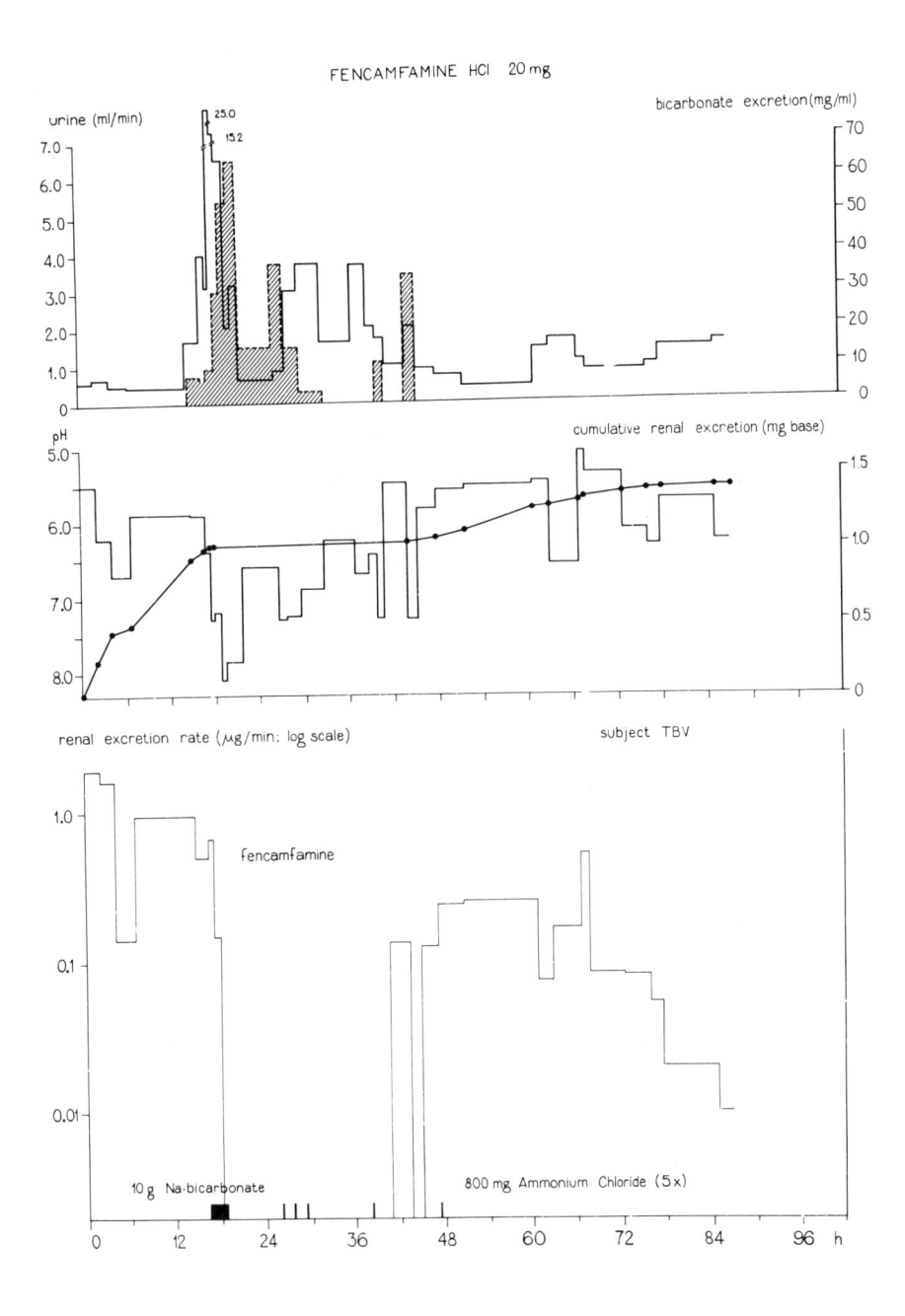

FIGURE 8. Renal excretion of fencamfamine as influenced by pH changes in the urine. Increase of the pH by sodium bicarbonate injection causes the excretion rate to drop drastically. Reacidification with ammonium chloride brings the excretion rates back to normal. (From Vree, et al., 1969.)

excreted in the urine depend on the dose of parent drug the total and renal clearance of the metabolite to

$$Q_{mr} = D \bullet f_m \bullet Cl_{mr} / Cl_m \qquad (11)$$

Depending on the parent drug and metabolite clearances, it may occur that the metabolite is excreted in a larger amount than the parent drug.

Metabolite profiles will give little relevant information for pharmacological action of the parent drug, but they may be of importance for monitoring drugs of abuse. In studying metabolites more variability is introduced.

IX. CONCLUSIONS

The concentration profile of drugs of abuse depends on

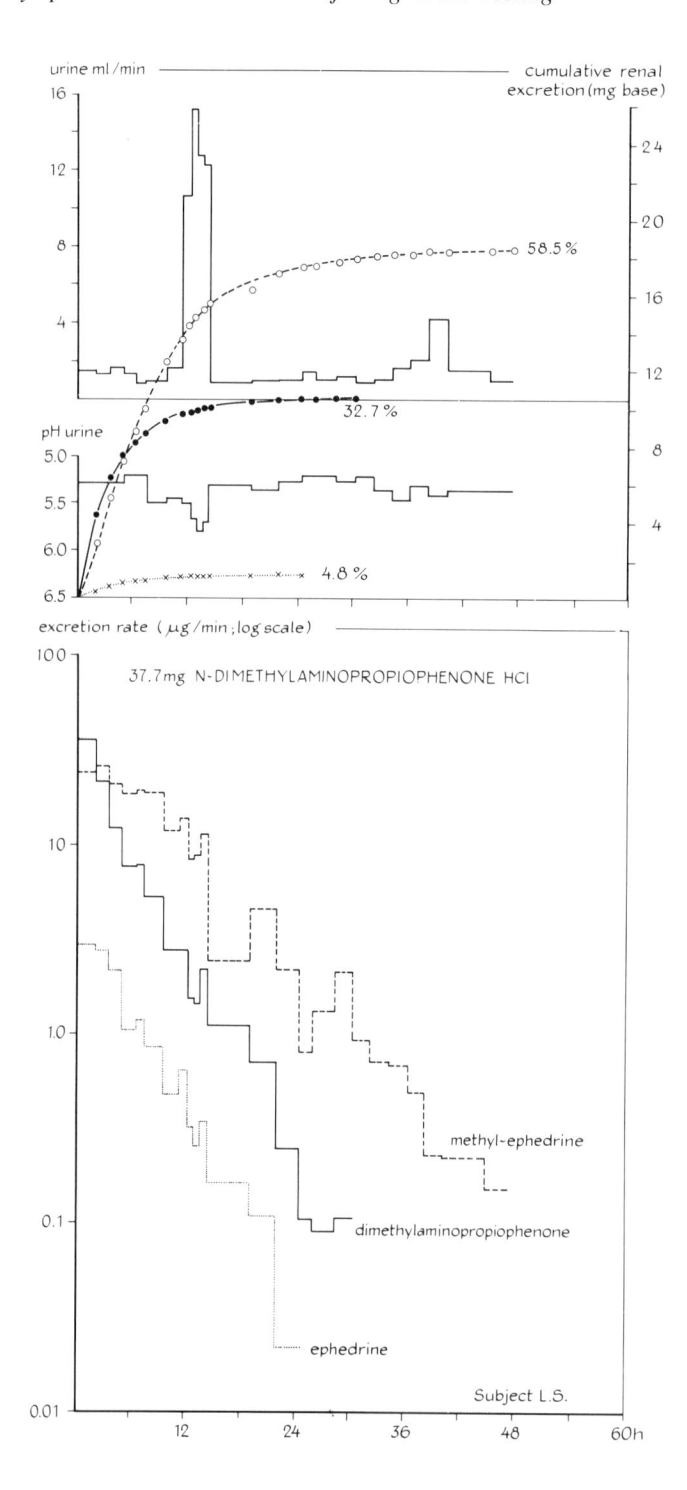

FIGURE 9. Renal excretion of dimethylcathinone and its metabolites. The major metabolite is methylephedrine which contributes to about 60%. Note also that the kinetics of this metabolite is slower than of the parent compound. From (Vree, 1974.)

a number of factors such as the pharamacokinetic disposition curve, $\psi(t)$, the absorption profile, and the observation site (blood, urine). These three factors vary for drugs and for individuals. The urine concentration, in addition, depends on the urine pH, the water intake, and the concommitant use of other drugs.

By setting a cutoff limit, all these factors are to be taken into account. Pharmacokinetic information, including variability among individuals, should be taken into account for interpretation of results of drug of abuse control.

REFERENCES

1. **Barnett, G.,** Relationship between pharamacokinetics and pharmacodynamics, in *Current Issues in Drugs of Abuse Testing*, Segura, J. and de la Torre, R., Eds., CRC Press, Boca Raton, FL., 1990.
2. **van Rossum, J. M., Burgers, J., van Lingen, G., and de Bie, J. E. G. M.,** Pharmacokinetics: a dynamic systems approach, *TIPS*, 4, 27–30, 1983.
3. **van Rossum, J. M., van Lingen, G., and Mensink, R.,** Kinetics of drug action: control systems dynamics of abuse drugs, in *Pharmacokinetics of Psychoactive Drugs*, Barnett, G. and Chiang, C.N., Eds., NIDA Research Monographs, Bethesda, MD, 1985.
4. **van Rossum, J. M. and de Bie, J. E. G. M.,** Perspectives in pharmacokinetics: pharmacokinetics from a dynamical systems point of view, *J. Pharmacokin. Biopharm.*, 17(3), 365–392, 1989.
5. **van Rossum, J. M. and de Bie, J. E. G. M.,** Pharmacokinetics of Drug Metabolism, *Eur. J. Drug Rehab. Pharmacokin.*, 1990, in press.
6. **Vree, T. B. and van Rossum, J. M.,** Suppresion of renal excretion of fencamfamine in man, *Eur. J. Pharmacol.*, 7, 227–230, 1969.
7. **Vree, T. B., Muskens, A. Th. J. M., and van Rossum, J. M.,** Metabolism of N-alkyl substituted aminoproprophenones in man, *Arch. Int. Pharmacodyn. Ther.*, 197, 392–395, 1972.
8. **Vree, T. B.,** Pharmacokinetics and Metabolism of Amphetamines, PhD. thesis, University of Nijmegen, The Netherlands, 1973.

Chapter 28

RELEVANCE OF PHARMACOGENETICS AND DRUG-DRUG INTERACTIONS

Rafael de la Torre

TABLE OF CONTENTS

I. Introduction 184

II. Relevance of Pharmacogenetics on Drugs of Abuse Testing 184

III. Polymorphic Metabolizing Enzymes Involved in the Metabolism of
 Drugs of Abuse 184
 A. S-Mephenytoin Hydroxylase 184
 B. Pseudocholinesterase 184
 C. Acetyltransferase 184
 D. Debrisoquine Hydroxylase 185

IV. Drug Interactions 185

V. Conclusions 187

References 190

I. INTRODUCTION

Genetic polymorphisms related to certain metabolic enzymes can be the dominant cause of interindividual variations in the elimination of several drugs.[1] This could lead to clinically significant differences in the pharmacological responses of some patients.[2]

The increasing knowledge of specific substrates and inhibitors of the different polymorphic metabolic pathways allow precise predictions of drug-drug interactions. This will be the case of dextropropoxyphene, a potent metabolic inhibitor of debrisoquine phenotype substrates, or the potent inhibitory effect of neuroleptics on tricyclic antidepressants metabolism.[2]

Additionally, the development of drug testing programs around the world highlights the need for taking into account interethnic differences in drug metabolism.[3-5]

II. RELEVANCE OF PHARMACOGENETICS ON DRUGS OF ABUSE TESTING

There is a reduced number of substances related to the world of drugs of abuse where there is a relationship with currently described genetic polymorphisms and their metabolism. Nevertheless, new and old drugs are regularly added to the list of those showing a genetic polymorphism in their biotransformation. Interindividual variations in metabolizing enzymes, to date nonpolymorphic, probably have a genetic basis,[6] and we should be in the look out further.

Examples will be given of some common abused drugs where it is known that some metabolic pathways are under control of different oxidative polymorphisms like codeine (debrisoquine phenotype) and diazepam (S-mephenytoin phenotype). Other genetic factors are also regulating nonoxidative enzymes important in the metabolism of drugs as would be the case of N-acetyltransferases (flunitrazepam) and pseudocholinesterase (cocaine).

III. POLYMORPHIC METABOLIZING ENZYMES INVOLVED IN THE METABOLISM OF DRUGS OF ABUSE

A. S-MEPHENYTOIN HYDROXYLASE

In the metabolism of mephenytoin, it has been shown that S- but not its R-enantiomer, is hydroxylated in a polymorphic manner.[7] The isozymes involved in this polymorphism belong to the cytochrome P450IIC subfamily. The number of substrates with which metabolism is regulated by this polymorphism is quite low and includes such drugs as desmethylmephenytoin, mephobarbital, propranolol, diazepam, and nordiazepam, and to a certain extent (50%) the N-demethylation of imipramine.[8]

The incidence of poor metabolizers (PM) is less than 5% in the caucasian population.[9] A higher incidence is observed in orientals where, according to population studies, the rate of PM is between 15 and 22%.[10]

From those drugs showing this polymorphism, benzodiazepines have some interest in drug of abuse testing as they can be subjected to abuse or used as a therapeutic agent. The oxidative demethylation of diazepam to nordiazepam and the oxidation of nordiazepam to oxazepam are impaired in poor metabolizers of mephenytoin. Pharmacokinetic studies in healthy volunteers after the administration of 10 mg of both substances show a reduction by one half in the clearance of the drug and a twice longer half-life in poor metabolizers of mephenytoin.[11]

B. PSEUDOCHOLINESTERASE

Human plasma cholinesterase hydrolyzes a number of drugs, some of them related with drugs of abuse, e.g., cocaine[12] and heroine.[13] The enzyme is defined by two genetic loci, E_1 and E_2. E_1 is the main loci responsible for the enzymatic activity clinically relevant. One form of this gene, the E_1^a is responsible for the enzymatic activity of the atypical cholinesterase or pseudocholinesterase. The frequency of the abnormal enzyme in the caucasian population is around $1/2500$, and lower incidences have been shown in other populations.[4]

Cocaine, a substrate of cholinesterase, is rapidly eliminated from the body by minimal urinary excretion but mostly by metabolism. While one of the main metabolites, benzoylecgonine, is formed nonenzymatically, ecgoninemethylester is formed by cholinesterases in liver and serum.[12,14] It has been suggested that a deficiency in cholinesterase activity might be the responsible in some cases for the acute toxicity of cocaine in drug abusers.[15]

C. ACETYLTRANSFERASE

Two arylamine N-acetyltransferases contribute to the biotransformation of drugs. They are encoded by two genes designated NAT1 and NAT2. Two mutant alleles have been identified for NAT2, which is the target of the observed common polymorphism. Individuals homozygous slow acetylators show a severely decreased or absent NAT2 liver enzyme protein.[16] The frequency of the poor acetylator condition is around 60% in caucasians and negroes and much lower in oriental populations, between 10 and 20%. The metabolism of arylamine drugs (e.g., isoniazid, procaine, dapsone, caffeine, ...) and arylamine carcinogens is affected by this polymorphism.[17]

One drug of some interest in the world of drugs of abuse is the benzodiazepine flunitrazepam. One of its main metabolites 7-aminoflunitrazepam is subsequently acetylated. Because acetylation is a secondary pathway of this drug, it is unlikely for the appearance of side effects related with this polymorphism. The use of acetylation has been proposed in some analytical chromatographic methods as a derivatization technique for its detection.[18] Laboratories doing drug testing, if pretending to interpret metabolic profiles, must be aware of the fact that a certain percentage of this metabolite, depending on the phenotype, is biologically acetylated and that inconsistent results could appear if this derivatization is used in urine samples.

D. DEBRISOQUINE HYDROXYLASE

There is a monogenic deficiency of the capacity for debrisoquine hydroxylation in 5 to 10% of different caucasian populations. Studies in oriental populations show a lower incidence of this phenotype 0.5 to 2.5%.[2] The isozyme of the cytochrome P450 enzymes group involved in this polymorphism is the cytochrome P450IID6, and mutations on the gene encoding such protein, CYP2D6, can explain the poor metabolizer phenotype.[19] There is an important number of drugs regulated by this polymorphism including some of those belonging to the groups of tryciclic antidepressants, β-blockers, antiarrythmics, neuroleptics, and opiates.

Several of these drugs are involved in drugs of abuse because of their use as therapeutic agents, e.g., trycyclic antidepressants and neuroleptics. From a pharmacodynamic point of view, the main concern with these drugs is that they can lead to clinically relevant metabolic interactions when they are co-administered or when associated with other drugs that co-segregate with this polymorphism, as will be the case with codeine.[2] Other therapeutic agents, like d-propoxyphene, where a polymorphic regulation in its metabolism has not been demonstrated, can act as very potent inhibitors of substrates co-segregating with debrisoquine polymorphism.[20]

Some opiates are under the same polymorphic genetic control as debrisoquine, e.g., dextrometorphan,[21] and codeine.[22,23] Dextrometorphan is used in therapeutics as an antitussive drug and has some interest in pharmacogenetics because it has been proposed as a probe drug for population phenotyping of debrisoquine polymorphism. Figure 1 shows the plasma concentration-time curve of dextrorphan, the main metabolite of dextrometorphan, in a study in healthy volunteers (n = 12) receiving a dose of 30 mg of dextrometorphan hydrobromide by the oral route.[24] As can be observed, one of the volunteers has this metabolic pathway impaired and later has been phenotyped as a poor metabolizer of debrisoquine. This same poor metabolizer was subjected to an excretion study with codeine (30 mg of codeine phosphate given by the oral route). When comparing its metabolic excretion profile (Figure 2B) with that of an extensive metabolizer of debrisoquine (Figure 2A), the absence of morphine, one of the main metabolites of codeine, and subsequently, normorphine can be observed.

IV. DRUG INTERACTIONS

As has been stated by Dr. San in Chapter 30, opiate drug addicts in different therapeutic schemes, like methadone maintenance programs, are in fact abusers of more than one substance. In addition to substances specifically involved in the world of drugs of abuse, the fact that most drug abusers are suffering from other diseases and treated with other drugs must be taken into account.

Most probably, there are not big differences between the kind of drug-drug interactions that can be observed within the normal population and within the drug addict population. In Table 1 there is a list of drug interactions between drugs of abuse and some other drugs. This table has been elaborated with data from Griffin and D'Arcy[25] and other authors cited in the text. What is specific of the drug addict population are the doses of some drugs ingested and the number of drugs concomitantly administered as misused drugs or therapeutic agents.

The case of ethanol deserves special mention. This substance, frequently consumed concomitantly with other drugs of abuse, leads to well-documented pharmacodynamic interactions enhancing the depressing effects over the central nervous system of most of these compounds. Sometimes ethanol gives rises to the formation of some compounds like cocaethylene (ethylcocaine) in the presence of cocaine that can be relevant from a pharmacodynamic point of view and in the interpretation of analytical results.[26] Figure 3 shows the excretion metabolic profile of one individual receiving 100 mg of cocaine intranasally and 1 g/kg of ethanol by the oral route (Figure 3A). When comparing this profile with that obtained in the same individual in the absence of alcohol (Figure 3B), we can observe the presence of a new compound identified as cocaethylene (benzoylecgonine, one of the main metabolites of cocaine, is not present in these particular chromatograms because of the analytical method used). Two facts are relevant in the detection of cocaethylene.

FIGURE 1. Plasma concentration-time curve of dextrorphan in healthy volunteers after the administration of dextrometorphan.

It has been recently reported that cocaethylene is a metabolite of cocaine in the presence of ethanol with a pharmacological profile very close to the profile of cocaine.[26] Thus from a pharmacodynamic point of view, its detection is very relevant. From an analytical point of view, the detection of benzoylecgonine by chromatographic techniques using its ethyl derivative must be avoided, because artifactually cocaethylene is being synthesized.

Quite frequently, when doing drug testing, there is a lack of information about the drugs ingested by the individual. When interpreting analytical results, neither the biochemist nor oftenly the physician considers the fact that the individual is treated with other drugs, sometimes because they are used as a therapeutic agent for the addiction or for a disease. It is possible to imagine some cases, exemplified with codeine, where it would be very difficult to interpret results.

Case 1

An individual is under treatment with imipramine, a known inhibitor of substrates that co-segregate with debrisoquine polymorphism,[2] and he has a cold and receives a treatment where codeine is administered. He is subjected to drug testing at the work place. When screened for drugs of abuse the test for opiates is positive, and when this result is confirmed codeine is identified in high concentrations and morphine in minute amounts.

Case 2

An heroine ex-addict is under treatment with d-propoxyphene, a known inhibitor of substrates that co-segregate with debrisoquine polymorphism.[2] Analytical controls are performed routinely to verify the abstinence. When screened for opiates the result is positive and the analytical confirmation of the presumptive test shows the presence of codeine in high concentrations and morphine in minute amounts.

The laboratory responsible for the drug testing was unaware of the ingestion of imipramine and d-propoxyphene by the individual, and when interpreting analytical results two possibilities were considered for these cases:

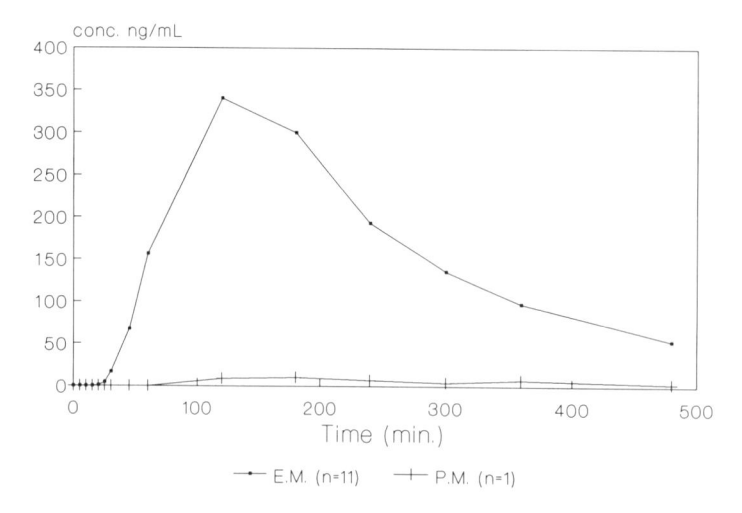

1. The individuals are poor metabolizers of debrisoquine, and that explains the small amounts of morphine in the urine being possible the use of codeine.
2. Because of the high concentrations of codeine in urine, the individuals are suspected of abuse.

The individual under treatment with imipramine furnished a medical prescription for codeine. Even though codeine was prescribed, abuse cannot be excluded because of the high amounts of codeine. If you take into account the ingestion of imipramine, the use of codeine for the treatment of a cold becomes more plausible. The individual under treatment with d-propoxyphene claimed an ingestion of codeine and a medical prescription was provided. If you take into account the ingestion of d-propoxyphene, the use of codeine for the treatment of a

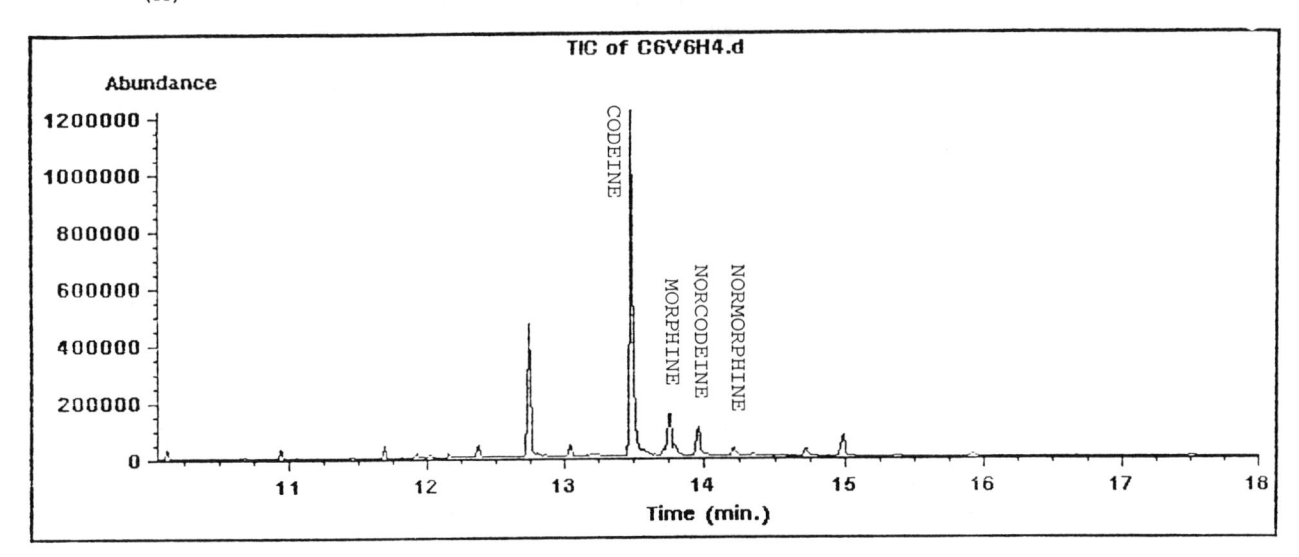

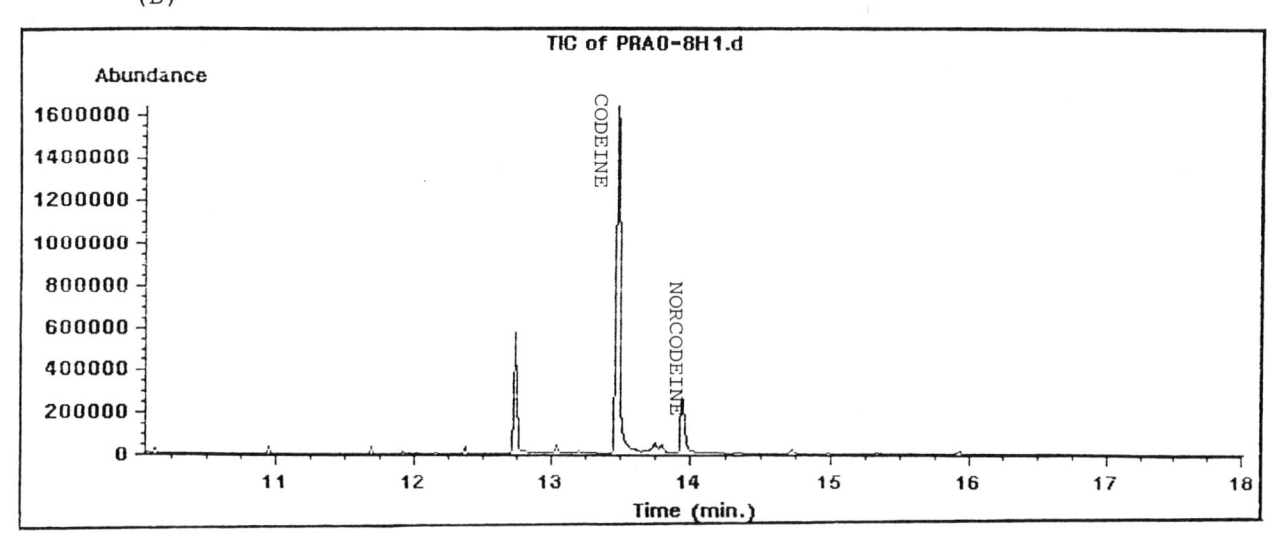

FIGURE 2. Metabolic urinary profile of codeine in a poor metabolizer (B) and in an extensive metabolizer (A) of debrisoquine. Urine collection period 0 to 8 hours. Chromatograms obtained by gas chromatography coupled to mass spectrometry.

cold becomes more plausible, but because of the preceding abuse of opiates, the abuse of codeine cannot be excluded on the basis of a single spot check of urine.

Probably these examples are limited cases, but when conducting drug testing the interpretation of results must be done in the broadest way, taking into account every factor because of the consequences of a positive test for the individual.

V. CONCLUSIONS

When doing drugs of abuse testing, three facts must be taken into account when interpreting analytical data.

1. The metabolism of some drugs is under genetic control.
2. There are interethnic differences in drug metabolism.
3. Drug-drug interactions can interfere in the interpretation of results.

TABLE 1
Drug-Drug Interactions Described in Substances Related with Drugs of Abuse

Drug	Interaction
Alcohol	
Analgesics	
Acetaminophen	Increased liver damage
Aspirin	Increased bleeding time
Anticoagulants	Metabolic inhibition
Anticonvulsivant	
Phenytoin	Metabolic induction
Antidepressants	
MAO inhibitors	Hypertensive reaction (tyramine)
	Metabolic inhibition of alcohol (nonspecific)
Tricyclics compounds	Enhanced sedation
	Behavioral disorders
Antidiabetic agents	Severe hypoglycemia
Metformin	Lactic acidosis
Tolbutamide, Chlorpropamide	Metabolic induction
	Facial flush
Antihypertensive agents	Enhanced hypotensive effects
Antihelmintics	
Tetrachloroethylene	Enhanced liver toxicity
	CNS-depressant side effects
β-Lactam antibiotics	Antabuse-like effects
Bromocriptine	Enhanced toxicity
CNS-depressants	
Anticonvulsivant, antihistaminics, barbiturate and non-barbiturate sedatives, hypnotics and minor tranquilizers as benzodiazepines, narcoleptics	Enhanced CNS-depressant effect
Disulfiram and disulfiram-like agents	Antabuse effects
Opiates	
Drugs with oxidative phenotype linked to Debrisoquine	
Dextropropoxyphene	Metabolic inhibition (codeine)
Cimetidine	Metabolic inhibition (methadone morphine, pethidine)
Barbiturates	Metabolic induction (pethidine)
Tricyclic Antidepressants	Enhanced CNS depression

TABLE 1 (continued)
Drug-Drug Interactions Described in Substances Related with Drugs of Abuse

Drug	Interaction

Barbiturates

Drug	Interaction
Dextropropoxyphene	
Valproate	Metabolic inhibition
(barbiturates)	
Alcohol	Increased intoxication
Amidopyrine	
Oral anticoagulants	
Tricyclic Antidepressants	
Chloramphenicol	
Doxycilline	
Corticosteroids	
Oral contraceptives	
Metronidazole	
Phenylbutazone	
Griseofulvin	Metabolic induction
IMAO Antidepressants	Metabolic inhibition
Cannabinoids	Metabolic induction/inhibition

Benzodiazepines

Drug	Interaction
Aminophylline	Antagonism diazepam sedation
Cimetidine	Metabolic inhibition
Dextropropoxyphene	
Oral contraceptives	
Valproate	
Drugs with oxidative phenotype linked to S-mephenytoin	Metabolic inhibition (diazepam, flurazepam)

Amphetamine-like compounds

Drug	Interaction
IMAO antidepressants	Hypertensive episodes

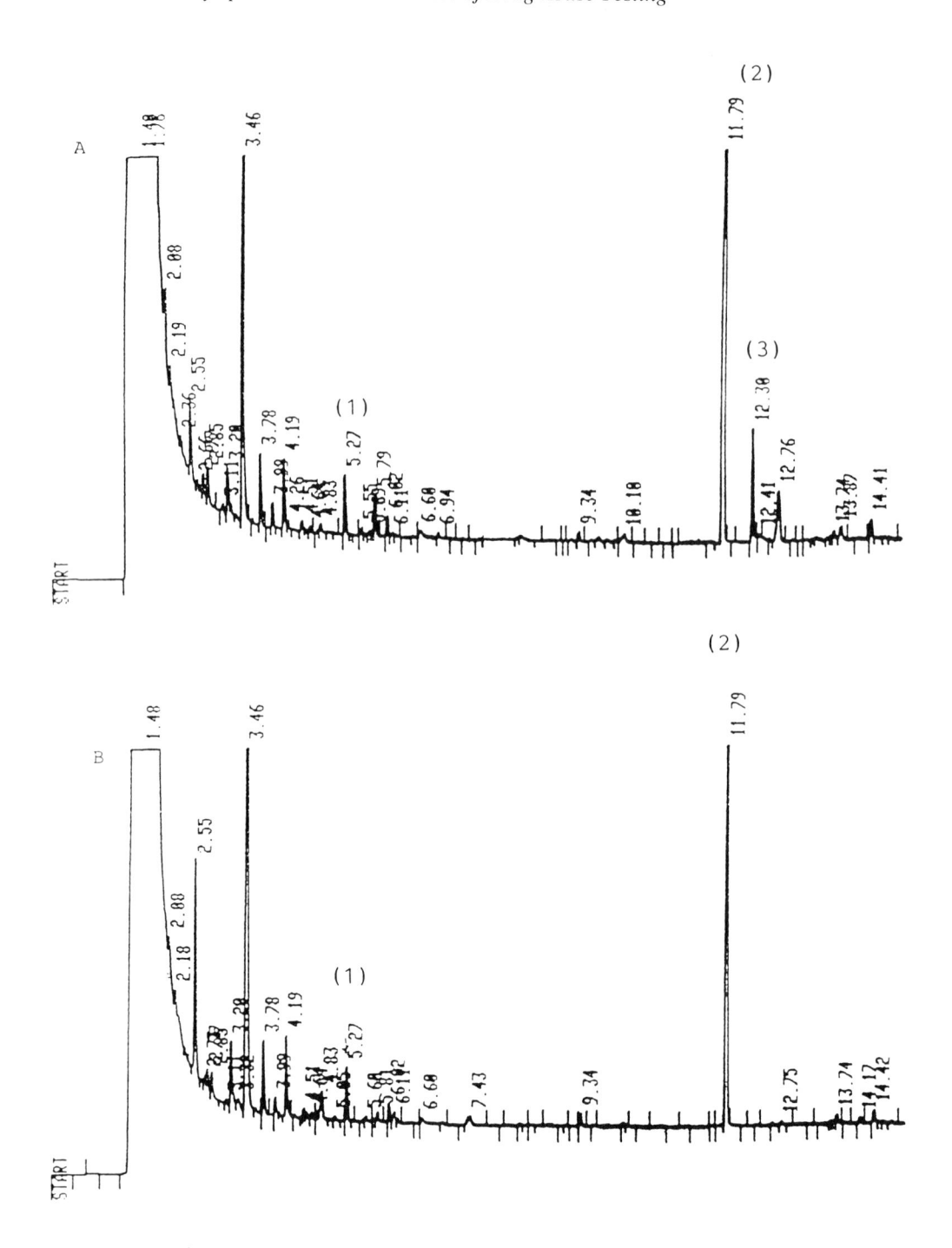

FIGURE 3. Metabolic urinary profile of cocaine in the presence (A) and in the absence of ethanol (B). Urine collection period 0 to 4 hours. Chromatograms obtained by capillary gas chromatography with nitrogen phosphorous detection (GC/NPD). (1) ecgoninemethylester, (2) cocaine, and (3) cocaethylene.

REFERENCES

1. **Balant, L. P., Gundert-Remy, U., Boobis, A. R., and von Bahr, Ch.,** Relevance of genetic polymorphism in drug metabolism in the development of new drugs, *Eur. J. Clin. Pharmacol.*, 36, 551–54, 1989.

2. **Brosen, K. and Gram, L. F.,** Clinical significance of the sparteine/debrisoquine oxidation polymorphism, *Eur. J. Clin. Pharmacol.*, 36, 537–47, 1989.

3. **Kalow, W., Goedde, H. W., and Agarwal, D. P., Eds.,** Ethnic differences in reactions to drugs and xenobiotics, *Progress in Clinical and Biological Research*, Vol. 214, Alan R. Riss, New York, 1986.

4. Kalow, W., Ethnic differences in drug metabolism, *Clin. Pharmacokin.* 7, 373–400, 1982.
5. Yue, Q. Y., Svensson, J.-O., Alm, C., Sjoqvist, F., and Sawe, J., Interindividual and interethnic differences in the demethylation and glucuronidation of codeine, *Br. J. Clin. Pharmacol.*, 28, 629–637, 1989.
6. Alvan, G., Balant, L. P., Bechtel, P. R., and Boobis, A. R., Eds., *European Consensus on Pharmacogenetics*, COST B1 Medicine, Brussels: Commission European Community, Office for Official Publications of the European Communities, Luxembourg, 1990.
7. Kupfer, A. and Preisig, R., Pharmacogenetics of mephenytoin: a new drug hydroxylation polymorphism in man, *Eur. J. Clin. Pharmacol.*, 26, 753–59, 1984.
8. Skjelbo, E., Hallas, J., Brosen, K., and Gram, L. F., The mephenytoin polymorphism is partially responsible for the N-demethylation of imipramine, in *Drug Metabolizing Enzymes: Genetics, Regulation and Toxicology*, Ingelman–Sundberg, M., Gustafsson, J–A., and Orrenius, S., Eds., 8th International Symposium on Microsomes and Drug Oxidation, Stockholms Projektgrupp, Stockholm, 1990, 51.
9. Sanz, E. J., Villen, T., Alm, C., and Bertilsson, L., S-mephenytoin hydroxylation phenotypes in a swedish population determined after co-administration with debrisoquine, *Clin. Pharmacol. Ther.*, 45, 495–99, 1989.
10. Horai, Y., Nakano, M., Ishizaki, T., Ishikawa, K., Zhou, H. H., Zhou, B. J., Liao, C. L., and Zhang, L. M., Metropolol and mephenytoin oxidation polymorphisms in Far Eastern oriental subjects: Japanese versus mainland Chinese, *Clin. Pharmacol. Ther.*, 46, 198–207, 1989.
11. Bertilsson, L., Henthorn, T. K., Sanz, E., Tybring, G., Sawe, J., and Villen, T., Importance of genetic factors in the regulation of diazepam metabolism: relationship to S-mephenytoin, but not debrisoquine, hydroxylation polymorphism, *Clin. Pharmacol. Ther.*, 45, 348–54, 1989.
12. Stewart, D. J., Inaba, T., Lucassen, M., and Kalow, W., Cocaine metabolism: cocaine and norcocaine hydrolysis by liver and serum esterases, *Clin. Pharmacol. Ther.*, 25, 464–68, 1979.
13. Lockridge, O., Mottershaw-Jackson, N., Eckerson, H. W., and LaDu, B. N., Hydrolysis of diacetylmorphine (heroine) by human serum cholinesterase, *J. Pharmacol. Exp.Ther.*, 215, 1–8, 1980.
14. Inaba, T., Stewart, D. J., and Kalow, W., Metabolism of cocaine in man, *Clin. Pharmacol. Ther.*, 23, 547–552, 1978.
15. Devenyi, P., Cocaine complications and pseudocholinesterase, *Ann. Intern. Med.*, 110, 167–68, 1989.
16. Blum, M., Grant, D. M., Demierre, A., McBride, O. W., Heim, M., and Meyer, U. A., Human acetylation polymorphism: characterization of two N-acetyltransferases (NAT) genes, including the gene encoding the polymorphic enzyme, in *Drug Metabolizing Enzymes: Genetics, Regulation and Toxicology*, Ingelman-Sundberg, M., Gustafsson, J.-A., Orrenius, S., Eds., 8th International Symposium on Microsomes and Drug Oxidation, Stockholms Projektgrupp, Stockholm, 1990, 40.
17. Webber, W. W. and Hein, D. W., N-acetylation pharmacogenetics, *Pharmacol. Rev.*, 37, 26–79, 1985.
18. Maurer, H. and Pfleger, K., Identification and differentiation of benzodiazepines and their metabolites in urine by computerized gas chromatography/mass spectrometry, *J. Chromatogr.*, 422, 85–101, 1987.
19. Kagimoto, M., Heim, M., Kagimoto, K., Zeugin, T., and Meyer, U. A., Debrisoquine/sparteine polymorphism: characterization of the mutations of the CYP2D6 causing deficient P450IID6 protein, in *Drug Metabolizing Enzymes: Genetics, Regulation and Toxicology*, Ingelman-Sundberg, M., Gustafsson, J.-A., Orrenius, S., Eds., 8th International Symposium on Microsomes and Drug Oxidation, Stockholms Projektgrupp, Stockholm, 1990, 46.
20. Sanz, E. and Bertilsson, L., D-propoxyphene is a potent inhibitor of debrisoquine, but not S-mephenytoin 4-hydroxylation in vivo, *Ther. Drug Monitor.*, in press, 1990.
21. Schmid, B., Bircher, J., Preisig, R., and Kupfer, A., Polymorphic dextrometorphan metabolism: co-segregation of oxidative O-demethylation with debrisoquine hydroxylation, *Clin. Pharmacol. Ther.*, 38, 618–624, 1985.
22. Yue, O. Y., Svensson, J.-O., Alm, C., Sjoqvist, F., and Sawe, J., Codeine O-demethylation co-segregates with polymorphic debrisoquine hydroxylation, *Br. J. Clin. Pharmacol.*, 28, 639–45, 1989.
23. Mortimer, O., Persson, K., Ladona, M. G., Spalding, D., Zanger, U. M., Meyer, U. A., and Rane, A., Polymorphic formation of morphine from codeine in poor and extensive metabolizers of dextrometorphan: relationship to the presence of immunoidentified cytochrome P450IIDI, *Clin. Pharmacol. Ther.*, 47, 27–35, 1990.
24. Caturla, M. C., de la Torre, R., Congost, M., and Segura, J., Plasma dextrometorphan metabolites and relation to urinary phenotyping: pilot study, *Eur. J. Clin. Pharmacol.*, 36(A149), 1989.
25. Griffin, J. P. and D'Arcy, P. F., Eds., *A Manual of Adverse Drug Interactions*, John Wright & Sons Ltd., Bristol, 1989.
26. Jatlow, P., Heary, W. L., Elsworth, J., and Roth, R., Cocaethylene inhibits uptake of dopamine and can reach high plasma concentrations following combined cocaine and alcohol, CPDD, Richmond, VA, 1990.

Chapter 29

TECHNICAL ISSUES TO BE POTENTIALLY STANDARDIZED AT INTERNATIONAL LEVEL: INTERPRETATION AND REPORTING OF RESULTS

Robert Wennig

TABLE OF CONTENTS

I.	Analytical Interpretation of Results	194
II.	Toxicological Interpretation	194
III.	If the Result Is Positive?	195
IV.	If the Result Is Negative?	195
V.	Sources of Error in Testing Urine Specimens for Drugs of Abuse	195
VI.	Medical Interpretation	196
VII.	Reporting of Results	196
VIII.	Future Developments	196
IX.	International Standardization	196
X.	Conclusions	197
	References	197

As it has been stressed several times by many of the previous speakers until now and reviewed in a report of the U.S. Substance Abuse Testing Committee,[1] analytical toxicology is not easy, but interpretation of the toxicological findings will be even more difficult. First of all, we have to consider different kinds of interpretations, which are sometimes overlapping: analytical interpretation; toxicological interpretation; medical interpretation; and, in some instances, we may even add legal interpretation, if there are legal limits, like in the case of ethanol, for instance, in many countries. It must also be borne in mind for which purposes the drugs of abuse testing has been performed (Table 1).

If only the use of a drug of abuse has to be detected, the identification of the drug(s) by qualitative analysis in urine will be sufficient in most cases. But there may be some problems if metabolism and origin of the drug is ambigious to find, e.g., benzphetamine or amphetamine, opiates (codeine and/or morphine) THC-carboxylic acid from therapeutic use as antiemetic in cancer patients or from cannabis abuse. A qualitative analysis is not sufficient, if an influence of drugs on the behavior of an individual is the aim of the investigation. In these cases, quantitative assays in order to obtain tissue concentrations, at least in blood, are necessary.

I. ANALYTICAL INTERPRETATION OF RESULTS

The analytical interpretation is among the most difficult issues arising in litigation or arbitration. It requires, accordingly, the greatest expertise in scientific consultants and expert witnesses. It requires also a multistage process as follows:

1. Verifying actual laboratory findings
2. Establishing validity or not of findings taking internal and external quality control (QC) results into account
3. Significance of the findings
4. Resolving inconsistent results or findings

This process is only valid if collection and storage of the specimens is performed according to the state-of-the-art.

The investigator has to have a basic understanding of the performing characteristics of the test assays, like appropriate detection limits, cutoff levels, and specificity of the assay for drugs, its metabolites and interfering substances.

The result may not be the last piece in the drug of abuse puzzle, the laboratory may have stopped at one drug (time pressure, lack of sample, etc.) and so another drug may have been overlooked. The investigator may also be aware of some common pitfalls, e.g., a patient in a drug treatment center may introduce different drugs in the food of other patients or even staff in order to discredit the laboratory.

II. TOXICOLOGICAL INTERPRETATION

The investigator has to take into account the following factors.

- The dose administered.
- The frequency of use.
- The routes of administration (Table 2) as route of administration has influence on the pharmocokinetics and thus on the detectability in the body fluids.
- The absorption, distribution, metabolism, and elimination of drugs.
- The drug interactions.
- The knowledge of clinical pharmacology and toxicology are also essential for understanding, selection, maintenance of assay procedures, with adequate detection limits and accuracy, as well as the estimation of drugs detectability duration after its use.
- Interindividual variations, e.g., 100 mg phenobarbital per liter in serum is a concentration compatible with coma. However, it may be a therapeutic concentration for an epileptic patient. Morphine concentrations in pain relief can be different from the expected values in cancer patients.[2] This stresses the importance of the case history.
- Tolerance and cross-tolerance, e.g., a 100 mg methadone dose for an addict may have no effect at all, but a normal individual may be killed. It is also known that prolonged exposure to one drug may predispose a tolerance to high doses of another similar drug or other similar drugs. Recently, an interesting case of cocaine tolerance has been published.[3]
- Individual idiosyncracy (due to genetic factors) may explain hypo- or hyperreactions in some instances.

Knowledgeable drug abusers may exploit the pharmacokinetic behavior of certain drugs, e.g., bicarbonate in-

TABLE 1
Purposes for Drugs of Abuse Testing

Samples from   **Samples to be analyzed**

Acute intoxications

Intensive Care Unit patients   Urine for screening
Blood (serum or plasma) for quantitative assays, if available

"Drug free" proof

Drug addict treatment institutions   Urine only
Prisons
Work places
Court cases (compulsory "clean-proof")

Impairment estimations

Crime scenes   Urine for screening
Driving under the influence (DUI cases)   Blood for quantitative assays
Work places (job performance)

---

gestion to increase the time of excretion of amphetamines and decrease their concentration in urine.

As most drugs are distributed to the site of action (brain) by blood, drug concentration in this body fluid provides the best information as to the potential effect on behavior, such as driving impairment or on psychological high. However, due to wide individual variations in the pharmacokinetics and pharmacodynamics, the use of plasma drug concentration for the estimation of impairment has not been established for most drugs. Only for very few drugs is sufficient data available.[4]

III. IF THE RESULT IS POSITIVE?

The following questions must be asked.

- Is it a real (confirmed) positive finding?
- Is the subject using the identified drug chronically or intermittently?
- Is she or he an addict?
- Was it a prescribed drug?
- Was she or he under the influence of a drug when the urine specimen was collected?
- Was she or he a passive smoker of cannabis?
- Was the morphine from poppy seed food?

Some of these questions may be answered through a confidential interview.

IV. IF THE RESULT IS NEGATIVE?

It may be as follows:

- The subject never used drugs.
- She or he stopped long enough before colleting the urine specimen.
- The specimen was diluted or altered.
- The drug was not detected.
- The dose was not high enough to be detectable.
- The specimen was substituted.
- Skill and training of laboratory technicians is not high enough.
- The analytical method has not an adequate detection limit or is inappropriate.

V. SOURCES OF ERROR IN TESTING URINE SPECIMENS FOR DRUGS OF ABUSE

The following may cause error in testing uring specimens for drugs of abuse:

- Substitution of urine by apple juice or beer or from a nondrug-using individual. (Advertising for lyophilized drug free urine from Texas!)[5]
- Adulterants:
  - Some are well known[6]

TABLE 2
Major Route of Drug Administration

Intravascular administration (heroin, cocaine, methamphetamine)
  Bolus injection
    Infusion
Extravascular Administration
  Smoking (cannabis, cocaine, phencyclidine)
  Inhalation (heroin, cocaine, solvents)
    Variable absorption
    Rapid rate to "high"
  Intranasal (cocaine)
    Quick absorption
  Oral Ingestion (LSD, MDMA, mescaline, etc)
    Sometimes incomplete absorption
    Degradation
    Food interactions
    First-pass metabolism

- Sodium hypochlorite[7]
- Interferences in immunoassays
- Unclean containers (old drug bottles)
- Collection or storage errors:
  - Failure to filter cloudy urine
  - Storage at room temperature (less than 25°C) for more than 4 days or refrigerator for more than 7 days
  - Exposure to strong light for LSD
  - Insufficient quality control
  - Contamination or carry-over
  - Faulty transcription

VI. MEDICAL INTERPRETATION

The medical interpretation of toxicological findings by a physician familiar with clinical toxicology is more orientated to patients personal data, as follows:

- Existing pathology, e.g., renal diseases or liver injury
- Genetic factors, like lack of enzymes
- Age
- State of tolerance
- Interactions with other (prescription) drugs
- Patient in metatoxic phase: drug used but already excreted
- Paratoxic situations, like heat or cold, which can influence the toxicity of drugs

VII. REPORTING OF RESULTS

When reporting the results of toxicological findings the investigator should

- Give all test results, e.g., screening tests and confirmation tests. (Quality assurance data must be reviewed before certifying that a test result is accurate.)
- Indicate in the report the drugs or/and metabolites tested whether positive or negative, as well as the detection limits and the cutoff levels for each drug or metabolite.
- Store all records at least for 2 years at a safe place.
- Compare quantitative tissue concentrations only to literature values which were generated by comparable analytical methodology and used for interpretations under similar conditions.[8,9]
- The results should be reported in an unambiguous way, e.g., in avoiding misinterpretation like expressing the results in nanograms per milliliter instead of nanograms per milligrams creatinine in the case of THC-carboxylic acid.[10]
- As long as drugs are used in mass quantities, the results should be expressed in mass units and not in molar units.[11,12]

VIII. FUTURE DEVELOPMENTS

It may well be that in the future, specimens other than urine for screening could be used, like saliva[13] or hair.[14] But for the moment, however, the data available are incomplete to be used for routine purposes.

IX. INTERNATIONAL STANDARDIZATION

It will be very difficult to find an international consensus for interpreting and reporting test results in this field. So at least, I would like to suggest some minimum requirements for testing as follows:

- Efforts should be focused on the most commonly abused drugs, like heroin and cocaine (bearing in mind all the other possibilities), and maybe amphetamine and methamphetamine. It is quite clear, after many discussions with colleagues from other European countries, that including THC-carboxylic acid in the screening procedures will not be accepted, as the legal situations are somewhat different from one country to another.
- Reporting should be done in mass units with full description of methods' performance, as previously described.
- Reporting should be done with explanations and warnings in cases of confusing origin of codeine and morphine, for instance, or that opiate immunoassays only cover morphinane-like structures by cross-reactivity, etc.

X. CONCLUSIONS

The toxicologist must have some concern with the scope of testing and should not express his results in a one-sheet "form" expert's report. He must know what is done with the results, because there is a big difference between a false positive acetone finding in a patient's urine for a physician and a false positive PCP in urine for a person's employer. A physician never bases his diagnosis only on a single laboratory test.[15] Toxicologists must be careful that there is a reasonable use of the tests made and make use of their normal common sense and not to sponsor a "big brother is watching you" situation by their knowledge. So let us not forget that drug of abuse testing is not only a technical and a business feature, but also a big intrusion in a human's individual privacy.

REFERENCES

1. **Substance-Abuse Testing Committee,** Report of the Substance-Abuse Testing Committee, Critical issues in urinalysis of abused substances, *Clin. Chem.*, 34, 605–632, 1988.
2. **Hassan, F. M., Pesce, A. J., Warner, A., and Denson, D. D.,** Morphine monitoring for an anaesthesic pain service, *Clin. Chem.*, 35, 1182, 1989.
3. **Howell, S. L. and Ezell, A. L.,** An example of cocaine tolerance in gunshot wound fatality, *J. Anal.Toxicol.*, 14, 60–61, 1990.
4. **Barnett, G. and Willette, R. E.,** Feasibility of chemical testing for drug-impaired performance, in *Advances in Analytical Toxicology*, Vol. 2, Baselt, R.C., Ed., Year Book Medical Publishers, Chicago, 1989, 218–250.
5. **Anon.,** *Actuel-Magazine*, January 1990, 15.
6. **Mikkelsen, S. L. and Owen Ash, K.,** Adulterants causing false negatives in illicit drug testing, *Clin.Chem.*, 34, 2333–2336, 1988.
7. **Wennig, R.,** Personal experience, 1988.
8. **Baselt, R. C.,** *Disposition of Toxic Drugs and Chemicals in Man*, Biomedical Publications, Davis, CA, 1982.
9. **Curry, A. S., Ed.,** *Analytical Methods in Human Toxicology*, Part 1, Verlag Chemie, Weinheim, 1985, 54–61.
10. **Manno, J. E.,** Interpretation of urinalysis results, in *Urine Testing for Drugs of Abuse*, Hawks, R.L. and Chiang, C.N., Eds., NIDA Monograph, 73, 1986, 59.
11. **Uges, D. R. A.,** Establishment and interpretation of therapeutic and toxic serum concentrations, in *DFG-Rundgespräche und Kolloquien, Klinisch-Toxikologische Analytik bei Akuten Vergiftungen und Drogenmissbrauch*, 1989.
12. **Prescott, L. F., Widdop, B., Vale, J. A., Griffin, J. P., Proutfoot, A. T., Volans, G. N., Whiting, B., and Wells, F. O.,** Who needs molar units for drugs?, *Lancet*, May 16, 1127–1129, 1987.
13. **Cone, E. J. and Weddington, W. W., Jr.,** Prolonged occurence of cocaine in human saliva and urine after chronic use, *J. Anal. Toxicol.*, 13, 65–68, 1989.
14. **Cone, E. J.,** Testing human hair for drugs of abuse, *J. Anal. Toxicol.*, 14, 1–7, 1990.
15. **Caplan, Y. H.,** Drug testing in urine, *J. Forensic. Sci.*, 34, 1417–1421, 1989.

Chapter 30

INTERPRETATION OF RESULTS OF URINE DRUG TESTING IN CLINICAL PRACTICE

L. San

TABLE OF CONTENTS

Summary 200

I. Introduction 200
    A. Diagnostic Confirmation of Acute Intoxication and/or Dependence 200
    B. Test of Reliability of the Information Provided by the Patient 200
    C. Monitoring Changes in Drug Consumption Patterns Among Patients Seeking Treatment 201
    D. To Assess Patient's Compliance With Therapeutic Regimens 201
        1. Antagonist Maintenance Programs 201
        2. Methadone Maintenance Programs 202
    E. To Monitor Drug Consumption During Detoxification Treatment 203
    F. Follow-Up of Patients Enrolled in Therapeutic Programs 205
    G. Promote Contact between Patients and Health Workers at Treatment Centers in Outpatient Treatment Programs 205

III. Health Care Repercussions 205
    A. Impact of the Most Frequent Errors 206
        1. False Positives 206
        2. False Negatives 206
        3. Voluntary Fraud 207

Acknowledgments 207

References 207

SUMMARY

In clinical practice, urine screening tests are carried out for different reasons.

1. To confirm the diagnosis in cases of acute intoxication and/or doubtful dependence
2. As a test of reliability of the information provided by the patient
3. To monitor changes in drug consumption patterns in patients seeking treatment
4. To assess patient's compliance with therapeutic regimens established (essential in, for example, methadone or naltrexone maintenance programs)
5. To monitor drug consumption during detoxification therapy
6. In the follow-up of patients enrolled in therapeutic programs
7. To keep patients on outpatient treatment in close contact with health workers in treatment centers

Urine drug testing has also been shown to have a dissuasive effect on drug consumption and to influence acceptance/rejection reactions in both patients and health workers engaged in urine testing. Finally, a study of the impact that false negative or false positive results and voluntary fraud have on clinical practice would appear to be necessary.

I. INTRODUCTION

Urine drug testing is not a new technique. It has been used in methadone maintenance programs since their inception in the mid-1960s. Although testing techniques have improved over the past 20 years, limitations in their use, accuracy, and the interpretation of results do, however, still exist. The issue of testing people for substance abuse via urine drug screening as a means to combating drug abuse in society is increasingly a subject of debate.[1]

Drug testing is no longer limited to health care centers, but has become a means for controlling substance abuse in several sectors, such as schools, the work place, and the army. This has provoked discussion about these kinds of tests as to whether or not they violate the rights of the individual.

Drug testing is not a new approach to monitoring subjects suspected of being drug abusers, and it is certainly not a panacea for the epidemics of drug abuse today.

Opinion is divided as to where, why, and who should carry out the tests. Most people think that the police should conduct tests in cases of reasonable doubt, but only a minority would accept employers instituting pre-employment or in-service drug screening programs.

From the clinical practice point of view, close cooperation between detoxification centers and laboratories is needed to improve the reliability of analytical results; those who are responsible for providing clinicians with tests results must do everything in their power to ensure that the results obtained are absolutely reliable.

A. DIAGNOSTIC CONFIRMATION OF ACUTE INTOXICATION AND/OR DEPENDENCE

Positive screening results for a given drug do not necessarily indicate that the subject is addicted to or dependent upon the drug; it merely indicates that the drug in question is present in the urine sample tested.

In cases of acute intoxication of known etiology, laboratory results confirm the presence or absence of the drug being tested and confirm the anamnesis and clinical symptoms presented by the subject. In cases of intoxication of unknown etiology, laboratory analysis is essential. The symptoms the patients present are of greatest importance in helping to determine which drugs are the most likely to be causing the condition. Here it is vital that a good working relationship exists between clinicians and analysts. In cases where symptoms are not clearly defined, screening should begin with the drugs most frequently consumed according to epidemiological data available at the time.

The presence of a drug in urine can also confirm certain diagnostic criteria in doubtful cases.[2] The most commonly used diagnostic criteria are DSM-III-R.[3] These do not require urine drug testing because diagnosis is established on the basis of dependent behavior.

B. TEST OF REALIABILITY OF THE INFORMATION PROVIDED BY THE PATIENT

Occasionally, urine tests have been used to confirm the veracity or reliability of information previously provided by the patient. Thus we have recently conducted a study to determine the presence of drugs in urine in a group of heroin abusers undergoing detoxification treatment.[4] The group was asked about their previous consumption of buprenorphine (Table 1). Only buprenorphine was investigated because many patients know that this drug cannot be detected in routine analysis conducted at detoxification centers. Some discrepancies might therefore be expected between information provided by patients and test results.

TABLE 1
Results of Questioning on Previous Consumption of Buprenorphine and Positivity of Urine Tests

Positivity (%)	MMP[a] (no. 134)	AMP[b] (no. 21)	DFP[c] (no. 33)	Total (no. 188)
According to the patient	4.5	0	6.1	4.2
According to urine test	5.4	0	12.1	6.7

[a] MMP: methadone maintenance program.
[b] AMP: antagonist maintenance program.
[c] DFP: drug-free program.

When patients were asked to say what they thought the results of tests for buprenorphine would be, 4.1% said they thought they would be positive. This figure was similar to the actual result of 6.7% (prevalence point). In the antagonist maintenance program group, no positive results were observed. This coincided with information given by patients. Previous consumption of buprenorphine was lowest in the drug-free program group, whereas the proportion of positive test results was the highest (Table 1).

C. MONITORING CHANGES IN DRUG CONSUMPTION PATTERNS AMONG PATIENTS SEEKING TREATMENT

During recent years, marked changes in the pattern of prescribing of psychotropic drugs and the availability of illicit drugs, particularly heroin and cocaine, have occurred. It has been suggested that a close relationship exists between the availability of drugs and drugs used in overdosing.[5]

A follow-up of the records of admissions to emergency wards of general hospitals[6] is a useful tool for obtaining information about the characteristics of consumption and abuse of licit and illicit drugs, as well as constituting a sensitive and early indicator of new consumption profiles amongst the general population.[7]

Between January and May 1990, systematic drug screening tests were carried out on all patients seeking treatment for the first time in an attempt to monitor the different drugs being consumed by patients at the time of seeking treatment. Figure 1 shows the results obtained for a series of drugs. Most subjects were heroin addicts, although heroin was found in only 65.3% of the samples tested. This was because many patients had already undergone detoxification treatments with methadone, dextropropoxyphene, or buprenorphine. The presence of these drugs was detected. The high frequency of positive results to cannabis is particularly striking and is probably related to its frequent consumption among drug addicts, as well as the fact that it takes several days for the substance to be eliminated through the urine. The large number of urine samples that test positive to amphetamines was also striking since none of the patients interviewed admitted dependence on or abuse of amphetamines; a fact that prompts us to suspect their possible use as adulterating agents.

D. TO ASSESS PATIENT'S COMPLIANCE WITH THERAPEUTIC REGIMENS

This point is of particular importance when the correct compliance with pharmacologic treatment directly influences the outcome of therapy, such as methadone maintenance programs and antagonist maintenance programs. The intake of disulfiram or calcium cyanamide in the treatment of alcoholism would be another interesting modality in such a way that incorrect intake of medication does not constitute a bias factor in the results obtained.

1. Antagonist Maintenance Programs

We present some results from a controlled, double-blind clinical trial comparing the efficacy of treatment with naltrexone and with placebo in a group of 50 heroin addicts on an outpatient and inpatient basis.[8]

After detoxification treatment, patients began naltrexone induction on an inpatient basis. They then left the hospital, returning daily for 1 week to the outpatients department for a 50 mg/day dose of naltrexone (days 4 to 7). From week 2 to week 4, patients attending the department received a single dose of 100 mg on Monday, 100 mg on Wednesday, and 150 mg on Friday. From

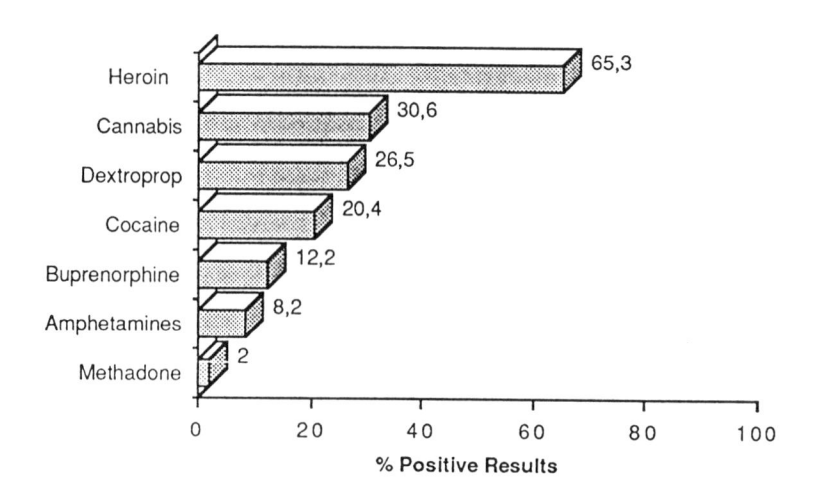

FIGURE 1. Results of urine testing for a series of drugs. Percentage of positive results.

Drug	% Positive Results
Heroin	65,3
Cannabis	30,6
Dextroprop	26,5
Cocaine	20,4
Buprenorphine	12,2
Amphetamines	8,2
Methadone	2

month 2 on, patients were randomly assigned to treatment with naltrexone or placebo. Treatment was administered in a double-blind fashion and vitamin B_2 (15 mg) was added to the capsules as a urine marker to check compliance. To preserve additionally the double-blind nature of the trial, quinine (10 μg) was added to placebo capsules to ensure that organoleptic characteristics of both types of capsules were the same. The total period of treatment was 6 months (6 months of active substance for the naltrexone group, and 1 month of active substance plus 5 months on placebo for the placebo group). During this period of time, urine samples were obtained three times per week in order to check the consumption of opiates, cocaine, and cannabis, as well to monitor compliance with treatment. After pharmacologic treatment, outpatient clinical control was continued for 6 months.

To evaluate the overall efficacy of treatment, four criteria were combined: degree of treatment acceptance, percentage of relapse in heroin consumption, presence of untoward effects, and overall rate of treatment retention.

Treatment was considered to have been successful if patients had regularly taken medication over a period of 6 months, had attended all scheduled appointments from the start of naltrexone induction, and had presented no untoward effects or symptoms of toxicity which would have necessitated the discontinuation of treatment. Treatment was considered a failure when at least one of the aforementioned conditions was not fulfilled.

In this study, all patients followed the same treatment program as far as frequency of visits, dosage and compliance evaluation, blood and urine tests, etc. were concerned. Of the 50 patients included in the study, 28 were randomly assigned to the naltrexone group and 22 to the placebo group.

When comparing both treatment groups, a higher success rate and a lower rate of failures and dropouts were recorded in the placebo group. Retention rates at 6 months of treatment were 17.4% in the naltrexone group and 40% in the placebo group. Although differences between both groups were clinically important, they were not statistically significant (Figure 2).

The conclusions drawn from this comparative study of naltrexone vs. placebo were verified by confirming compliance with the therapeutic regimens established by measuring B_2 in urine (Table 2).

2. Methadone Maintenance Programs

In Spain, where implementation of methadone maintenance programs is still recent, we have found no studies evaluating the degree of compliance with pharmacologic treatment. Only one study exists on urine screening tests, carried out on patients on methadone maintenance programs in Asturias, in which the presence of methadone in urine was tested.[9] Tests were carried out on 331 patients in 1987 and 329 patients in 1988 to determine the presence of opiate in urine, and only in those cases in which consumption of other drugs was suspected were other tests conducted. As far as the presence of methadone in urine was concerned, it should be noted that of 946 tests performed, 276 (29.2%) were negative and, of these, only 60% could be attributed to the consumption of placebo or to tests being carried out before methadone was taken under supervision at the outpatients department.

In our study on urine tests in patients undergoing

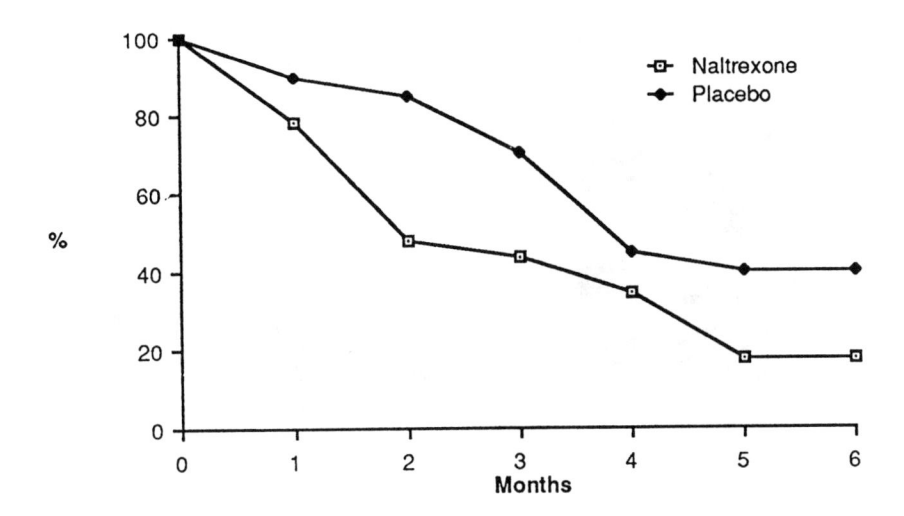

FIGURE 2. Retention rates at 6 months of treatment (17.4 vs. 20%).

TABLE 2
Compliance With the Therapeutic Regimens
(Naltrexone Vs. Placebo)

	Naltrexone group (no. 28)	Placebo group (no. 22)
Average of urine tests to assess compliance	3.9	5.0
% Correct compliance	94.4	82.2

detoxification treatment with methadone, most of the patients studied showed good compliance with methadone treatment.[4]

E. TO MONITOR DRUG CONSUMPTION DURING DETOXIFICATION TREATMENT

To ascertain the prevalence of drug consumption in a group of addicts undergoing detoxification treatment, a study was conducted on heroin addicts fulfilling DSM-III-R criteria[3] and undergoing different types of outpatient treatment: methadone maintenance programs (MMP), antagonists (naltrexone) maintenance programs (AMP), and drug-free programs (DFP). Patients were selected during one randomly chosen week in June 1988. Patients on MMP came from the only methadone dispensing unit in the city where patients were given daily doses of methadone. Patients on AMP and DFP came from the outpatients department of the Hospital del Mar in Barcelona.

The study was therefore a cross-sectional study comprising the total number of patients taking part that week in the MMP in Barcelona or reporting to the outpatients department of Hospital del Mar for follow-up visits. A total of 188 patients were included in the study: 134 in MMP, 21 in AMP, and 33 in DFP. A data collection questionnaire was administered to each patient before urine samples were obtained to check buprenorphine and other drugs consumption. All patients gave their informed consent.

Urine samples were analyzed by enzyme-multiplied immunoassay tests (Syva Co., Palo Alto, CA) to detect the presence of opiates (heroin), cocaine, methadone dextropropoxyphene, cannabis, and benzodiazepines, and radioimmunoassay (Diagnostic Products Corporation, Los Angeles, CA) to detect buprenorphine. Samples were processed at all times in accordance with protocols described for each technique by manufacturers. An index of positivity to drug consumption was drawn up by dividing the sum of the percentages of positivity for each drug by the six drugs under study.

Of the total number of patients, 65.9% said they had consumed buprenorphine at some time (prevalence period). The difference between the MMP group and the

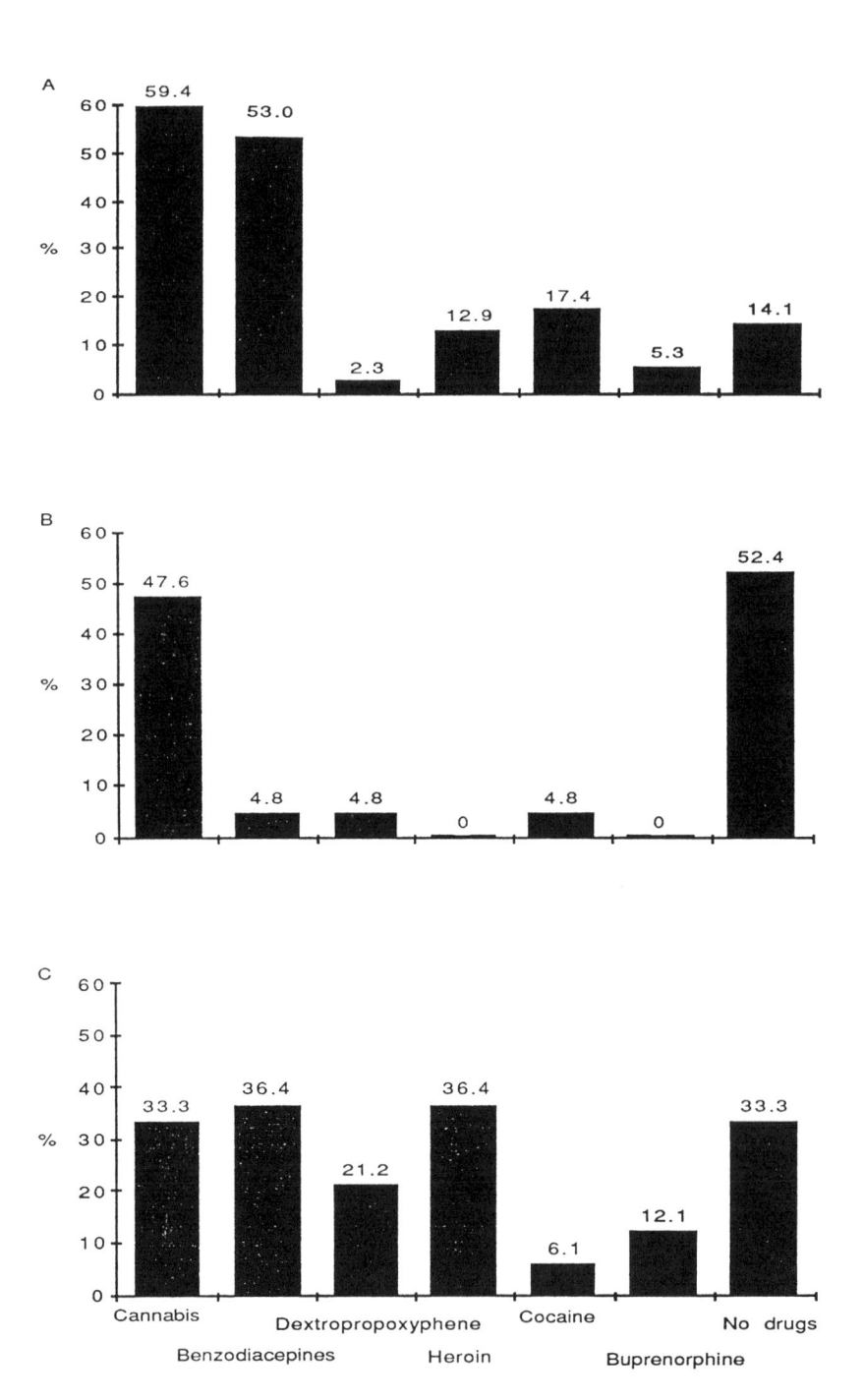

FIGURE 3. Results of urine tests for the three groups (A — mehtadone maintenance program; B — antagonist maintenance program; C — drug-free program).

remaining two groups was statistically significant ($p < 0.05$ in both cases). The overall results of urine tests for the three groups are shown in Figure 3. In the MMP group, results were positive to cannabis, benzodiazepines, cocaine, and buprenorphine. In the AMP group, positive results were obtained for cannabis, benzodiazepines, dextropropoxyphene, and cocaine, while negative results were obtained for heroin or buprenorphine. In the DFP group, results were positive to cannabis, benzodiazepines, dextropropoxyphene, heroin, cocaine, and buprenorphine. The most statistically significant differences for cannabis derivatives were found between the MMP and DFP groups;

for benzodiazepines between the MMP and AMP groups and the AMP and DFP groups; for dextropropoxyphene between the MMP and DFP groups; and for heroin between the AMP and DFP groups and between the DFP and MMP groups ($p < 0.05$ in all cases). No statistically significant differences were found for cocaine and buprenorphine between the three groups. Overall, the group presenting the lowest index of positivity in urine tests was the AMP group (10.3%) compared with the DFP group (24.2%) and the MMP group (25.1%). The average number of substances consumed by each group were MMP, 1.48; AMP, 0.62; and DFP, 1.45.

Prescription of benzodiazepines was also investigated in this group, and 52.6% of patients were found to be taken this substance on prescription. The average period of abstinence in heroin consumption was 4.5 months, excluding patients in MMP group. In the latter group, the average daily dose of methadone was 51.7 mg and the average period of maintenance treatment was 4.8 months.

The frequent consumption of cannabis derivatives and benzodiazepines in the three groups is particularly striking, although half of the patients said they took benzodiazepines under medical prescription. Overall, the largest groups of polydrug users were MMP and DFP groups. Patients in the AMP group did not consume as much cannabis, benzodiazepines, dextropropoxyphene, heroin, cocaine, and buprenorphine.

F. FOLLOW-UP OF PATIENTS ENROLLED IN THERAPEUTIC PROGRAMS

Few studies on the follow-up and assessment of success of treatment have been carried out on drug addicts in Spain. The only multicenter study carried out was the EMETYST project.[10] The study described a group of addicts who sought detoxification treatment, studied their subsequent time-course with respect to drug consumption, psychological status, productive activities, and other legal aspects. Its aim was to determine the efficacy of treatment, as well as attempt to identify prognostic factors.

The consumption of heroin, cocaine, traquilizers, cannabis, alcohol, and tobacco was studied over a period of 24 months. There was no statistically significant decrease in the consumption of cocaine, alcohol, and tobacco. Consumption of heroin, cannabis, and tranquilizers decreased at 6 months and stabilized at 12 and 24 months. Forty-two (32%) patients did not consume drugs for over 18 months.

Perhaps a drawback of urine tests in this kind of study is that no distinction can be made between drug consumption and drug dependence.

G. PROMOTE CONTACT BETWEEN PATIENTS AND HEALTH WORKERS AT TREATMENT CENTERS IN OUTPATIENT TREATMENT PROGRAMS

In certain instances, urine testing is used to keep patients and health workers in contact with each other. This is the situation in outpatient detoxification programs where patients receive treatment each time they go to the treatment center for drug testing and the assessment of the success of treatment. Clinicians are able to closely supervise the course of abstinence, as well as ensure compliance with therapeutic regimens.

When patients have completed detoxification treatment, urine testing three times a week helps maintain close contact with patients, so that if patients consume drugs, clinicians can intervene almost immediately and, if necessary, modify the treatment programs. Urine testing is carried out by nursing staff who can provide patients with information and develop health education programs specifically directed to the addict population (transmissible diseases, hepatitis B prophylaxis, tuberculosis, etc.).

II. HEALTH CARE REPERCUSSIONS

The interpretation of results at the health care level can have important repercussions and in most cases, it may well imply the discontinuation of treatment programs followed by the patient. This occurs when a patient is tested positive during inpatient detoxification or at the time of residential treatment programs (therapeutic community). In other cases, positive testing means that ongoing maintenance programs should be modified. This is why analytical results must be highly accurate and reliable since errors may lead to the discontinuation of treatment to the detriment of patients who might not have broken any of the rules relating to drug consumption during treatment.

Patients often say that urine testing has a dissuasive effect on drug consumption because, when systematic controls are carried out, any potential consumption can be immediately detected. Thus, treatment centers frequently systematically collect urine samples, but not all samples obtained are processed. For example, in hospital detoxification units, urine samples are collected daily (in the presence of nursing staff), but only samples from days 1, 5, and 12 after admission are analyzed and at any other time if patients are suspected of consuming drugs while in the hospital. When a patient presents a positive result, a retrospective analysis of urine samples is carried out to determine the possible day on which consumption most likely took place and this is contrasted with any note on the nursing records.

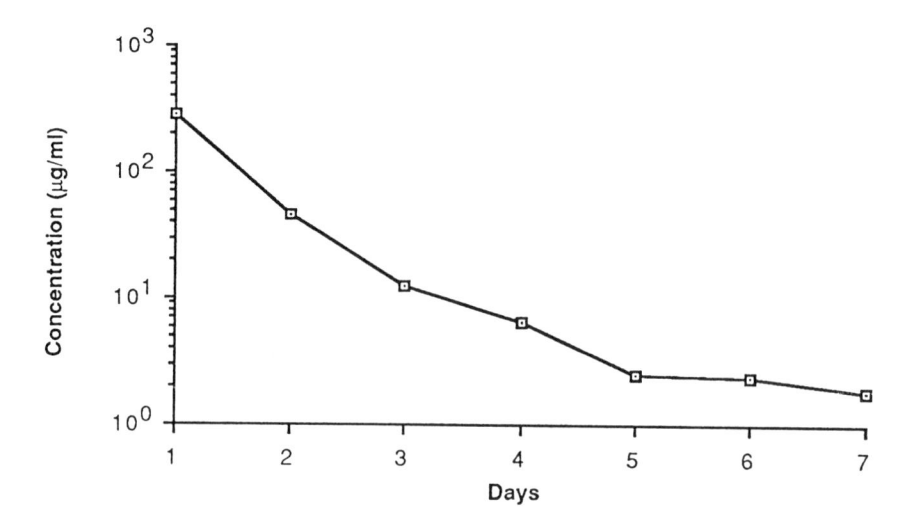

FIGURE 4. Decrease in opiate urine concentrations during hospitalization from day 1 to day 7.

One of the advantages of urine tests in the follow-up of patients is the rapid detection of any kind of drug consumption. This allows treatment programs to be modified.

The distrust of analytical results shown by clinicians must be overcome. It is not uncommon to find health care workers questioning laboratory results, preferring to believe the information provided by patients instead of laboratory results with reference to possible drug consumption. This often occurs when results are positive, as the efficacy of clinicians' professional activity may be questioned since positive testing may be regarded as a failure to achieve abstinence.

A. IMPACT OF THE MOST FREQUENT ERRORS

1. False positives

A false positive is a negative result reported as a positive one. It is known that certain drugs may give false positive results while others tend to accumulate (diazepam) although consumption has been discontinued.

As an example of a false positive result we report the case of a 25-year-old woman admitted to our unit for detoxification treatment for codeine dependence. On day 1, the patient underwent a routine search for codeine tablets and regular urine tests were carried out by enzyme immunoassay. The patient presented positive results during the first 7 days of detoxification. It was decided to discharge the patient because of the suspicion of heroin or codeine consumption while in the hospital. Subsequently, a quantitative analysis was carried out because of the reiterated denial of the patient. Urine specimens were anlyzed by fluorescence immunoassay (Opiates TDx® System, Abbott) and the results were the following: day 1, 280.9 µg/ml; day 2, 45.2 µg/ml; day 3, 12.4 µg/ml; day 4, 6.6 µg/ml; day 5, 2.5 µg/ml; day 6, 2.4 µg/ml; and day 7, 1.9 µg/ml.

The concentration of opiates in urine decreased from day 1 and there were no peaks indicating opiate consumption during that period. Figure 4 shows the decrease in opiate urine concentrations during hospitalization. Using gas chromatography/mass spectrometry, the presence of codeine was confirmed in all samples analyzed, as well the presence of morphine in samples from days 1, 2, 4, 5, and 6. As the patient was not a heroin consumer, it was considered that the morphine detected was a metabolic product of codeine.

The high concentration of opiates on day 1 after admission indicated a high tolerance to the substance when compared with data on acute intoxications in which lethal dose varies between 29.1 and 229 mg/kg. From initial data, it was decided that the patient might have consumed codeine tablets, but, subsequently, it was confirmed that this was not true. This kind of error must be avoided so that confirmation by different techniques is mandatory.[11]

2. False negatives

A false negative result occurs when consumption is not detected in urine tests. Generally, this situation has no direct clinical repercussions. However, its importance stems from the fact that patients learn that by consuming certain substances in certain ways that are not detected in routine analysis. This is the case when testing for buprenorphine in those centers with drug-free programs where health care workers have their doubts about whether patients are really off drugs. This kind of error can lead to the persistence of drug consumption and relapses are subsequently confirmed.

3. Voluntary fraud

It sounds too basic to mention, but it is extremely important that the urine to be tested is obtained from the subject being studied; in other words, that the urine sample is a certified specimen. It is not uncommon for patients attending centers for urine testing to bring specimens voided by family members, friends, or neighbors who are expected to live drug-free. No patient actively consuming drugs will bring a urine specimen for screening without some attempt to conceal drug use if he/she is aware of the serious consequences to be derived from it.[1]

ACKNOWLEDGMENTS

Acknowledgment is given to Marta Pulido, M.D., for editorial assistance, supported in part by the Institut Municipal d'Investigació Mèdica, Barcelona.

REFERENCES

1. **Dougherty, R. J.,** Controversies regarding urine testing, *J. Subst. Abuse. Treat.*, 458, 115–117, 1987.
2. **Gavin, D. R., Ross, H. E., and Skinner, H. A.,** Diagnostic validity of the drug abuse screening test in the assessment of DSM-III drug disorders, *Br. J. Addiction*, 84, 301–307, 1989.
3. **American Psychiatric Association,** *Diagnostic and Statistical Manual of Mental Disorders*, 3rd ed. (revised), APA, Washington, D.C., 1987.
4. **San, L., Tremoleda, J., Ollé, J. M., Porta Serra, M., and de la Torre, R.,** Prevalencia del consumo de buprenorfina en heroinómanos en tratamiento, *Med. Clin. (Barc.)*, 93, 645–648, 1989.
5. **Gohdse, A. H., Stapleton, J., Edwards, G., and Edeh, J.,** Monitoring changing patterns of drug dependence in accident and emergency departments, *Drug Alcohol Depend.*, 19, 265–269, 1987.
6. **Cohen, S.,** Narcotism, dimensions of the problem, *Ann. N.Y. Acad. Sci.*, 31158, 4–9, 1978.
7. **Camí, J., Alvárez, F., Monteis, J., Caus, J., Menoyo, E., and de Torres, S.,** Heroína, nueva causa de urgencias toxicológicas, *Med. Clin. (Barc.)*, 82, 1–4, 1984.
8. **San, L., Pomarol, G., Peri, J. M., Ollé, J. M., and Camí, J. M.,** Follow-up after six month maintenance on naltrexone versus placebo in heroin addicts, *Br. J. Addiction*, in press, 1990.
9. **Cabeza, J. M., Martín, M. A., Díaz, I., and Rodríguez, J. J.,** Estudio analítico del consumo de drogas en los centros de desintoxicación con metadona en el Principado de Asturias, *Rev. Toxicol.*, 6, 243–254, 1989.
10. **Sánchez-Carbonell, J., Brigós, B., and Camí, J.,** Evolución de una muestra de heroinómanos dos años después del inicio del tratamiento (proyecto EMETYST), *Med. Clin. (Barc.)*, 92, 135–139, 1989.
11. **Segura, J., de la Torre, R., Botet, C. R., Congost, M., Ventura, R., and Camí, J.,** Análisis de drogas de abuso, problemática asociada y control de calidad, *Comunidad y Drogas*, 11, 11–28, 1989.

Chapter 31

DISCUSSION ON THE INTERPRETATION OF RESULTS

Vereby: Two brief questions. One is that in drug metabolism it is believed that glucoronidation makes a compound more polar and therefore it is more easily excreted. Do you have any data on the partition coefficient of morphine-6-glucoronide?

Moore: I can tell you that I don't have the exact figure in my head, but the 6-glucoronide is very much like the 3-glucoronide, and it is not particularly lipophilic and acts in all systems that have been tested in as a very polar compound.

Vereby: The other thing — it was an outline on buprenorphine and I am very interested in that compound. I am very surprised to know it is abused because it is known to be an agonist/antagonist, and it would probably precipitate withdrawal. I am wondering what you think about it.

Moore: I spent a lot of time in the late seventies and early eighties developing assays for buprenorphine because in a previous existence in a hospital I was responsible for a lot of pharmacokinetics of buprenorphine. When looking to the pharmacological literature, all people say "yes". This is a partial agonist and it should produce an abstinence syndrome, and I think in all the time we used it we didn't actually see an abstinence syndrome produced by the use of buprenorphine together with large concentrations of methadone. However, as always, there is more in the literature that you are able to read. So, I went back to when I heard about some of the abuse that was taking place with buprenorphine, because as you, I was very sceptical. I read Nancy Melo's paper on it, and I also read Don Jazinski's paper on it, which are actually used frequently to suggest that buprenorphine is nonaddicting. And you will see phrases like (they are talking about heroin ex-abusers) buprenorphine could not be distinguished from heroin by these abusers. There is one particular case where they were given, I think, 8 mg of oral buprenorphine to heroin addicts and they produced a 50 or 70% fault in the amount of heroin that they were taking in the day and this represented a reduction of 300 or 400 mg reduction of heroin per day. And this was with buprenorphine given orally, which is not particularly a good route of administration for that drug. That is quite phenomenal. So, yes, I think we are all slightly misled and that may be why buprenorphine, which was an uncontrolled substance, is now controlled in many countries.

Cook: Just a comment on Dr. de la Torre's talk in the area of phencyclidine on metabolism. We did some studies some years ago where we measured the half-life of phencyclidine in several subjects and I believe that in two over sixteen subjects, we observed half-lives that were twice as long as the average subject. Unfortunately, we where not able to follow these studies in terms to link that fact to debrisoquine oxidation. But, I think it points out that there may be some other examples of drugs of abuse where perhaps there are genetic differences in people and we should be in the look out further.

Van Rossum: If we take into account the cutoff limits for individuals with a rapid metabolism in regards to those with a slow metabolism, is it just bad for them?

de la Torre: To our knowledge there is no drug like morphine or THC where the influence of genetics is significative. Codeine and the examples given are interesting for the interpretation of results but not in fact a drug of abuse. Diazepam and other benzodiazepines are in the border in much drug testing programs between their consideration as a therapeutic drug or drugs of abuse to be controlled. There is no significative drug where the influence of genetics is strong enough to influence cutoff limits of immunological techniques.

Baselt: We must be very careful in assigning any obvious differences in the rate of elimination strictly to genetics. There has been very few studies on pH dependence on codeine, morphine, even cocaine, and very limited studies on PCP. We work with subjects in which we do not routinely control their urinary pH. That is something that you may keep in mind as a possible contribution of variability.

Vereby: We are talking about individual differences in drug disposition and urinary drug testing in considering one single spot urine specimen, and what are the chances to be positive or negative. We have done a study with benzodiazepines. I'm not sure if Dr. Baselt is right in the hypothesis, but we had a very heavy fellow weighting 90 kg and another 60 kg and we gave a dose of 10 mg of diazepam for five days and nights. The EMIT cutoff that we set was 300 ng/ml and we did gas chromotographic studies with metabolites like nordiazepam and oxazepam. The heavy fellow was negative for benzodiazepams for three days under these conditions. The very light fellow was positive for the first day and a half. On the other hand, the heavier was negative by the seventh day; the other fellow was positive for about twelve days.

Baselt: We have some examples with cocaine and obesity in dermal studies of dermal absorption. When you apply cocaine base to the skin of relatively heavy individuals you can see very little excretion of benzoylecgonine in the urine. If you take thin individuals, they can excrete relatively high levels. Whether it has to be with absorption, distribution of transport across membranes, I don't know. There is definitely a difference.

Szendrey: How do you interpret the high level prevalence of THC consumption in your Spanish population of drug addicts and which is your experience with methadone maintenance programs?

San: In regards to the prevalence of THC consumption in heroin abuser. It is well known in our country (Spain) that THC is used widespread in such population. Often, in heroin abusers, many of them responding well to the treatment, are still consuming THC, because its consideration as a minor drug within such population. In regards to methadone programs in Spain, the situation is changing from 1983 when they started to today with the appearance of the problem of AIDS. Today, new legal rules are making easier the use of methadone and other opiates in treatment centers.

Szendrey: There have been some reports on methylation of morphine to codeine, which is their relevance?

Baselt: Just some comments on the metabolism of codeine to morphine. It has not been conclusively demonstrated that that occurs. Preliminary results suggesting that fact are based on the use of preparations of morphine where codeine is almost always present in pharmaceutical grade as an impurity. If you take highly purifed morphine, nobody has been able to demonstrate such conversion.

Cook: Just a comment on the statement of Dr. Baselt on phencyclidine metabolism. Phencyclidine is metabolized almost in 90% of the administered dose. It is unlikely to expect big variations on the clearance of the drug because changes in urinary pH.

Segura: Just one comment on the cross-reactivity reported on immunologic methods brochures. Usually, the data there has been obtained only with pure substances, but what we find in the urines is the results of metabolism. For instance, after taking diethylpropion (supposed not to cross-react with amphetamines EMIT antibody), a strong reaction is found. This is due to the presence of its metabolic products diethyl-norephedrine, N-ethyl-norephedrine, and so on. The point is that we should look very carefully to these tables and take into account the presence of metabolism and other processes.

Section IV
Aspects for Potential International Harmonization

Chapter 32

QUALITY CONTROL PROGRAMS

Jordi Segura

TABLE OF CONTENTS

I.	Introduction	214
II.	Internal Programs	214
III.	External Programs	215
IV.	Development of Proficiency Testing Programs	216
	A. United States	216
	B. Europe	216
V.	Future Developments	217
References		218

I. INTRODUCTION

The goal of any analytical process is to obtain objective and reliable data in order to make appropriate decisions. In some fields, however, the analytical result is not the major issue. In the domain of clinical biochemistry, for instance, the data for a parameter in a blood analysis is used by the physician, in addition to a set of other clinical data, before the suitable treatment is chosen. The sharp precision of the test result is of less importance because of the existence of normal "ranges" for the general population.

When dealing with drug abuse, we are confronted with a totally different situation. The detection of the drug or its metabolites in urine is usually the most important result in the decision-making process. The radical nature of the result (yes or no; presence or absence) stresses even more the need for reliability; no quantitative results are usually obtained and, if so, no clear relationship with dose, time of ingestion, or blood concentrations may usually be extrapolated.

The potential appearance of errors in any laboratory is, however, a known fact (Figure 1). The origin of such problems may be systematic and will affect all determinations carried out by the same instrument, reagent, methodology, or personnel. The appearance of accidental errors in a given sample or set of samples due to unexpected reasons should also be considered. Obviously any program for the quality of results should try to detect and correct all systematic errors and to minimize the appearance of these other unexpected sources of variations.

II. INTERNAL PROGRAMS

In order to achieve suitable reliability, a series of measures should be implemented to control different steps of the whole process: collection, transport and storage of the sample, allocating and sample preparation, instrument's performance, and results throughput.[1] In related fields such as doping control or animal toxicology, a set of regulations known as Good Laboratory Practices (GLPs) summarizes the expected requirements.[2-4]

A fundamental need is the existence of written Standard Operating Procedures (SOPs), where a complete and detailed description of all the laboratory steps to be followed to analyze a sample are described. The analysts should strictly follow those guidelines, which should have been revised and approved by the director of the laboratory. Some of the steps to be covered by SOPs follow:

- **Sample reception** to include the inspections of the seals and the recording of any additional information about the sample.
- **Internal chain of custody** to record all movements of the sample inside the laboratory, including allocated subsamples and storage.
- **Preliminary assays**, usually immunological methods, including the preparation of reagents, standard and controls. The procedure should assure the inclusion of blank urine(s), spiked urine(s) with drug or metabolites close to the cutoff level, and positive urine(s) for each batch of samples. Written procedures for setup and calibration of the instruments are also needed.
- **Confirmatory assays**, usually chromatography connected to mass spectrometry, including additionally those specific requirements for the specificity of the procedure and, where quantitation is applicable, for the linearity of the response. A basic requirement is a written description about the criteria to report a result as positive.
- **Administrative procedures and release of the results** includes a description of all archiving processes for both samples and results together with how, where, by whom, and to whom the results should be released from the laboratory.

The quality of the results generated by a laboratory is also directly related to the experience and skillfulness of the personnel involved (Figure 2). A written job description is necessary for all people including the director of the laboratory, the certifying scientist (if a different person), the analytical supervisors, and the technicians. A continuous education program at all steps is highly recommended.

In addition to setup the above-mentioned measures to improve the quality of the results, a quality assurance scheme to check the suitability of the above procedures for the planned objectives is necessary. Several different ways for internal quality assurance are possible. The simplest is the revision of those values obtained from control samples along different batches. Any deviation from common values due to systematic or randomized factors should be easily detected and corrected. Testing repeated aliquots of samples is more expensive and systematic errors may be disregarded when using the same instrument. It may be used from time to time but is not recommended as a routine quality assessment. The introduction of control samples not known to the analysts but only to the director appears as the method of choice to control that internal quality measures operate as desired.

ERRORS

SYSTEMATIC	RANDOMIZED
Instruments	Accidental
Reagents	Normal distribution
Personnel	Subject to statistics
Operatives	
Methodologicals	
Others	

FIGURE 1. Possible sources and characteristics of erroneous results in the analytical laboratory.

PERSONNEL

STAFF	NEEDS
Laboratory Director	Job description
Certifying Scientist	Education
Supervisors	Experience
Technologists	Performance monitoring
Quality Assurance Unit	Training records

FIGURE 2. Levels and overall requirements for the staff involved in drug analysis.

III. EXTERNAL PROGRAMS

The credibility of the reliability of drug testing facilities for the external clients (either private or public) should be established, however, by means independent of the internal laboratory organization. The information on the quality of a given center when compared to other laboratories involved in the same kind of work is also useful not only for the external clients but for the laboratory itself.

The objectives of different external quality control programs, also called Proficiency Testing Programs (PTPs), may differ substantially, although all of them may be classified into three different groups:

1. **Informative programs** to obtain information about the quality level of drug testing in a given group of laboratories. Sometimes these are referred to as "survey" programs. They are important to take further administrative decisions on how to improve quality if necessary.
2. **Educative programs** that furnish adequate information back to the laboratories thus allowing education and training of the personnel which in turn improves the overall quality of the further results.
3. **Accreditation programs** where the results of the tests are taken, usually together with *in situ* inspections, as criteria to authorize the performance of a given laboratory for a given area of drug testing. Contrary to the above cited programs, which are usually established on a voluntary basis, mandatory participation is established for accreditation programs.

Proficiency programs may be classified also according to the way of introducing samples into the laboratory scheme. *Open* and *blind* programs may be considered (Figure 3). The test samples are known to the laboratory personnel in open tests thus allowing "special" attention to those samples. In this case, the "best" performance of the laboratory is monitored which may not be representative of performance under routine operation. Samples on open programs do not monitor the whole process inside the laboratory (especially sample reception and results release) but only the analytical component. This fact is corrected by the blind tests where samples are introduced into the laboratory under the normal protocol for common samples without laboratory knowledge. Implementation of blind programs is difficult except for large laboratory structures working for large clients and not involved at all in sample collection process. In practice, it is nearly impossible for laboratories working in clinical and therapeutic networks.

PROFICIENCY TESTING

OPEN	BLIND
Known samples	Unknown samples
Special attention	Routine control
Monitors the analytical side	Monitors the whole process

FIGURE 3. Characteristics of open and blind proficiency testing programs.

NIDA Program
Some characteristics

- Mandatory for initial certification
- Mandatory to mantain cartification
- Only GC-MS for confirmation
- Quantitative results. Statistical criteria
- No false identification acceptable
  False positive may result in revocation
  Some flexibility for false negatives

FIGURE 4. Main trends included in the NIDA Proficiency Testing Program (see Reference 12).

IV. DEVELOPMENT OF PROFICIENCY TESTING PROGRAMS

A. UNITED STATES

Proficiency testing for drugs of abuse analysis in urine has a long tradition in the United States. Extensive experience was obtained by the Centers for Disease Control[5] during its 9-year national survey program. Other programs were conducted also, either by public research centers,[6,7] by professional associations like the American Association of Clinical Chemistry, the American Association of Bioanalysts or the College of American Pathologists,[1] and also by the Administration (Defense Department). Reviews of these and other initiatives have been described.[8,9]

Some conflicting results on the reliability of drug testing as obtained from PTPs were presented in 1985 to 1987. So, deception after inaccurate results when applying blind controls[10] was followed, however, by encouraging data for keeping on with the maintenance of proficiency testing programs.[11]

A major step forward on the development of PTPs at the maximum level (accreditation) has been issued after the NIDA Guidelines for Drug Testing[12] that includes the correct performance in a mandatory program to obtain and maintain accreditation (Figure 4). Preliminary results obtained in a pilot study with 50 laboratories have already been presented.[13] The difficulty in complying with the narrow limits established for quantitative reporting has been one of the major issues, although quantitative work appears to be a useful indicator of real capabilities of the laboratory.

B. EUROPE

The use of urine drug testing for purposes out of clinical or therapeutic implications has not a long tradition in Europe. In recent years, however, implications in the workplace and other areas are gaining acceptance. Consequently, the development of PTPs, specifically on drugs of abuse urinalysis, has followed important delays as compared to United States.

A program coordinated from the University of Padova covered 35 laboratories, mainly Italian, from 1980 to 1985.[14] Subsequently, some isolated results obtained in other countries in the form of informative survey programs suggested the need for improving the quality of this kind of testing. For instance, results obtained in 1984 in 12 laboratories[20] analyzing true urine samples containing morphine and codeine ranged extensively from the lower to the higher concentration reported.

A recent survey from United Kingdom[15] reported on 25 samples analyzed between April 1987 and December 1989 by an average of 95 laboratories. The samples contained morphine, methadone, amphetamine, and

EVOLUTION OF ERRORS

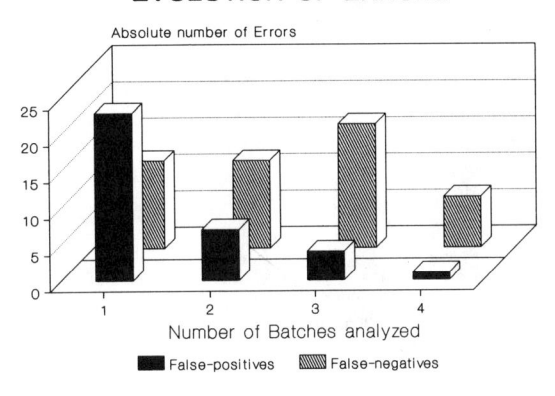

FIGURE 5. Evolution of errors in the Spanish Proficiency Testing Program along the first year of its implementation.

cocaine at concentrations of 0, 1, 2 and 5 mg/l, and benzoilecgonine at concentrations of 0, 0.4, 1, 2 and 4 mg/l. A significant inverse dose-related variation in the percentage of uncertain plus false negative reports was detected for morphine over the 1 to 5 mg/l range. There were significant increases in false positives plus uncertain reports in the presence of interfering substance for morphine and amphetamine. A significant lack of sensitivity for some chromatographic techniques at concentrations down to 1 mg/l was also detected. This is probably related more to some lack of skill than to the techniques themselves, but it is specially worrying when taking into account that 1 mg/l is in the upper range in drug addict urines for the majority of drugs or metabolites.

Since 1986, Spain has developed a Proficiency Testing Program coordinated from the Institut Municipal d'Investigació Mèdica de Barcelona under the sponsorship of the Ministry of Health (Plan Nacional sobre Drogas). The program has been planned to cover informative (status of drug testing in the country) and educative (improve experience and formation of analysts involved) purposes. Thirteen laboratories were included when the program was initiated and 46 were involved in 1990. Drug groups included are morphine-related opiates other opiates like methadone and dextropropoxyphene, cocaine metabolites (bencoylecgonine and ecgonine methyl ester), cannabinoids and its 9-COOH metabolite, amphetamines, barbiturates, and bezodiazepines. The laboratories may analyze the samples for groups of drugs or, when confirmatory techniques are available, for specific substances. Techniques used are identified by code. After evaluation of the results, a comprehensive report is prepared by the coordinating center that includes general and particular recommendations for the participating laboratories. Detailed methodology and results along the first year of the program have already been published.[16] In short, they demonstrated an important decrease for errors (specially false positives) and detected an important source of problems when using commercially available thin layer chromatography (Figures 5 and 6). In order to improve reliability of confirmatory techniques, reference standards for the main drugs and metabolites (including 6-acetyl-morphine, morphine-3-glucuronide, or ecgonine methyl ester) were synthesized and distributed. Intensive training periods for confirmatory techniques were also developed in the coordinating center. An extensive report of the program after 3 years of implementation is reported elsewhere in this book.[17] The extension toward a third level (i.e., accreditation) is now being considered.

V. FUTURE DEVELOPMENTS

Because of the widespread problem of drug abuse, coordinated initiatives at supranational or international levels appear necessary for the future. One of the first international bodies that is considering the problems associated with drug testing in urine and its social and individual consequences is the European Economic Community. A resolution approved in 1989[18] states the need for guaranties when this kind of analysis is performed and could evolve toward some way of coordinated approach for quality control in drugs of abuse testing in Europe.

Interest by other regional (Association of Southeast Asian Nations, ASEAN, personal communication) or worldwide organizations (United Nations[19]) have been mentioned, which in turn confirm that next years will probably see important efforts to improve the quality of drug testing in a cooperative international approach.

ERRORS / TECHNIQUES

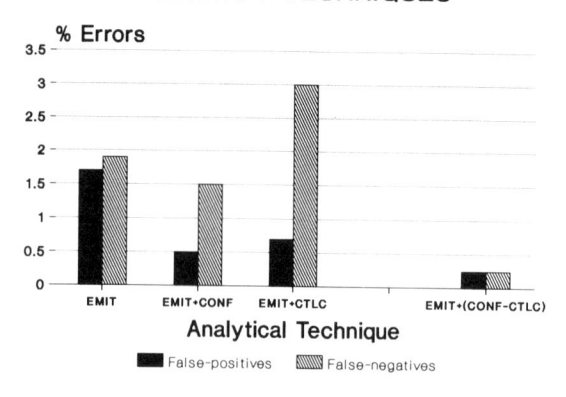

FIGURE 6. Relationship between the number of false results and the techniques used by the laboratories participating in the Spanish Proficiency Testing Program along the first year of its implementation. (EMIT — enzyme immunoassay technique, CONF — the whole confirmatory techniques, and CTLC — commercially pre-prepared thin layer chromatographhy.)

REFERENCES

1. **Substance Abuse Testing Committee,** Critical issues in urinalysis of abused substances: report of the substance-abuse testing committee, *Clin. Chem.*, 34(3), 605–632, 1988.
2. **Dugal, R. and Donike, M.,** Requirements for accreditation and good laboratory practices; presented by the IOC Medical Commission at the 2nd World Conference on Anti-Doping in Sport, Moscow, 1988.
3. Good Laboratory Practice Regulations for Nonclinical Laboratory Studies, *Fed. Reg.*, (21 CFR Part. 58), December 1978, 22.
4. *OECD Principles of Good Laboratory Practices*, May 12, 1981.
5. **Boone, D. J., Guerrant, G. O., and Knouse, R. W.,** Proficiency testing in clinical toxicology: program sponsored by the Centers for Disease Control, *J. Anal. Toxicol.*, 1, 139, 1977.
6. **Shoemaker, M. J., Klein, M., and Sideman, L.,** Drug Abuse proficiency testing in Pennsylvania 1972–76, *J. Anal. Toxicol.*, 1, 130, 1977.
7. **Dinovo, E. C. and Gottschalk,** Results of a nine-laboratory survey of forensic toxicology proficiency, *Clin. Chem.*, 22, 843, 1976.
8. **Willette, R. E.,** Drug Testing Programs, in *Urine Testing for Drugs of Abuse*, Hawks, R.L. and Chiang, C.N., Eds., NIDA Research Monogr. 73, Dept of Health and Human Services, (ADM)87-1481, Rockville, MD, National Institute on Drug Abuse, 1986, 6.
9. **McBay A. J.,** Problems in testing for abused drugs, *JAMA*, 255, 39, 1986.
10. **Hansen, H. J., Caudill, S. P., and Boone, J.,** Crisis in drug testing. Results of CDC blind study, *JAMA*, 253, 2382–2387, 1985.
11. **Frings, C. S., White, R. M., and Battaglia, D. J.,** Status of drugs-of-abuse testing in urine, an AACC study, *Clin. Chem.*, 33(9), 1683–1686, 1987.
12. **National Institute on Drug Abuse and Department of Health and Human Services,** Mandatory Guidelines for Federal Workplace Drug Testing Programs. *Fed. Reg.*, 53/69, April 11, 1988.
13. **Davis, K. H., Hawks, R. L., and Blanke, R. V.,** Assessment of laboratory quality in urine drug testing. A proficiency testing pilot study, *JAMA*, 260(12), 1749–1750, 1988.
14. **Ferrara, S. D. and Garcia, F. J. C.,** Psychotropic drugs, organization and role of the laboratory, in *Psychoactive Drugs and Health Problems*, Indäpään-Heikkila, J., Ghodse, H., and Khan, I., Eds., Helsinki, The National Board of Health, The Government of Finland, 1987, 100–139.
15. **Wilson, J. F., Williams, J., Walker, G., Toseland, P. A., Smith, B.L., Richens, A., and Burnett, D.,** Sensitivity and specificity of techniques used to detect drugs of abuse in urine, presented at the Association of Clinical Biochemists, Brighton, May 1990.
16. **Segura, J., de la Torre, R., Congost, M., and Camí, J.,** Proficiency testing on drugs of abuse, one year's experience in Spain, *Clin. Chem.*, 35, 879–883, 1989.
17. **de la Torre, R., Segura, J., Artola, A., Marrugat, J., Marraut, F., and Milessi, M.,** Spanish proficiency testing program (1986–1989), this volume.
18. Conclusions du Conseil et des ministres de la santé des États membres, réunis au sein du Conseil du 16 mai 1989 concernant la fiabilité des analyses de liquides corporels pour déceler l'usage de drogues illicites, *Journal Officiel des Communautés Européennes*, 89/C, 185/2, 22 Juillet 1989.
19. **United Nations Commission on Narcotic Drugs,** Guidelines for the Establishment of National Testing Programmes and Laboratories for Drugs Of Abuse in Body Fluids, 10th special session, Commission on Narcotic Drugs, Vienna, February 8–19, 1988.
20. **Möller, M. R.,** personal communication.

Chapter 33

SPANISH PROFICIENCY TESTING PROGRAM (1986–1989)

R. de la Torre, J. Segura, A. Artola, J. Marrugat, F. Manaut, and M. Milessi

TABLE OF CONTENTS

Definitions		220
I.	Introduction	220
II.	Menu of Substances and Preparation of Samples	220
III.	Results and Discussion	220
IV.	Conclusions	224
References		224

DEFINITIONS

Percentage of false negative results: number of false negative results compared to the total number of analyses for the detection of the substance when it was present in the control urine.

Percentage of false positive results: number of false positive results compared to the total number of analyses for the detection of the substance.

Global percentage of errors: the sum number of false positive and false negative results compared with the total number of analyses for the detection of substances of the menu independently if they were present or absent in the control urines.

I. INTRODUCTION

Since 1986, there has been a Proficiency Testing Program for the Analysis of Drugs of Abuse in Spain developed by the Department of Pharmacology and of Toxicology of the Municipal Institute for Medical Research (IMIM) in Barcelona in conjunstion with the Spanish National Plan on Drugs of Abuse (PNSD). The program has an advisory committee and it is coordinated with five reference laboratories from France, Germany, Norway, and the United States (see Acknowledgments).

Primary objectives are to have an accurate view of the state of this analytical field in Spain and to improve the educational level of people engaged in such a responsibility. The current number of participating laboratories is 45, nearly the double of those that started the program in the first year (n = 25). Most of them (80%) are public centers devoted to clinical diagnostic and assistance, while the others are involved in forensic, military, or workplace drug testing.

Laboratories have been provided with methanolic stock solutions of parent drugs and metabolites to be used as standards for confirmatory methods.

An on-site 2 week practical education program in the coordinating center (IMIM) has been implemented for participating laboratories (about 85% have already attended it) to learn and practice confirmatory techniques.

II. MENU OF SUBSTANCES AND PREPARATION OF SAMPLES

The menu of substances covered by the program has been evolving during the last 3 years. Table 1 lists analytes used currently for the preparation of control urines. While the eight groups of substances covered by the program have been essentially the same during this period of time, a big effort has been done to introduce gradually, when necessary and available, main urinary metabolites of substances belonging to each group. A total of 16 substances and metabolites are used at the present time. Amounts of drugs added to the urines have been reduced during the last 3 years to the cutoff levels to those equivalents or slightly above the EMIT assays (LOW calibrator), a technique widely used within participating laboratories. The concentrations of substances and ratios of metabolites have been adjusted to try to mimic real urine samples. Sterilized urine specimens are sent four times per year (six control urines per batch) by a courier service. Additional details on the preparation and control of the samples have been published previously.[1]

III. RESULTS AND DISCUSSION

Results generated by the different participating laboratories (see Figure 1) have been arranged, for evaluation purposes, depending on the number of years that each one has joined the program. For example, results of laboratories of the second year are all the results generated by laboratories engaged in the program for 2 or 3 years, but driving their second year of participation.

From the results of the last 3 years, some facts can be stressed. The global percentage of errors is between 3 and 4%, independent of the number of years that each laboratory has been involved in the program with a slight decrease from a 4% for the first 2 years to a 3.3% for year 3. One of the main reasons is that while there is a percentage of false positive results quite constant during the 3 years evaluated, around 1%, there is a decrease of the percentage of false negative results to 8.7% in year 3 from an initial 10.6% (mean of the first 2 years).

Interestingly, the global percentage of errors is higher when laboratories are trying to identify specific substances (4.6%) than when they are analyzing groups of substances (3.7%). This global figure can be reproduced when the percentage of false negative and false positive results are evaluated separately. The percentage of false negative results is 10.6% when analyzing groups of substances and 13.3% when identifying specific products involved. The same happens with the percentage of false negative results where the rate when analyzing groups of substances is 1% and when identifying substances is 1.8%.

Some substances have been introduced in the menu of the program for educational purposes (phenylpropanolamine and phenobarbital) or because their high prevalence of abuse in the Spanish drug addict population (flunitrazepam). The concentrations added to control urines for these substances added were such that they gave a positive

TABLE 1
Percentage of False Positive and False Negative Results According to Analyte

Menu	Least concentration (µg/ml) of drug potentially present[a]	False positive (%)	False negative (%)
Amphetamines		0.7	26.7
Amphetamine	0.3	2.1	17.4
Phenylpropanolamine	5.0	1.0	19.0
Barbiturates		0.8	23.3
Phenobarbital	5.0	2.0	18.4
Secobarbital	0.3	3.1	12.2
Benzodiazepines		1.2	13.1
Oxazepam	0.3	1.5	7.1
Nordiazepam	0.3	1.1	6.0
7-amino-flunitrazepam	5.0	6.9	25.0
Opiates		0.7	4.9
Morphine	0.3	1.5	15.2
Morphine 3-O-glucuronide	0.3[b]		
Codeine	0.3	2.3	16.5
6-monoacetyl morphine	0.3	4.1[b]	25.0
Methadone		0.5	5.7
Methadone	0.3	0.6	5.0
Propoxyphene		0.4	19.4
Propoxyphene	0.3	0.6	23.8
Cocaine		0.9	6.0
Benzoylecgonine	0.3	1.6	11.9
Ecgonine methylester	0.3	1.2	7.1
Cannabinoids		2.2	12.2
9-COOH-delta^9 THC	0.1	0.0	18.8

[a] Minimal concentrations never used. Always a 15% excess to the nominal concentration of the control urine was added to correct any loss during the preparation of samples.
[b] Never added alone but in conjunction with morphine.

result by commonly used presumptive tests. This was checked in the coordinating center when preparing batches of samples and in the reference laboratories. Nevertheless, some of these substances have well known analytical problems especially when screened by immunological techniques because of low cross-reactivity of the analytes toward the antibodies commonly in use. In fact, the higher rates of false negative results when analyzing groups of substances correspond to those found for the analysis of amphetamines (26.7%), barbiturates (23.3%), and benzodiazepines (13.1%) that match the substances mentioned before. If we delete the results from these analytes, the percentage of false negative results drops from an initial 10.6 to a 4.1% and the global percentage of errors from an initial 3.7 to a 2.1%. These rates can be more easily compared with results obtained by other proficiency testing programs. The high rate of false negative results for propoxyphene is due specifically to an inadequate use by some laboratories of commercial thin layer chromatography for its screening. In fact, the advisory committee has strongly recommended to the participating laboratories using this technique that they review their analytical procedures for the detection of propoxyphene and other substances of the menu or to substitute it by alternative techniques.

As expected, false negative results for the analysis of groups of substances are highly dependent of the concentrations of the analyte added to the control urine, as it can be observed in Figure 2. Differences when concentration in the control urine was higher or lower than 0.5 µg/ml were statistically significant for both morphine ($p = 0.02$) and benzoylecgonine ($p < 0.04$).

Most false positive and false negative results are attributable not to the application of immunological presumptive tests, as expected, but to the inadequate use of some chromatographic techniques. Figure 3 shows the global percentage of errors observed for the different analytical techniques used by participating laboratories in the program as presumptive test (Figure 3A) or with confirmatory purposes (Figure 3B). These rates are just

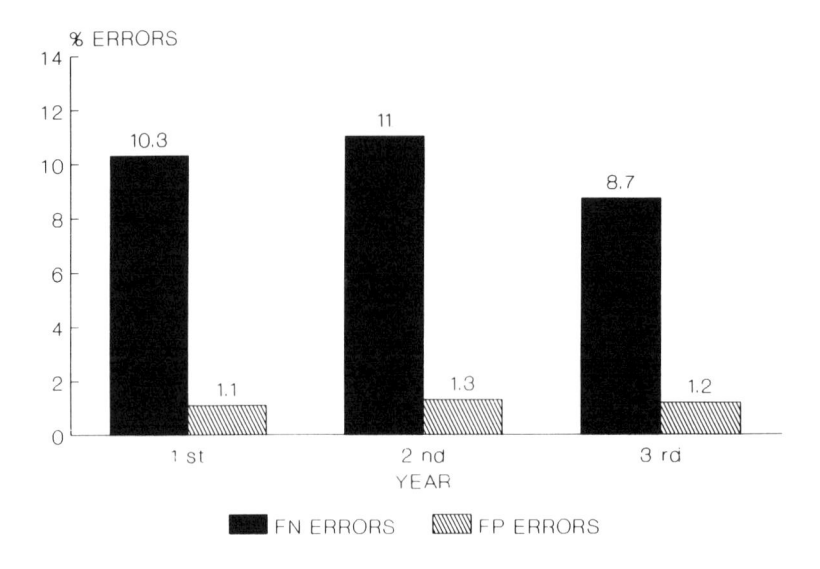

FIGURE 1. Evolution of the relative number of false negative and false positive results.

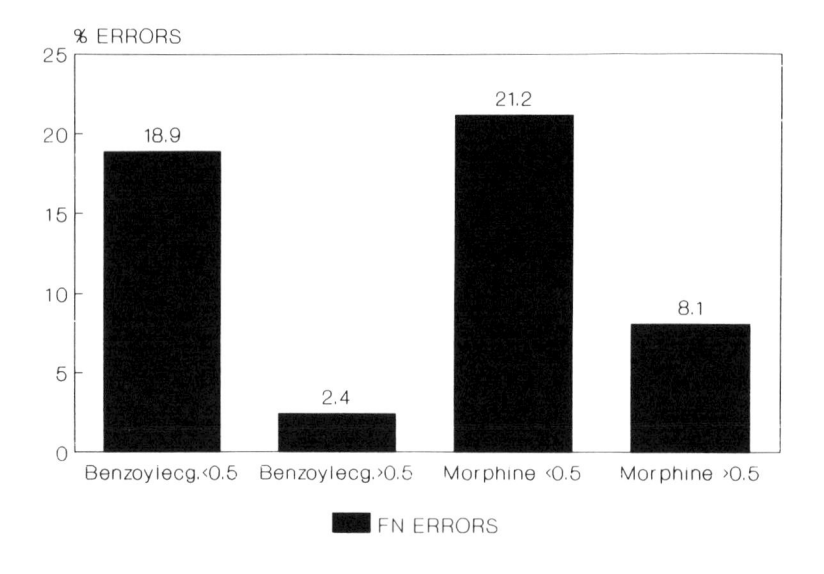

FIGURE 2. Rate of false negative results for morphine and benzoylecgonine depending of their concentration in urine (higher or lower than 0.5 µg/ml).

the expression of how the analytical techniques have been applied by participating laboratories. Results of immunological techniques, where most of the errors are of the false negative type, can be easily explained by the introduction in the menu of some substances as mentioned before. More difficult to justify are those errors generated by chromatographic techniques. In fact, most of the methodologies used with these techniques have not been fully developed in some laboratories or not tested before their application to routine and quality control samples. Additionally, larger number of errors are concentrated in a few number of laboratories.

The experience described here raises some questions when thinking in an hypotetical future Proficiency Testing Programs at supranational level: which is the most adequate menu of substances to be controlled in, for instance, the laboratories covering the European drug addict population? As it can be deduced from the Spanish

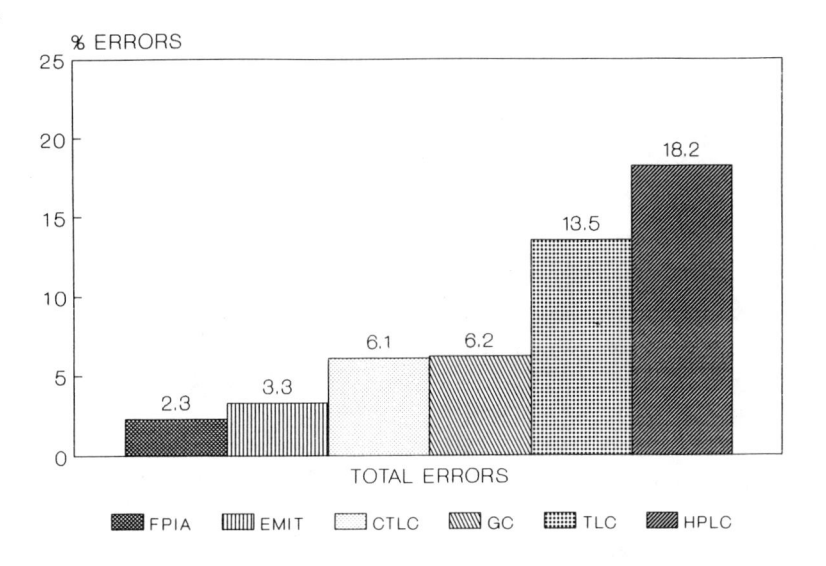

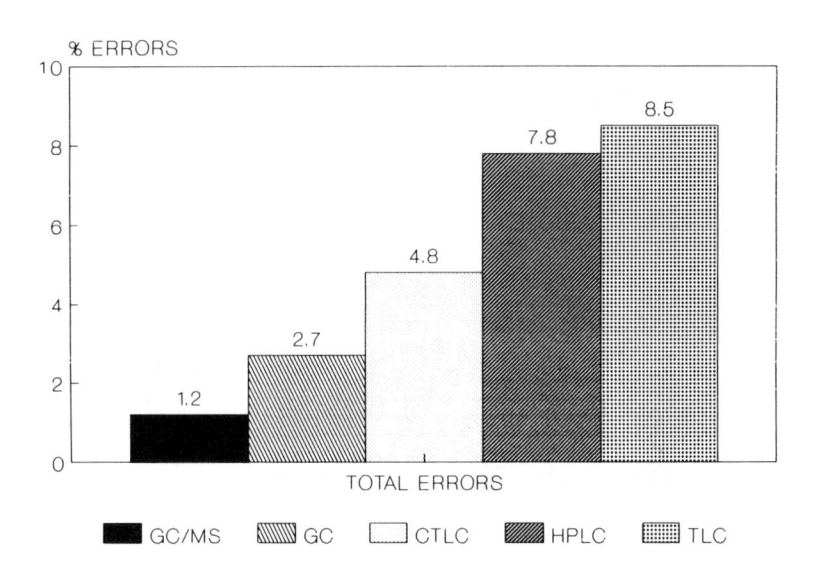

FIGURE 3. Global percentage of errors for analytical techniques applied as presumptive (A) or confirmatory (B) tests. EMIT = enzyme immunoassay, FPIA = fluorescence polarization immunoassay, GC = gas chromatography, GC/MS = gas chromatography coupled to mass spectrometry, TLC = thin layer chromatography, CTLC = commercial pre-prepared TLC, and HPLC = high performance liquid chromatography.

experience, results can be quite different if we introduce, or not introduce, 7-amino flunitrazepam in the menu of substances. Other substances with a high prevalence of abuse in Spain[2] and in some areas of Europe, like bu-

prenorphine, are not controlled at all. Are laboratories ready to control some synthetic derivatives of phenylalkylamines or other designer drugs becoming quite popular in some holiday places? The fact is that most commonly used screening techniques have some problems in detecting some of them. The menu of the substances controlled appears to influence the confidence of analytical reliability of laboratories and the reliability of drug testing itself.

IV. CONCLUSIONS

The Proficiency Testing program has a beneficial effect when adequate techniques are used. Nevertheless, still a considerable rate of error, even after 3 years of participation in the Proficiency Testing program, is present in some laboratories. Analytical errors can have serious consequences for the individual, therefore rates of errors must be reduced drastically. As a consequence, the development of confirmatory techniques must be mandatory, at least in such laboratories involved in drug screening in fields others than the therapeutic one (i.e., work place, military, etc.). For clinical laboratories, the actual scheme with a stronger focus on presumptive detection of substances might be adequate. In the case of laboratories doing drug testing for some occupational groups, and as a logical extension of this preliminary educational period, an accreditative scheme by the Spanish administration should be applied.

REFERENCES

1. **Segura, J., de la Torre, R., Congost, M., and Camí, J.,** Proficiency testing on drugs of abuse: one year's experience in Spain, *Clin. Chem.*, 35, 879–883, 1989.
2. **San, L., Tremoleda, J. M., Ollé, J. M., Porta, M., and de la Torre, R.,** Prevalencia del consumo de buprenorfina en heroinomanos en tratamiento, *Med. Clin.*, 93, 645–648, 1989.

Chapter 34

ACCREDITATION AND REACCREDITATION OF LABORATORIES BY THE IOC MEDICAL COMMISSION

Manfred Donike

TABLE OF CONTENTS

I.	Introduction	226
II.	Development of Dope Analysis	226
III.	The Concept of Accreditation and Reaccreditation of Laboratories	226
IV.	Requirements for Accreditation of Laboratories	227
	A. Letter of Support	227
	B. Essential Equipment	227
	C. Repertoire	227
V.	The Accreditation	227
VI.	The Reaccreditation and Proficiency Test	228
VII.	Implementation	228
VIII.	Summary	228

Annex 1: Standardization of Analytical Procedures and Quality Tests for Dope Control Laboratories (1980) 229

Annex 2: International Olympic Committee List of Doping Classes and Methods (1990) 230

Annex 3: Requirements for Accreditation and Good Laboratory Practices (1988) 232

References 237

I. INTRODUCTION

The accreditation system of the International Olympic Committee (IOC) Medical Commission is, to the best of my knowledge, worldwide the first accreditation system of analytical laboratories. The goal of this accreditation is to harmonize analytical methods, so that the same standards are applied for detection of dope agents in screening procedures as well as for confirmation analyses. It was designed in 1978 first by a small working group of the IAAF (International Amateur Athletic Federation). The IOC Medical Commission adopted this accreditation scheme to make it available for all sports, at Olympic Games, and in the years in between.

The original can be traced back to 1968, the Olympic Winter Games in Grenoble and the Olympic Summer Games in Mexico. The IOC Medical Commission, founded in 1966, had to realize that besides difficulties in organizing the sample-taking procedure, there existed a lack in analytical methods and also a lack in the knowledge of the pharmacokinetics and metabolism of the dope agents.

It is obvious that according to the rules, but also to common sense, the identification of a dope agent and/or its metabolites in an urine sample of an athlete is proof of a violation of the rule. So the question to answer was by which analytical methods can reliable results be obtained?

Looking back to the analytical possibilities of the 1970s, paper chromatography, thin layer chromatography, and a very preliminary kind of gas chromatography were available and used in forensic toxicological and clinical chemical laboratories.

II. DEVELOPMENT OF DOPE ANALYSIS

The first dope control which really earns the designation comprehensive was performed in 1972 at the Games of the 20th Olympiad in Munich. At that time, stimulants of the amphetamine type were the favorite drugs used to increase performance. The dramatic increase of the use of amphetamines can be explained by the fact that during World War II the amphetamines were applied to soldiers to increase alertness and performance. In this way, the "benefits" of amphetamine became known to a larger population. In this way amphetamines were introduced into sports.

Due to the development in analytical techniques and especially by the introduction of a long-term stable nitrogen specific detector (N-FID), it was possible to detect the amphetamine and other nitrogen-containing drugs effectively.[1]

Surprisingly, the easy detection of amphetamines led, at the same time, to the disappearance of narcotic drugs like morphine and pethidine. These narcotics have been used together with amphetamine, caffeine, and respiratory stimulants like nicetamid or micorene in the form of a cocktail. So the introduction of an effective test for one type of drug, the stimulants, hindered the use of the other one, the narcotics.

After 1972, Olympic Sports were confronted with a new problem — the misuse of anabolic steroids, which now can be detected by a comprehensive screening procedure.[2]

III. THE CONCEPT OF ACCREDITATION AND REACCREDITATION OF LABORATORIES

Between Munich 1972 and 1976, it became known to the IOC Medical Commission that in some cases false positive results have been reported to the sport authorities, e.g., the Medical Commissions of International Federations or National Federations.

There is consensus in sports that false positive results cannot be tolerated, and all means should be taken to avoid false positive results. One measure should be mentioned here without going into the details: the "B" analysis performed on a second aliquot of urine, coded and sealed as the first, the A, sample.

Further there were rumors on false negative analyses. When athletes realize that the results of a urine analysis was negative, even in spite of the fact that they have taken drugs, they are encouraged to use a dope agent. To overcome this apparent problem, the IAAF Commission drafted a paper in 1978 under the name "Requirements for Accreditation of Laboratories and Standardization of Analytical Methods" to avoid, in the field of sports, the above-mentioned accusations of false positive and false negative results. This paper was taken over by the IOC Medical Commission in 1980 in preparing the Olympic Games in Moscow (Annex 1). Here, it was especially one aspect — the international distrust in the capability, but also in the intent of this socialistic country to fight against doping. So an international accreditation has been performed under supervision.

Until 1984 the number of accredited laboratories increased to ten. One chapter of the paper mentioned before "Requirements for Accreditation ..." foresaw the reaccreditation in time intervals of 2 years to insure the competence of the IOC accredited laboratories. This has been done under the aspect that it is relatively easy to provide a budget for staff and instrumentation at an occasion like the Olympic Games, but afterwards the support of such laboratories decreased. A fundamental aspect to running a laboratory is that the budget should be in reasonable relation to the task which the authorities stipulate. The first reaccreditation of IOC Medial Commission including stimulants, narcotics, and anabolic steroids was performed 1985. Since then the demand and workload increased by the addition of the groups of β-blockers, diuretics, and some peptide hormones to the doping definition of the IOC Medical Commission. This definition (Annex 2) bans the application of substances belonging to certain classes of pharmacological active compounds.

Examples are given illustrating which substances are belonging to each class of banned substances, but this should not be regarded as a definite list. So each enumeration ends with the expression "and related compounds". The lists of examples represent fairly well the repertoire of the doping control laboratories. As over the years the list of examples was extended more and more today, it seems to be more or less comprehensive.

The intention to create specialized laboratories for this kind of work is due to fact that the analytical competence, capability, and experience was not found in existing forensic toxicological laboratories. For example, in dope control laboratories the techniques of combined gas chromotography, mass spectrometry, and N-FID detection were introduced several years before the use in forensic toxicological analysis. Further, the problems occurring in sports often are quite different from the problems encountered in forensic toxicological analysis. In the case of the detection of anabolic steroids, a high retrospectivity is demanded to detect drugs which have been applied months before the competition.

Another factor is the background information you must have available to successfully analyze the samples which are collected out at sport events. Another important aspect should also be mentioned: during events like Olympic Games or tournaments like ice hockey, basketball, and fencing, the IOC Medical Commission expect the results within 24 hours after the collection of the samples. In some areas we find parallels between the tasks of a forensic toxicological laboratory and a dope control laboratory, e.g., in the detection of controlled substances, like the amphetamine and narcotics.

IV. REQUIREMENTS FOR ACCREDITATION OF LABORATORIES

A. LETTER OF SUPPORT

The IOC Medical Commission asks for a letter of support of a national authority, e.g., the National Olympic Committee or the corresponding centralized support organization. This is based on the argument mentioned before, the connection with sport and the authorities.

B. ESSENTIAL EQUIPMENT

In this paragraph, the essential analytical equipment which is necessary to run a dope control laboratory is described. It includes gas chromatograph, high pressure liquid chromatograph, equipment for thin layer chromatography, modern mass spectrometer, and for the determination of peptide harmones, (radio) immunoassay equipment, or at least access to it.

C. REPERTOIRE

The capability of the applied screening procedures should cover the examples listed under the classes of banned substances. Today, we can divide them into screening procedures designed to detect the forbidden substances according to the chemical/biochemical properties as described in Annex 3.

Additional immunoassay techniques should be applied for the detection of peptide hormones like HCG, which are on the list of banned classes.

Note: The intention of the IOC Medical Commission to initiate excretion studies is more or less educational. In performing excretion studies, the laboratory staff will learn to handle the biological samples and how to trace the low concentrations near the detection limit.

V. THE ACCREDITATION[3]

The accreditation of analytical laboratories will be performed as outlined in the requirements (Annex 3). The laboratories have to provide a list of reference substances of drugs and their metabolites and a list of excretion studies performed.

The pre-accreditation procedure is the time period prior to accreditation when the laboratories will be asked to analyze three sets of ten samples. The results will be discussed with the head of the laboratory. This period of pre-accreditation will last 6 to 12 months. A longer period will be granted only under exceptional circumstances as the experience shows that if a laboratory needs a longer time to acquire the necessary competence, it will never achieve accreditation.

The accreditation procedure by itself consists of analyzing ten control samples under the observation of a delegate of the subcommission Doping and Biochemistry of the IOC Medical Commission. It is mandatory that the test be performed within 3 days and the comprehensive documentation including the literature be submitted within 3 weeks.

The control samples will contain substances which are on the list of examples of the banned classes so that nobody can claim to be tested with an unknown sample. Blank urines may be included as well as samples containing up to three dope agents. Most of these test samples will be excretion studies which will contain the drugs applied or their metabolites in a reasonable concentration, this means that in agreement with the concentrations you have to expect in a real dope case. Further, the samples are pretested in a reference laboratory. These measures insure that the laboratory will receive a fair set of samples. The documentation of the results obtained in the reference laboratory will be made available to the delegate of the subcommission observing the accreditation.

VI. THE REACCREDITATION AND PROFICIENCY TEST

In the reaccreditation procedure designed to check the competence of a laboratory after a certain period of time, the IOC Medical Commission has agreed to challenge the laboratory yearly with up to ten samples. The samples are composed following the same scheme as outlined above for the accreditation.

In addition, the IOC Medical Commission introduced a proficiency testing program with four samples every 4 months. The first goal of the proficiency test is that the IOC Medical Commission gets information about the performance of the different screening procedures the year under routine conditions. The laboratories are informed that they should introduce these samples in routine analyses. The reasons to perform a proficiency test in the way it is done is that it is very difficult to introduce blind samples into a dope control laboratory. Sometimes at major sport events it may be possible, but also there exists some difficulties. At the occasion of sport events, normally the number of samples to be collected and sent is known in advance to the laboratory, so if an additional sample arrives, the staff in the laboratory will become alert. Even at Olympic Games some problems occurred when the IOC Medical Commission tried to introduce blind samples at the dope control station. By change, somebody who is involved in the procedure at the national level will inform the laboratory.

The IOC Medical Commission, through the IOC Medical Subcommission on Doping and Biochemistry, reserves the right to inspect an IOC accredited laboratory when special circumstances are given, e.g., multiple failure at reaccreditation tests. Till now, the subcommission has not yet used this right. Further, special requirements must be fulfilled by laboratories seeking accreditation for future Olympic Games. These laboratories have not only to perform an accreditation procedure in the described way for, e.g., a sample load of up to 30 or 50 per week, but in addition they have to demonstrate their capability to deal with up to 200 samples per day under a situation which is known to be a stress situation.

VII. IMPLEMENTATION

For the purpose of evaluation of the data, the IOC Medical Subcommission on Doping and Biochemistry acts as review committee. For the proficiency tests, the review committee will consist of the secretary of the subcommission, a member of the subcommission, and one head of an IOC accredited laboratory.

In the reaccreditation procedure, the IOC Medical Commission will not tolerate a false positive result. In a false negative case, special procedures are foreseen to give the laboratory the possibility to correct it, and for the quantitative results which are asked for in the case of the determination of the caffeine concentration and the testosterone/epitestosterone ratio, the commission is asking for a result close to the mean of all laboratories. Two standard deviations will be the tolerable range of ± 15% of the mean.

Laboratories failing reaccreditation are submitted to restrictions so that they cannot analyze samples for international federations and must ask for confirmation of positive A-samples (Annex 3) by a fully accredited IOC laboratory.

VIII. SUMMARY

To summarize, the system of accreditation, reaccreditation, and proficiency has been created to serve the needs of the international sport community. It was updated several times based on the experiences made to meet the necessary scientific standards and also to meet the requirements of the sport federations. The goal of the IOC Medical Commission is to protect the health of the athletes, to insure fair not pharmacological manipulated competitions, and to protect the ethics of the sport. But doping in sports should not be regarded as isolated from the misuse of drugs in society. The misuse of anabolic steroids is so widespread that it is no longer a problem only of a high-performance sport, it is a problem of society.

ANNEX 1: MEDICAL COMMISSION OF THE INTERNATIONAL OLYMPIC COMMITTEE: REQUIREMENTS FOR ACCREDITATION OF LABORATORIES (1980) (UPDATED, SEE ANNEX 3)

STANDARDIZATION OF ANALYTICAL PROCEDURES AND QUALITY TESTS FOR DOPE CONTROL LABORATORIES (1980)

The IOC Medical Commission considers it essential to test the work of dope control laboratories. The Commission therefore proposes the following rules for analytical procedure and quality tests, which are required for the accreditation program.

I. ESSENTIAL EQUIPMENT FOR

1. Gas chromatography (GC)
2. High pressure liquid chromatography (HPLC)
3. Thin layer chromatography (TLC)
4. Mass spectrometry (MS) in combination with gas chromatography (GC) and computer evaluation (COM)

II. ANALYTICAL PROCEDURES

The IOC Medical Commission requires the following procedures:

1. For "Volatile Doping Agents": GC screening with a nitrogen specific detector (N-FID) and capillary column cross-linked with a moderate polarity phase, e.g., SE 54. Alternative suitable GLC systems may be used.
2. For "Doping Agents excreted as conjugates": GC screening after hydrolysis and extraction at pH 9.5, derivatization, cross-linked capillary column, detection with a nitrogen specific detector (N-FID), or by mass fragmentography (mass specific detection).
3. For "Pemoline, Caffeine and Diuretics": screening with high pressure liquid chromatography.
4. For "Anabolic Steroids":

    a. For free steroids: After extraction at ph 9.0, derivatization and detection by mass fragmentography (mass specific detection).
    b. For conjugated steroids: After enzymatic hydrolysis, extraction, trimethylsilylation, and detection by mass fragmentography (mass specific detection). Alternatively an extraction of the free and the conjugated fraction, e.g., with XAD-2 may be performed, followed by a separation of the two fractions, treated and analyzed as described above.

5. For "Acidic Substances", e.g., diuretics and probenecide: Extraction at, e.g., pH 2 or lower, and derivatization, GC with nitrogen specific detection, or by mass fragmentography (mass specific detection).

Note: Definite identification of a doping substance requires analysis by mass spectrometry.

III. ACCREDITATION OF ANALYTICAL LABORATORIES

Analytical laboratories which request accreditation must fulfill the following requirements and answer the enclosed questionnaire:

1. Provide a list of substances which the laboratory is able to detect. The minimum repertoire will be the list of examples enumerated in the dope definition of the IOC Medical Commission under the different classes of forbidden substances.
2. Provide a list of available reference substances (dope agents and metabolites).
3. Minimum concentration, which can be detected following the administration of the drugs to humans.
4. The maximum time required to obtain a result after receipt of the sample for analysis:

    a. for anabolic steroids
    b. for other doping agents

5. The control samples are to be analyzed in the presence of a member of the IOC Medical Subcommission on Doping and Biochemistry of Sport or a designated expert ("delegate"). The control samples will be made available under the direction of the above subcommission.
6. The laboratory seeking accreditation will be re-

quired to analyze and report its results on the ten control samples to the IOC Medical Subcommission on Doping and Biochemistry of Sport. The report, of which six copies are to be sent to the secretary of the Subcommission on Doping and Biochemistry of Sport within 3 weeks after completing the accreditation, should include:

a. Complete description of the analytical procedures
b. Copies of the GC-, MS-, and COM-protocols

After considering the results, the above subcommission will announce its decision.

7. In the presence of the delegate, the laboratory seeking accreditation must establish correctly the positive samples and identify the dope agents and their metabolites within a period of 3 days.
8. The control samples will contain up to six steroids, up to six stimulants, up to three β-blockers, up to two narcotics, and up to two diuretics. A blank urine may be included as well as samples containing more than one dope agent.
9. Prior to visiting the laboratory, the delegate will be provided with all the documentation on the samples to be used in the accreditation of the laboratory concerned. If the laboratory produces a correct result within 3 days of the visit of the delegate, the delegate will then discuss the result with the laboratory staff. Upon receipt of the official report, the delegate will present a formal written report to the subcommission.
10. Every year, accredited laboratories will be required to analyze up to ten new control samples as part of the continuing accreditation program and report their results to the secretary of the IOC Subcommission on Doping and Biochemistry of Sport. The details of the procedures of reaccreditation will be sent to the laboratory concerned 3 months prior to the test.

ANNEX 2: INTERNATIONAL OLYMPIC COMMITTEE LIST OF DOPING CLASSES AND METHODS (1990)

I. DOPING CLASSES

A. Stimulants
B. Narcotics
C. Anabolic steroids
D. β-blockers
E. Diuretics
F. Peptide hormones and analogs

II. DOPING METHODS

A. Blood doping
B. Pharmacological, chemical, and physical manipulations

III. CLASSES OF DRUGS SUBJECT TO CERTAIN RESTRICTIONS

A. Alcohol
B. Marijuana
C. Local anaesthetics
D. Corticosteroids

Note: The doping definition of the IOC Medical Commission is based on the banning of pharmacological classes of agents. This definition has the advantage that also new drugs, some of which may be especially designed for doping purposes, are banned.

The following list represents examples of the different dope classes to illustrate the doping definition. Unless indicated all substances belonging to the banned classes may not be used for medical treatment, even if they are not listed as examples. If substances of the banned classes are detected in the laboratory, the IOC Medical Commission will act. It should be noted that the presence of the drug in the urine constitutes an offense, irrespective of the route of administration.

LIST OF EXAMPLES TO THE DIFFERENT CLASSES OF BANNED SUBSTANCES

A. STIMULANTS, e.g.,

- Amfepramone
- Amfetaminil
- Amiphenazole
- Amphetamine
- Benzphetamine
- Caffeine*
- Cathine
- Chlorphentermine
- Clobenzorex
- Clorprenaline

*For caffeine the definition of a positive depends upon the following: if the concentration in urine exceeds 12 µg/ml.

- Cocaine
- Cropropamide (component of "micoren")
- Crotethamide (component of "microren")
- Dimetamfetamine
- Ephedrine
- Etafedrine
- Etamivan
- Etilamfetamine
- Fencamfamin
- Fenetylline
- Fenproporex
- Furfenorex
- Mefenorex
- Methamphetamine
- Methoxyphenamine
- Methylephedrine
- Methylphenidate
- Morazone
- Nikethamide
- Pemoline
- Pentetrazol
- Phendimetrazine
- Phenmetrazine
- Phentermine
- Phenylpropanolamine
- Pipradrol
- Prolintane
- Propylhexedrine
- Pyrovalerone
- Strychnine
- And related compounds

B. NARCOTICS ANALGESICS, e.g.,

- Alphaprodine
- Anileridine
- Buprenorphine
- Codeine
- Dextromoramide
- Dextropropoxyphen
- Diamorphine (heroin)
- Dihydrocodeine
- Dipipanone
- Ethoheptazine
- Ethylmorphine
- Levorphanol
- Methadone
- Morphine
- Nalbuphine
- Pentazocine
- Pethidine
- Phenazocine
- Trimeperidine
- And related compounds

C. ANABOLIC STEROIDS, e.g.,

- Bolasterone
- Boldenone
- Clostebol
- Dehytdrochlormethyltestosterone
- Fluoxymesterone
- Mesterolone
- Metandienone
- Metenolone
- Methyltestosterone
- Nandrolone
- Norethandrolone
- Oxandrolone
- Oxymesterone
- Oxymetholone
- Stanozolol
- Testosterone*
- And related compounds

*Testosterone: the definition of a positive depends upon the following: the administration of testosterone or the use of any other manipulation having the result of increasing the ratio in urine of testosterone/epitestosterone to above six.

D. β-BLOCKERS, e.g.,

- Acebutolol
- Alprenolol
- Atenolol
- Labetalol
- Metoprolol
- Nadolol
- Oxprenolol
- Propranolol
- Sotalol
- And related compounds

E. DIURETICS, e.g.,

- Acetazolamide
- Amiloride
- Bendroflumethiazide
- Benzthiazide
- Bumetanide

- Canrenone
- Chlormerodrin (heroin)
- Chlortalidone
- Diclofenamide
- Ethacrynic acid
- Furosemide
- Hydrochlorothiazide
- Mersalyl
- Spironolactone
- Triamterene
- And related compounds

F. PEPTIDE HORMONES AND ANALOGS

- Chorionic Gonadotrophin (hCG, human chorionic gonadotrophin)
- Corticotrophin (ACTH)
- Growth Hormone (HGH, somatotrophin)
- Erythropoietin (EPO)

ANNEX 3: INTERNATIONAL OLYMPIC COMMITTEE MEDICAL COMMISSION

REQUIREMENTS FOR ACCREDITATION AND GOOD LABORATORY PRACTICES (1988)

PART A: REQUIREMENTS FOR IOC ACCREDITATION

A. REQUIREMENTS FOR IOC ACCREDITATION

1. Letters of Support

Laboratories seeking accreditation are requested to provide a letter of support of a national authority, e.g., NOC, sports governing body, etc., and any other letter of support that they would wish the Medical Commission to consider. The final decision regarding the acceptance of the letters of support will be made by the IOC Medical Commission, taking into account such factors as continuity, volume of workload, long-term financial support, administrative commitment of the host institution, and research activities and accomplishments such as publication records of senior staff.

2. Essential Equipment

2.1 Gas chromatography (GC)
2.2 High pressure liquid chromatography (HPLC)
2.3 Thin layer chromatography (TLC)
2.4 Mass spectrometry (MS) in combination with gas chromatography (GC) and computer evaluation
2.5 Access to radioimmunoassay equipment

3. Summary of Analytical Procedures

The IOC Medical Commission requires, *as a minimum*, the following procedures:

3.1 For nitrogen-containing doping agents excreted free: GC screening with a nitrogen specific detector (NPD) and capillary column, cross-linked with a moderate polarity phase, e.g., SE 54. Alternative suitable GC systems may be used.

3.2 For nitrogen-containing doping agents excreted as conjugates: GC screening after hydrolysis and extraction at pH 9.5, derivatization, cross-linked capillary column detection with a nitrogen specific detector (N-FID), or by selected ion monitoring (mass specific detection).

3.3 For pemoline, caffeine, and diuretics: screening with high pressure liquid chromatography.

3.4 For anabolic steroids:

  3.4.1 For free steroids: after extraction at pH 9.0 derivatization and detection by selected monitoring (mass specific detection).

  3.4.2 For conjugated steroids: after enzymatic hydrolysis, extraction, trimethylsilylation, and detection by selected ion monitoring (mass specific detection). Alternatively an extraction of the free and the conjugated fraction, e.g., with XAD-2 may be performed, followed by a separation of the two fractions, treated and analyzed as described above.

3.5 For acidic substances, e.g., diuretics and probenecid: extraction at, e.g., pH 2 or lower, and derivatization, GC with nitrogen specific detection after derivatization, or by selected ion monitoring (mass specific detection), or by high pressure liquid chromatography.

3.6 For β-blocking agents: GC and/or GC/MS screening.

3.7 For hCG: a suitable immunoassay to detect and quantitate hCG.

Note: Definite identification of a doping substance requires analysis by mass spectrometry.

Note: For hCG, a second suitable analytical method must be used before declaring a sample positive for hCG. This method will be recommended by the subcommission on doping and biochemistry of sport as soon as possible.

4. Accreditation of Analytical Laboratories

Analytical laboratories which request accreditation must fulfill the following requirements and answer the questionnaire (Part C of this document):

4.1 Initial requirements

4.1.1 Provide a list of substances which the laboratory is able to detect and identify. The minimum repertoire will be the list of examples enumerated in the dope definition of the IOC Medical Commission under the different classes of forbidden substances (and their metabolites).

4.1.2 Provide a list of available reference substances (dope agents and metabolites).

4.1.3 List of the excretion studies (dose, etc.) that have been performed on human volunteers. Whenever possible, state the minimum concentration which can be detected (based on an excretion study with a reasonable number of serial collections). The post-administration time at which this concentration was detected (and confirmed) should also be stated.

4.1.4 For each screening procedure, state the maximum time required to obtain a result after receipt of a single sample for analysis.

Note: Reference urines for which it is not possible to conduct volunteer studies (such as heroin) can be obtained with the cooperation of drug addition rehabilitation clinics.

4.2 Preaccreditation procedures

4.2.1 Prior to the official accreditation tests, laboratories seeking accreditation will be requested to analyze three sets of ten samples successively over a period which can vary from 6 to 12 months. The corresponding documentation (raw data) of the results shall be sent to the secretary of the doping subcommission.

4.3 Accreditation procedures

4.3.1 The laboratory seeking accreditation will be required to analyze ten control samples in the presence of a delegate of the IOC Subcommission on Doping and Biochemistry of Sport.

4.3.2 The laboratory must establish correctly and identify the dope agents and their relevant metabolites within a period of 3 days.

4.3.3 The report, copies of which should be sent by express courier to the chairman of the IOC Medical Commission and to each of the five members of the IOC Subcommission on Doping and Biochemistry of Sport within 3 weeks after completing the accreditation test, should include:

4.3.3.1 Protocols: complete description of the analytical procedures, with literature references.

4.3.3.2 Copies of the screening and confirmation raw data used in generating the results.

Note: The control samples will contain substances which are examples of the list of classes of banned substances. Blank urines may be includes as well as samples containing more than one (but not more than three) dope agent. For example, a sample may contain a diuretic and a metabolite, plus the metabolites of an anabolic steroid excreted mostly or entirely as biotransformation products.

4.3.4 Prior to visiting the laboratory, the delegate will be provided with all the documentation on the samples to be used in the accreditation of the laboratory concerned. If the laboratory produces correct results within the three days, the delegate will then discuss the results with the laboratory staff. The delegate will present a formal written report to the subcommission, using Part D of the present document. A copy of the confidential report will be sent to the laboratory.

4.3.5 After considering the data as well as other factors, the subcommission will announce its decision through the Chairman of the IOC Medical Commission. The laboratory will be informed by letter with 2 months of the submission.

Note: (1) For Olympic Games and major regional and area games, special requirements must be fulfilled as outlined in paragraph 4.7 below. (2) A temporary accreditation may be granted according to the conditions described in Annex 1.

4.4 Reaccreditation procedures — A document outlining the details of the procedure and conditions of reaccreditation will be sent to the laboratories 3 months prior to the test. Part of the reaccreditation procedure will be (1) the request to analyze up to ten control samples and reporting their results to the chairman of the IOC Medical Commission with copies to the secretary of the Subcommission on Doping and Biochemistry of Sport, (2) provide a fully documented report including raw data, and (3) sending a filled questionnaire. The questions will be such that the present status of the laboratory regarding personnel, instrumentation, space, etc., will be documented. Decisions regarding reaccreditation will be made on those factors as well as other available data.

4.5 Proficiency testing program — After accreditation, laboratories will be challenged with one set of four samples, every 4 months (excluding the reaccreditation period), representing a total of two cycles per year. The accredited laboratories must participate in the IOC Proficiency test (PT) which will be performed at regular intervals between the reaccreditation. Results and documentation are to be sent to the Secretary of the Subcommission.

4.6 Review mechanisms — Under certain circumstances, such as those indicated under 4.8 below, the Subcommission on Doping and Biochemistry of Sport reserves the right to inspect an accredited laboratory. The announcement of such an inspection will be made in writing by the Chairman of the IOC Medical Commission to the director of the laboratory concerned.

4.7 Special requirements — Laboratories seeking accreditation for forthcoming Olympic Games and Regional or Continental Games must first pass the accreditation 12 months before the event. Second, as part of the accreditation process, 4 months before the actual event, the laboratory must provide the following information (in writing) to the IOC Medical Commission of the progress made in preparing the laboratory for the Olympic Games and/or large international events, e.g., Regional or Continental Games:

4.7.1 Identification of external scientists (if required)

4.7.2 List of the staff (with qualifications) who will be working in the laboratory

4.7.3 Information on the number of samples which can be analyzed

4.7.4 Protocol of analytical methods (procedure manual)

4.7.5 A summary of the decision-making process to be used during the games, in the case both of positive and negative results.

Based on this information, the IOC Subcommission on Doping and Biochemistry of Sport will decide whether it will grant a special accreditation for the time period of the Olympic Games or important international events.

4.8 Reaccreditation and proficiency testing: policy, education, and consequences

4.8.1 In addition to the yearly reaccreditation procedures, the IOC Medical Commission has deviced a proficiency testing (PT) program, which is a part (in conjunction with laboratory inspection) of the initial evaluation of a laboratory seeking accreditation and of the continuing assessment of laboratory performance necessary to maintain this accreditation. For the purposes of reaccreditation, the IOC Medical Commission's Subcommission on Doping and Biochemistry of Sport will act as the review committee, chaired by the chairman of the IOC Medical Commission. For the PT, the review committee will consist of three members (secretary of the subcommission, one member of the subcommission and the head of an IOC accredited laboratory or a recognized scientist in the field of biochemical analysis). All procedures associated with the handling and testing of the proficiency test specimens after receipt by the laboratory should be carried out in a manner identical to that applied to normal laboratory specimens. The proficiency testing program will be implemented in early 1989 and its main purpose is educational. It is conceived, on an experimental basis until 1990, as performance assessment program on a regular basis, to correct deficiencies and to provide statistical interlaboratory comparisons. Therefore, the sanctions described under 4.8.3 will not be applied until the first proficiency cycle of 1990.

4.8.2 (a) For all banned drugs in the official IOC List, no false drug identifications are acceptable. A false positive will generally result in suspension of accreditation until the laboratory passes successfully the next reaccreditation. False negatives may lead under circumstances to suspension of accreditation. (b) Quantitative results (caffeine, sympathomimetic amines, etc.) and testosterone/epitestosterone ratios must fall within two standard deviations (or ±15% whichever is lager) of the calculated group mean resulting from all participating laboratories testing a given drug, excluding those results which hare outside the 95% confidence interval of all results.

Note: A higher concentration than that defined by these standards will be regarded as a false positive, while a lower concentration will be considered a false negative.

4.8.3 In the proficiency testing program, the procedure for dealing with a false negative or a false positive report from a laboratory will be the following:

4.8.3.1 Immediate notice to the laboratory.
4.8.3.2 Allow the laboratory 10 working days to respond to the error. This response should include the submission of data from the batch of specimens in which the error occurred, unless the error is to be explained as an administrative error.
4.8.3.3 Ten working days will be allowed for review of the response. The response will be reviewed by members of the review committee which will have the authority to decide whether the laboratory explanation can be accepted as an error which was beyond its control (such as a clerical error where the laboratory can document that the analysis which it submitted was not the one attributed to it). If the error is determined to be attributable to the laboratory and that it is (a) *an administrative error* (clerical, sample mix-up, etc.), the review committee will have the option of recommending corrective action to minimize the occurrence of the particular error in the future and if necessary to review and request previously run specimens to be reanalyzed if there is reason to believe that the error might have been systematic. If it is (b) *a technical or methodological error* the laboratory must submit all data from the batch of specimens which included the test specimen with the erroneous analysis. In addition, the laboratory will be required to test additional specimens. The exact procedure, including the number of samples to be reanalyzed, will be determined by the review committee after consideration of the results and the analytical data. The review committee will have the option to recommend (1) no further action other than the above (in the case of less serious error with associated corrective action which reasonably assures the unlikelihood of reoccurrence), or (2) suspension of accreditation until the next reaccreditation procedure as described in 4.8.4.
4.8.3.4 During the time required to resolve the error, the laboratory would remain on the IOC registry but with a designation that a (some) false negative(s) result(s) is (are) pending resolution. If the review committee recommends that the laboratory should undergo reaccreditation, suspension will then become the official status of the laboratory until that reaccreditation takes place.

4.8.4 For yearly reaccreditation, ten samples, the composition of which is described under 4.10, the following will apply in the case of false negatives. The percentage as listed below will be based on the number of substances present in the test samples. For example, if each of the ten samples contains two substances, 90% correct results will mean the correct identification (and/or quantitation where appropriate) of 18 substances.

100% correct results: reaccreditation
90% correct results: as described under 4.8
80% correct results: as described under 4.8
70% correct results: the accreditation of the laboratory will be suspended. Reinstatement may be achieved conditional to success in two proficiency testing cycles and the following year accreditation procedure. An inspection, as described under review mechanisms, is possible. During the time that the accreditation is suspended, the laboratory *must* abstain from accepting samples from international federations, national olympic committees, and national federations. Noncompliance with this requirement may lead to irreversible revocation of accreditation.

4.8.5 Once accreditation is suspended, a laboratory must participate in two additional consecutive proficiency testing cycles and the next reaccreditation procedure. If deemed necessary, it must also agree to an inspection before reinstatement as an accredited laboratory can be considered.

4.8.6 In the case of false positive(s), the same procedure as described above (4.8.5) for 70% correct results will apply.

4.9 Code of ethics — In order to maintain the status of IOC accredited laboratory, its director must agree in writing to comply with all the dispositions of the IOC Medical Commission Code of Ethics for accredited laboratories.

4.10 Specimen composition for accreditation and proficiency testing — Samples appropriate for proficiency testing, accreditation, and reaccreditation purposes will be obtained after administration of one or more doping agents at the doses listed in Annex IV. Each sample may contain one or more compounds (but possibly several metabolites). In addition, nicotine and caffeine may be present in low concentrations. After ingestion of a pharmaceutical dose, the urines will be collected and the cumulative urines combined in such a way that the following range of concentrations (in weight units/ml urine) will be achieved.

a. Stimulants: 0.5 to 50 µg/ml (except strychnine at 0.2 µg/ml and Pipradol at 0.1 µg/ml)
b. Narcotics: 0.5 to 50 µg/ml
c. Anabolic steroids: about 10 ng/ml for the main metabolite
d. β-blockers: 0.5 to 50 µg/ml
e. Diuretics: 0.1 to 2 µg/ml
f. Urine with a high caffeine concentration will be a spiked urine.

These concentration ranges have been chosen to allow detection of the drug and/or metabolites) by IOC recommended screening techniques. These levels are generally in the range of concentrations which might be expected in the urines of athletes using banned drugs. For some drugs, the specimen composition will consist of the parent drug as well as major metabolites as noted above. In some cases, more than one drug class may be included in one specimen, but generally no more than three will be present in any one specimen to more reasonably represent the type of specimen which a laboratory normally encounters. Within a particular proficiency testing cycle, the actual composition of specimens going to different laboratories will vary. It is presumed that these concentrations and drug types will be changed periodically due to factors such as changes in detection technology and patterns of drug abuse. Annex IV reproduces the current list of banned classes of drugs with examples. Finally, it should be noted that the concentration ranges listed above represent ranges of concentration expected, under realistic circumstances, after the administration of banned drugs to or by athletes. They should not be interpreted as cutoff values, or as limits of detection and/or quantitation.

REFERENCES

1. **Donike, M.,** Erfahrungen mit dem Stickstoffdetektor (N-FID) bei der Dopingkontrolle, *Medizinische Technik*, 92, 153, 1972.
2. **Donike, M., Zimmermann, J., Bärwald, K. R., Schänzer, W., Christ, V., Klostermann, K., und Opfermann, G.,** Routinebestimmung von Anabolika in Harn, *Deutsche Zeitschrift für Sportmedizin*, 35, 14–24, 1984.
3. Medical Commission of the International Olympic Committee, Requirements for Accreditation and Good Laboratory Practices, 1988.

Chapter 35

POSSIBILITIES AND ACHIEVEMENTS OF THE BCR PROGRAM

B. Griepink

TABLE OF CONTENTS

I.	Introduction	240
II.	State-of-the-Art of Chemical Analysis	241
III.	Means to Improve Measurement Quality	241
	A. Within Laboratory Measures	242
	1. QA Manual	242
	2. Statistical Control and Use of Control Charts	243
	3. Verification of Results by Using Other Methods	243
	4. Application of Certified Reference Materials (CRMs)	245
	B. Between Laboratory Measures	246
	1. Aims of Intercomparisons	246
	2. Results of Intercomparisons	247
IV.	Improvement of Measurement Quality Using the BCR Program	247
	A. Examples of Achievements Obtained in BCR Intercomparisons	247
V.	Certified Reference Materials (CRMs)	249
	A. Requirements	249
	1. Homogeneity	249
	2. Stability	249
	3. Similarity with the Real Sample	251
	4. Accuracy, Uncertainty, and Traceability	251
VI.	Some Examples of Current BCR Projects	251
	A. Biomedical Analysis	252
	B. Examples of Projects Related to Food and Agricultural Products	252
	C. Environmental Analysis	252
	D. Example of a Project in Metrology	253
VII.	Possibilities to Participate in BCR Work	253
	A. Proposals	253
	B. Selection Criteria	254
	C. Financial Support to Projects	254
References		255

I. INTRODUCTION

The aim of the Bureau Communitaire de Reference of the European Economic Communities (BCR) program is to improve accuracy in the methods of measurement, and thereby to bring harmony to the results obtained throughout the community. The task consists essentially of bringing together, for each project, laboratories of possibly all the member states for collaborative work to improve the measurement or analysis concerned.

The participants in such an exercise all receive the same sample (stability and homogeneity have been verified prior to the exercise) and determine the chosen components. Afterward, all results are examined in a meeting in which all participate and conclusions can be drawn on each laboratory's performance and on the errors and their sources in the method or its application in the particular laboratory. If necessary, a second exercise (intercomparison) can be held to verify the conclusions and estimate the effect of the changes or adaptations made as a consequence of the conclusions arrived at before.

In some cases, where the measurements are of a complicated nature, this "intercomparison" exercise is repeated several times, each time to verify another part of the whole chain of measurement (e.g., extraction, cleanup, separation, identification, and quantitations) with improvements made at each step until a satisfactory agreement is reached. The results are then disseminated not only by reports and publications, but also by means of reference materials or by the calibrations provided by metrology laboratories. The transfer of know-how is the essence of the program both during and after the execution of the projects.

Among the projects that were proposed to the commission and then accepted for support, a large proportion concerned written standards or *community directives*. They originated from laboratories in the member states which had experienced measurement difficulties and where it was realized that norms and directives would have little harmonization effect if measurements were not satisfactory.

The program was requested, for example, to work on problems related to the *directives* on water pollution, heavy metals in blood, dangerous chemicals (e.g., carcinogens, dioxins), sulfur in fuels, and protection against noise and measurements related to the quality of agricultural products (e.g., flour, cereals, meat, milk, wine, fruit juice).

The BCR program does not produce any written standard; it helps the process of standardization by providing the technical support needed for the correct implementation of methods of measurements (in particular by establishing reference materials when necessary).

In addition, it also aims to solve, through collaborative activities, the challenging measurement problems important to industry, whether they are for classical applications (e.g., thermal conductivity), advanced technologies (e.g., electronics, high frequency telecommunications, etc.) or environmental (e.g., food or biomedical analyses).

In the current BCR program the priority areas are

1. *Biomedical analyses* giving priority to:

   - The determination of enzymes and hormones (in human serum)
   - Hematological tests (e.g., blood coagulations)
   - Analyses related to cardiovascular diseases
   - Analyses of tumor markers and drugs in the human body

2. *Analyses related to food and agriculture*, in particular,

   - Analyses related to health of farm animals (feedstuffs, hormones, antibiotics, etc.) and to the quality of cereals, fruits, and vegetables
   - Analyses related to the quality of processed food (nutritional properties, presence of dangerous substances, bacterial contamination)

3. *Analyses related to the environment*, in particular,

   - The determination of pollutants in water
   - The determination of traces of heavy elements in various matrices
   - The determination of traces of dangerous compounds in various matrices
   - The determination of air pollutants at the work place
   - The mutagenicity of chemical substances

4. *Analyses of metals*, essentially nonferrous metals and surface analysis of materials.

5. *Applied metrology*. The emphasis will be placed upon the measurement and calibration of quantities which are the most important for testing laboratories and for laboratories in industry, in particular for quality control purposes.

This list is not exclusive. Other topics can be taken into

TABLE 1
Results of Analysis of Spiked Milk Powder for Chlorinated Pesticides (BCR, 1981)

Compound	Range (mg/kg)	Factor (highest value: lowest value)	Added contents (mg/kg)
HCB	0.001–0.22	220	0.28
α-HCH	0.009–0.60	67	0.11
γ-HCH	0.00114–0.18	158	0.20
DDE	0.0043–0.47	109	0.54
op'DDT	0.003–0.24	80	—
β-HCH	0.01–0.13	13	0.08
β-HEPO	0.001–0.13	130	0.12
Dieldrin	0.01–0.104	10	0.10
pp'DDT	0.005–0.36	72	—

account, provided that they meet the criteria of solving a measurement problem of community interest, i.e., implementation of a directive or removal of trade hindrances.

II. STATE-OF-THE-ART OF CHEMICAL ANALYSIS

The introduction and wide-spread use of modern automated instruments has certainly allowed to determine determinants at much lower levels and to achieve a high sample throughput. This, however, has not *ipso facto* led to accurate results; on the contrary, the many sources of error possible, of which the analyst is hardly aware (e.g., software is often not given by the manufacturer), can cause large errors of analysis.

Estimations made in FRG of the direct costs caused by such errors amount to a value of 10^9 ECU per annum;[1] the indirect costs are at least an order of magnitude higher.

Trace element analysis may show variations in results of up to a factor of 10 or more; e.g., in 1983, for seawater analysis on Cd, Pb, and Hg spreads were observed of 0.0001 to 0.123, 0.001 to 0.036, and 0.0004 to 0.002 μg/l respectively. In the determination of polycyclic aromatic hydrocarbons (PAHs) in spiked coconut oil (1987, BCR) carried out by very experienced laboratories typical spreads of a factor of 2 to 3 were obtained at levels of 30 to 600 μg/kg. In an exercise of laboratory proficiency testing for trace metals in an aqueous solution (mg/l), Einerson et al.[2] found for As values between 0.025 and 1200 (target value upon dissolution: 1) and for Hg values between 0.395 and 1.23 (target 0.5).

Table 1 gives an impression of the spread between some 40 experienced laboratories in the determination of chlorinated pesticides in spiked milk powder (BCR, 1983).

These and many other examples in the open literature clearly demonstrate that large errors may occur in relatively simple cases.[3-11]

III. MEANS TO IMPROVE MEASUREMENT QUALITY

Measurement quality can be improved and assessed at two levels.

1. Within the laboratory (e.g., quality manual, control charts, use of certified reference materials)
2. Between laboratories (e.g., participation in intercomparisons, proficiency testing by an independent organization).

Two basic parameters should be considered when discussing results of analysis: the accuracy (absence of systematic errors) and uncertainty (coefficient of variation: confidence interval) as caused by random errors and random variations in the procedure. In this context, accuracy is of primary importance, but if the uncertainty in a result is too high, it cannot be used to come to any conclusion about the outcome of an experiment or to judge the quality of the environment or of food, nor can it be used for the diagnosis of a patient's illness. An unacceptably high uncertainty renders the result useless.

In the analysis, all basic principles of the calibration, the elimination of sources of contamination and losses, the correction for interferences, etc. should be followed.[12-16] Owing to a vast extent of automation calibration is paramount. Modern equipment often does not allow the analyst to follow the actual performance in analysis. Therefore, he should carefully consider that the basis of all results, i.e., the calibration, is done properly. Various calibration methods have all their advantages and drawbacks. It is the art and the skill of the specially trained analytical chemist to make the proper choice considering, e.g., linearity verification, bracketing standards, matrix matching, standard addition, presence of internal and external standards, verification of purity, identity and stoichiometry of calibrants used, etc.

Modern equipment often requires calibration with a similar matrix (e.g., solid sampling Zeeman ETAAS). In such a case, a calibration with more than one reference material to be verified by a calibration with a pure solution is recommended.

A. WITHIN LABORATORY MEASURES

Within laboratory quality assurance[17-21] involves, among others,

1. Implementation of a detailed quality assurance (QA) manual
2. A regime of statistical control of results from daily routine
3. Analysis for verification (e.g., use of reference methods)
4. Application of certified reference materials

1. QA Manual

Good laboratory practice (GLP) is one of the manifestations of the increased attention paid to the achievement of good quality results. GLP involves quality assurance (QA), although QA can and should be applied in cases where the formal GLP system is not required. GLP is therefore the system with direct legal implication (e.g., [eco]toxicology). The need for a QA- or GLP-framework of guidelines to bring the quality of a laboratory to such a level that it meets predefined standards, arises from the economic, scientific, or political implication of laboratory results.

GLP guidelines have been laid down in written form by the OECD,[22] the principles of GLP as developed by the FDA and EPA were adopted by U.S. law in 1979. GLP describes the way the laboratory should work, its organization, and the way to produce valid results. Analytical methods are not mentioned. GLP guidelines are implemented in a laboratory through a QA program which is delineated in a QA manual. This comprises a detailed description of the items listed next in order to assess and monitor the quality of the analytical results.

The summary given below was compiled by Vijverberg and Cofino.[18]

1. Test facilities, organization, and personnel

   - Location of the laboratories and safety aspects
   - Structure of the organization and allocation of responsibilities
   - Education
   - Management

2. Quality Assessment

   - Interlaboratory and intralaboratory testing programs
   - Reference material

3. Statistical quality control

   - Control charts

4. Apparatus, chemicals, reagents, and blank

   - Apparatus
     - Preventive maintenance and maintenance calibration
     - Cleaning glassware and nonglassware
   - Chemicals
     - Registration
     - Quality control checks
     - Rules for storage of waste
     - Handling and storage
   - Reagents
     - Standard solution
   - Blank

5. Sampling and storage

   - Sampling strategy
   - Way of sampling
   - Storage and preservation
   - Sample identification

6. Documentation

   - Study
   - Methods

- Work sheets
- Notebook

7. Reporting of results

    - Not computerized
    - Computerized

8. Archiving of results

In the framework of this paper, most attention will be paid to those aspects of the above listing where the BCR can be of help or play a role: inter- and intralaboratory testing programs, materials for use for control charts, and certified reference materials.

2. Statistical Control and Use of Control Charts

When a laboratory works at a constant level of high quality (i.e., in the absence of detectable systematic errors), fluctuations in the results become random and can be predicted statistically.[23]

This implies, in the first place, that limits of determination and detection should be constant and well known;[24] rules for rounding off final results should be based on the performance of the method in the laboratory. Furthermore, if such a situation of absence of systematic fluctuations exists, normal statistics (e.g., regression analysis, t-, and F-tests, analysis of variance, etc.) can be applied to study the results wherever necessary.[24]

Besides these checks, control checks should be used as soon as the method is in control in the laboratory. A control chart provides a graphical way of interpreting the method's output in time, so that the repeatability of the results and the method's precision over a period of time can be evaluated at a glance. To do so, one or several standards of good homogeneity and stability should be analyzed with each batch of unknown materials. Some 5 to 10% of all samples should be used for this purpose.[25] In a SHEWHART control chart[25] the laboratory plots for each standard analyzed at a time the obtained value (X) or the difference between duplicate values (R). The X-chart additionally presents the lines corresponding to a risk of five, respectively, 1% that the results are not comprised in the whole population of results. These lines are for "warning" and "action", respectively (Figure 1). Figure 2 presents an example of the determination of the chemical oxygen demand using dichromate (COD_{Cr}) of a control solution, taken from the quality handbook of the Nordish Council of Ministers.[26]

The results of a method are considered to be out of control if

1. The upper or lower control limit is exceeded ("action")
2. The same "alarm line" is exceeded twice in succesion
3. Eleven successive measurements are on the same side of the line

X- and R-chart systems are also being tested in which the weighing factor for each point of the curve decreases according to a geometric progression (e.g., let the value at moment i be X_i, then the value plotted in a chart for a moment is

$$X_i + (X_{i-1})\, 0.2 + (X_{i-2})\, 0.16 + ...)$$

This gives an earlier detection of an upward or downward trend.

Cumulative sum ("cusum") charts are frequently used, particularly as an early detection of a drift in the results. In these charts, the cumulative sum of the differences between found value and probable value are plotted against the result obtained at moment i

$$s_i = \sum_{i=1}^{i}(X_i - X_{ref})$$

in which s_i is the cumulative sum, X_i is the measured value, and X_{ref} is the reference value which should be accurately known. Dewey and Hunt[27] presented a practical evaluation of the use of cusum charts. It should be emphasized that good results can only be obtained if the value of X_{ref} is accurately known. A certified reference material of good quality should therefore be used. The evaluation of a cusum chart is done using the V-mask method.[28-30]

In laboratories with a high throughput of analyses of various kinds, such monitoring of performance can be done in an automated way controlled by computer. Software packages may become available soon.

3. Verification of Results by Using Other Methods

The use of control charts as discussed in the previous chapter allows to detect the introduction of sources of systematic errors following changes of equipment, etc. (e.g., new reagents or solvents, new technician, new capillary column, etc.). They, however, are not able to detect

X – CHART

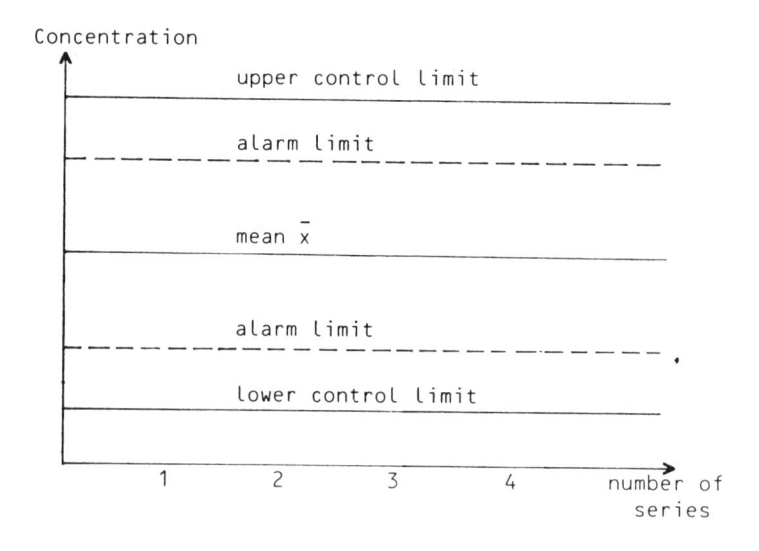

[Chart showing Concentration on y-axis with horizontal lines for upper control limit, alarm limit, mean x̄, alarm limit, lower control limit; x-axis labeled number of series 1–4]

R – CHART

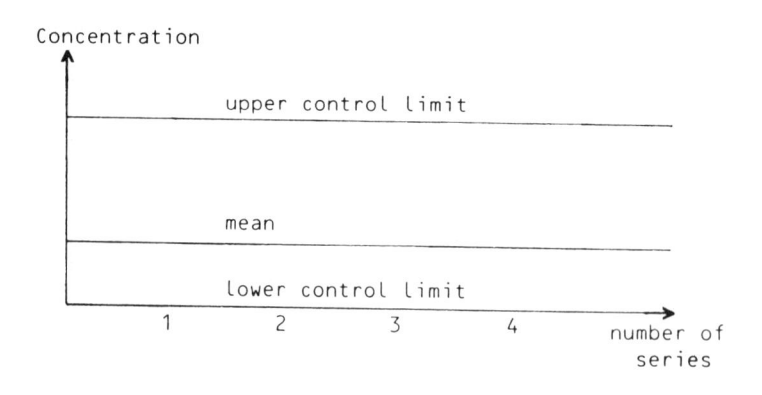

[Chart showing Concentration on y-axis with horizontal lines for upper control limit, mean, lower control limit; x-axis labeled number of series 1–4]

FIGURE 1. Example of X- and R-charts.

a constant systematic error present at the introduction of the quality performance charts. To detect such sources of error in order to eliminate them, two possibilities exist which can be regarded as being complementary:

1. Verification using a different method
2. Application of a certified reference material

No method exists which is principally free of sources of error be it human failures or methodological or instrumental insufficiencies. Comparison of results obtained by two entirely different techniques (e.g., a destructive and a nondestructive technique or MS/MS and GC/ECD) often allows to detect errors in the methods as applied by the laboratory. The more different the measurement principles of the two methods are, the more evidence for presence or absence of systematic methodological errors can be obtained.

If the method of confrontation is a method of which the sources of error and the effects of the various steps are well known and if this method is relatively insensitive with respect to human failures, one can call it a "reference method".

The application of such a reference method, if possible, belongs to a good quality control system. However, good reference or independent methods do not always exist. Furthermore, if the technician using this reference method is not sufficiently experienced with the method,

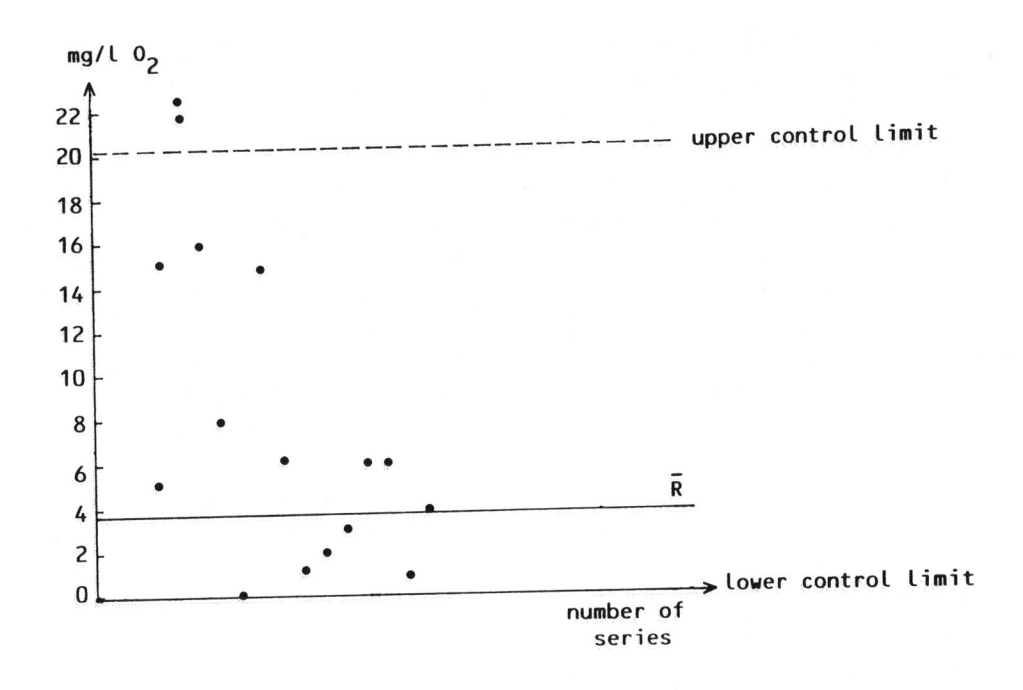

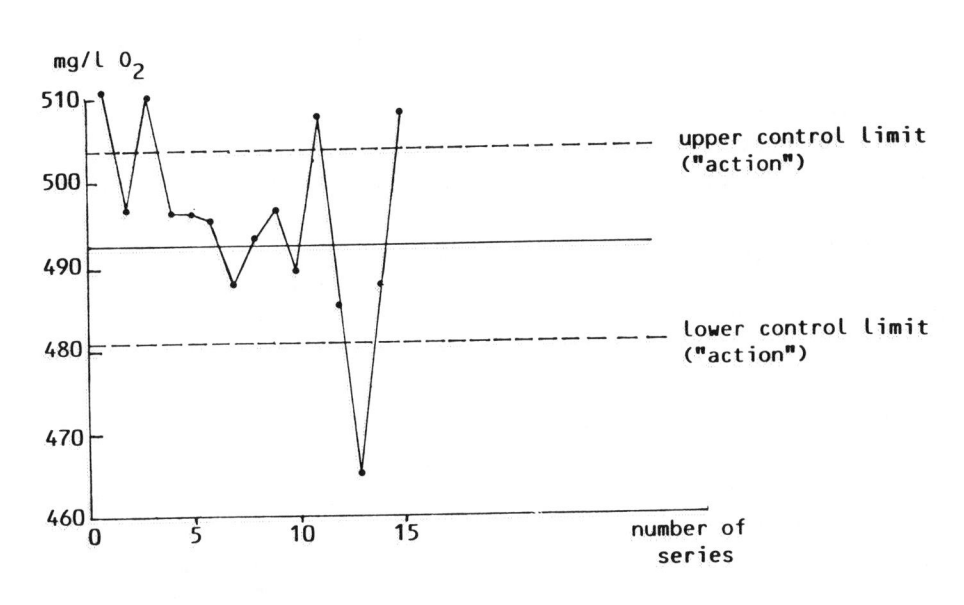

FIGURE 2. R- and X-chart of a COD-determination.[26]

the application may even create errors. The results of a method are not only dependent on the method, but also on the person who uses it.

Good reference methods for trace element determinations are isotope dilution mass spectrometry (IDMS) (provided that the digestion takes place in a closed system after addition of the spike) and activation techniques.

For organic compounds, isotope dilution mass spectrometry, if applicable, is a technique to be used for the development of a reference method, as shown by Siekmann at various occasions[31,32] and in BCR-certification campaigns.[33,34] IDMS is the proper method for the determinations of, e.g., cortisol, oestradiol, or progesterone in human serum.

4. Application of Certified Reference Materials (CRMs)

Results can only be accurate and comparable worldwide if they are traceable. By definition, traceability of a measurement is achieved by an unbroken chain of calibrations connecting the measurement process to the fundemental units. In the vast majority of chemical analysis, the chain is broken because the sample is physically destroyed by dissolutions, calcination, etc. To ensure the full traceability, it is necessary to demonstrate that no loss or contamination has occurred in the course of the sample treatment.

Indeed the physical calibration of all measuring instruments is not always of great importance for the chemist. The manner in which the calibration curve is established for the particular assays is of prime importance (it has to take into account all possible interferences) as well as the conditions of sample treatment.

The only possibility for any laboratory to ensure traceability in a simple manner is to verify the analytical procedure by means of a so-called matrix reference material certified in a reliable manner.

The laboratory which measures such a reference material by its own procedure and finds a value in disagreement with the certified value is thus warned that its measurement includes an error of which the source must be identified.

Besides the aspect of achieving traceability, certified reference materials having well-known and well-documented properties should be used for the following:

1. Demonstrate the accuracy of results obtained in a laboratory
2. Monitor the performance of the method (e.g., cusum charts)
3. Calibrate equipment which requires a calibrant similar to the matrix (e.g., optical emission spectrometry, X-ray fluorescence spectrometry)
4. Demonstrate equivalence between methods
5. Detect errors in the application of standardized methods (e.g., ISO, ASTM, ECCLS, ...)

B. BETWEEN LABORATORY MEASURES

If sufficient CRMs of similar composition as the unknowns are available or if an accurate (free of systematic errors) method is operated in the laboratory, good evidence of accuracy of results can be given. However, such ideal conditions hardly exist in most laboratories for most tasks. Therefore intercomparisons are frequently conducted.

Most analytical methods comprise the following two steps:

1. Sample (pre)treatment (e.g., extraction, cleanup, digestion, separation, preconcentration, ...)
2. Final measurement (spectrometry techniques, voltammetry, mass spectrometry, gas chromatography, ...)

Specific sources of error are connected to each of these steps. As pointed out before, sources of error can be detected by comparing results obtained by many widely differing techniques which are only available in a group of several laboratories. Moreover, intercomparisons allow the detection of a source of error not mentioned so far — the typical attitude of the laboratory (personnel) itself, e.g., the way to calibrate, to avoid contamination or loss, the attitude toward the demands of the work, the degree of training and responsibility of the laboratory worker, etc. That is the reason that laboratories with different methods cover well the aspects 1 and 2 mentioned above still are keen to participate in intercomparisons. This way they can test and compare the performance of their laboratory for a special test.

When different laboratories participate in an intercomparison, different sample pretreatment methods and different techniques of final determination are in discussion as well as these laboratories. If results of such an intercomparison are in good and statistical agreement, the collaboratively obtained value is likely to be the best approximation of the truth. If such an exercise is properly designed for the purpose of certification (e.g., selection of competent laboratories, work under a strict QA regime, and achievement of traceability of a measurement) the intercomparison may lead to a certification.

1. Aims of Intercomparisons

Before conducting an intercomparison, the aims should be clearly defined. An intercomparison can be held

1. To detect the pitfalls of a commonly applied method and to ascertain its performance in practice
2. To measure the quality of a laboratory or a part of a laboratory (e.g., audits for accredited laboratories)
3. To improve the quality of a laboratory in collaborative work with mutual learning processes
4. To certify the contents of a reference material

In the ideal situation, where the results of all laboratories are in control and systematic errors have been eliminated, intercomparisons of type 2 and 4 will be held only. For the time being, however, types 1 and 3 play an important role. The organization of the collaborative trial, the sort of samples, and the laboratories invited depend strongly on the aim of the exercise.

The evaluation of the results submitted should be done accordingly. The basic principles are given in norms and ISO guidelines.[35]

2. Results of Intercomparisons

Horwitz generalized experiences obtained over many years in intercomparisons in the U.S. FDA. As a rule of thumb, he indicates[36,37] that the agreement between laboratories (expressed as the interlaboratory coefficient of variation, CV [%]) depends on the content of the analyte:

$$CV(\%) = 2^{(1-\frac{1}{2}\log C)}$$

in which C is the content expressed as g/g. The curve representing this equation is commonly called the "Horwitz-trumpet".

This rule of Horwitz is not a law of nature. When participating laboratories have not been in quality exercises before, the results most likely are worse than indicated; well-trained and experienced laboratories with a good history in quality control, which therefore may be selected for certification purposes, may do better. Figures 3A and B illustrate this.

To certify chlorinated biphenyl congeners in various matrices (e.g., fish), a special group has been formed in the BCR framework. In a carefully designed sequence of intercomparisons of the type given in Section III.B.1, (3) in which all aspects of the determination were checked in consequence, participating laboratories improved their performance.[39] In 1985, an intercomparison was held and the interlaboratory CV (%) for the seven congeners (IUPAC Nrs: 28, 52, 101, 118, 138, 153, and 180) is plotted in Figure 3A. It can be seen that the CV (%) is slightly better than expected from the above equation. However, this was considered to be insufficient for certification and further studies were made. Then in 1987, different fish oils were analyzed and the CV (%) was considerably improved (Figure 3B). After such improvement, certification was done.[39]

IV. IMPROVEMENT OF MEASUREMENT QUALITY USING THE BCR PROGRAM

As pointed out before basically the BCR program follows two routes to improve the quality of measurement

1. Intercomparisons, to detect sources of error and consequently remove them

2. Certification of reference materials (once a sufficient quality of measurement has been achieved by a pilot group) to disseminate the obtained quality

A. EXAMPLES OF ACHIEVEMENTS OBTAINED IN BCR INTERCOMPARISONS

Intercomparisons are a useful and important means to avoid systematic errors in laboratories, to assess the quality of work done in the laboratory, to motivate laboratory workers, and to demonstrate the quality of a laboratory's result to its "customers" (e.g., public authorities).

The following will give some experiences obtained in the BCR program. Participants discussed thoroughly the reasons for discrepancy after an intercomparison and charged and improved their methods in the light of the outcome of the discussion before embarking on a new exercise with a different sample. The determination of various hormones in human plasma is not easy because most methods lack selectivity. It is likely that too high values are obtained with techniques such as RIA.

Intercomparisons have shown discrepancies in the order of magnitude of a factor of 20; even very experienced laboratories did not agree better than by a factor of 2 between means of results obtained by the same techniques.[40] This is unacceptable for diagnostic but certainly for therapeutic reasons.

It was decided to use IDMS as the method of certification of cortisol in serum, since this method is not prone to a bias toward too high values.[40] Indeed, after a series of intercomparisons among users of GC/MS equipment, the between laboratory CV became smaller than the within laboratory CV (typically 0.4 and 1.2%, respectively).[33]

Figure 4A (top) presents the results for CB 118 obtained in a quality improvement exercise on chlorinated biphenyl congeners.[38] Occupational health laboratories determine the amounts of organic vapor sorbed on a suitable reagent attached to the worker's dress. At the end of a working day, the sorbers are analyzed to investigate whether the worker's exposure has been within the legal limits.

A group of industrial and official laboratories was formed and over a few years time some intercomparisons were held to improve the measurement quality. Figure 4A (bottom) presents the successive improvements necessary for the certification.

Many other similar examples could be given to illustrate the improvements made in a series of intercomparisons. Some other examples can be found in the literature.[41]

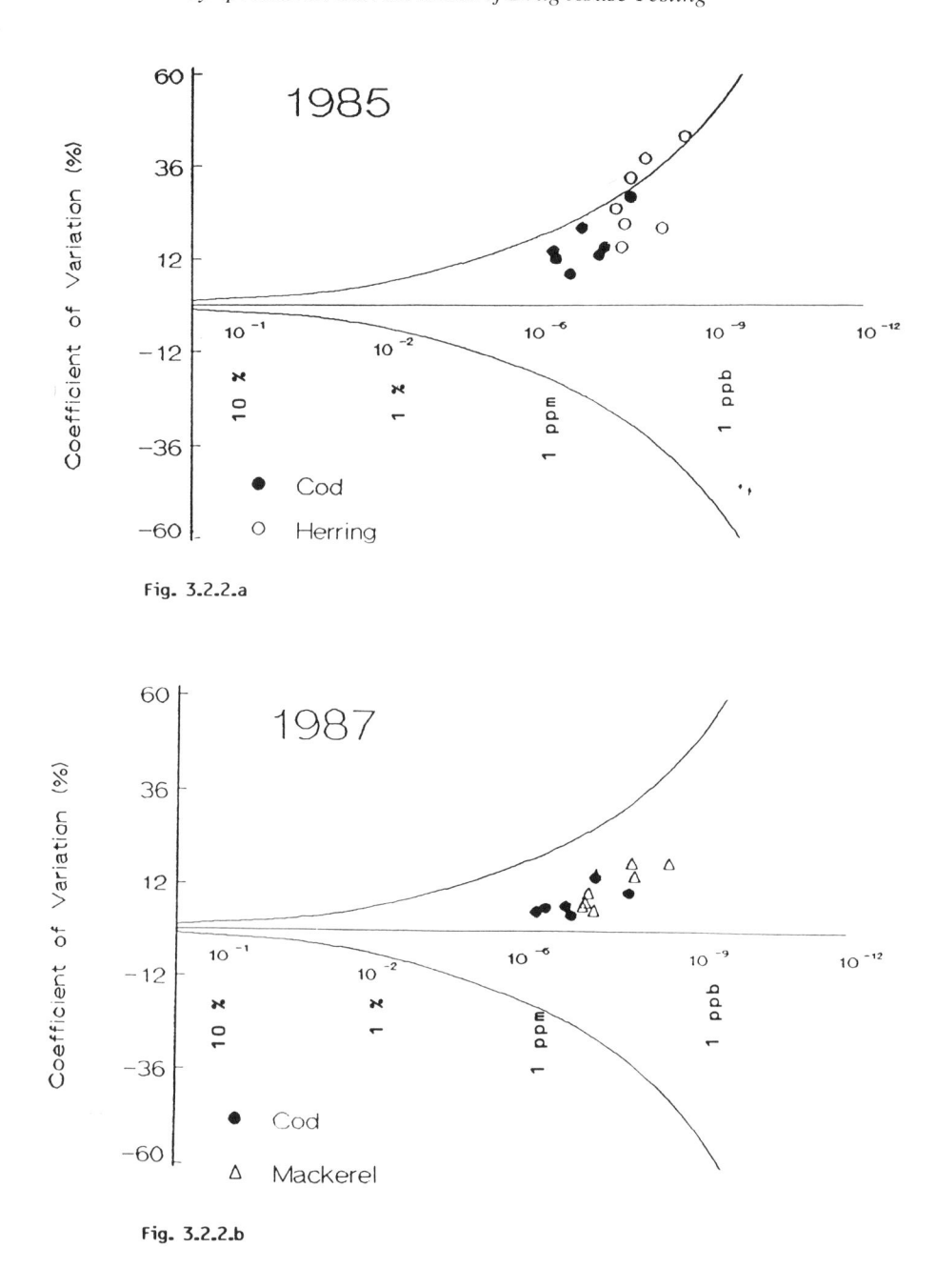

FIGURE 3. (A and B) Interlaboratory mean values for seven chlorinated biphenyl congeners in two fish oils analyzed in 1985 and 1987.

Experiences of various control schemes (e.g., AOAC [U.S.], VDLUFA [D], EPA [U.S.], WRC [U.K.], TNO [NL], and others) all point in the same direction; participation in intercomparisons is a useful tool if the laboratory intends to improve the quality of work or to demonstrate this quality.

In intercomparisons for the improvement of the quality of the participants' results, wherever possible, two similar samples with different contents should be studied. The results of each laboratory can be presented in a so-called Youden plot.[42,43] The abcissa (x) is used for the first sample, the ordinate (y) for the second. Thus each laboratory is represented by one point. When the laboratory is situated in the vicinity of the point representing the most accurate values of the two samples, its performance is good. If the laboratory is in good control but has systematic errors (e.g., calibration), their position can be found close to the line y = x. In case the within laboratory consistency is poor their results are in the lower right and upper left quadrant.

The evaluation becomes more difficult if the contents differ more widely or if the matrix varies. However, in cases where such exercises were carried out on a regular basis, a definite improvement of the performance of the participants could be indicated.[44]

Figure 4B gives an example of such a plot obtained in a BCR intercomparison for the determination of methylmercury in fish extracts, showing that most of the results of all laboratories are consistent (i.e., good control, although not always accurate), but that some of them still suffer from systematic errors (e.g., labs 12 and 13).

V. CERTIFIED REFERENCE MATERIALS (CRMs)

The use of certified reference materials has been indicated previously in this paper. This part will deal in more detail with the requirements for CRMs.[45-47]

IUPAC defines that the value of a certified reference material (NIST: "standard reference material") is being "based on the consistent results obtained by using indepedent analytical techniques". In the view of the BCR this definition should be enlarged to: "based on the consistent results obtained by using different analytical techniques which are likely to give accurate results for the particular matrix and which are applied by different independent laboratories". The last addition gives tribute to the important factor of the laboratory.

The following categories of CRMs can be mentioned.

1. Pure substances
2. Matrix materials
3. CRMs for the calibration of relative methods (e.g., mass spectrometry of solid materials, XRF, ...)
4. Biological CRMs used for the measurement of biologically defined parameters (e.g., vitamin content in food, thromboplastins in serum)

CRMs should have the same traceability to the primary units as the transfer standards used for physical measurements.

A. REQUIREMENTS

CRMs have to fulfill many requirements which in practice are often contradictory. Therefore, compromises are necessary. A CRM "fresh strawberries" can never exist; ground and dried strawberry powder would be the best approximation.

1. Homogeneity

Standards in physics that are not destroyed when applied can be unique. CRMs in chemistry can be used once only, when taken out of their ampule, bottle, or other container. Therefore the amount of starting material should be high. This high amount (e.g., 20 to 50 kg of dried and powderized material) must be homogeneous to assure that every sample out of this bulk should have the same composition. But even in a sample (e.g., bottle with 40 g) there should be homogeneity, as normally laboratories take subsamples for analysis of about 100 to 1000 mg.

Homogeneity decreases with decreasing subsample size. The producer of a CRM therefore gives the minimum amount of sample for which the homogeneity is sufficient, i.e., for which the uncertainty caused by inhomogeneity does not exceed the uncertainty of the certified values.

Suitable techniques to study matrix homogeneity for trace elements are XRF, INAA, ICP, etc. Their standard deviation should be small as compared to the final uncertainty aimed at in the certification. In a homogeneity study, all care is applied to obtain a good repeatability; in this stage the accuracy of the techniques is of less importance.

The homogeneity of a sample is investigated by repeated analysis at different levels of intake and comparing the coefficients of variation of the obtained results with those expected from the analytical methods themselves.[38,39] This approach involves many individual repetitions, but various techniques of analysis (e.g., INAA, ICP, [ET]AAS) can be applied. Whenever a method is in full statistical control for a given matrix, the sampling constants method[40-43] can be followed.

Segregation is always possible if the CRM is not a pure compound. Matrix CRMs and biological CRMs usually contain more phases of different particle size of different density. Segregation will occur even upon standing on a laboratory bench. Rehomogenization before taking the analytical subsample is required.

2. Stability

The user of a CRM should know how long he can use his samples. The manufacturer of the CRM therefore makes all necessary investigations to obtain the necessary information on the stability or even find a date of expiration.

Long-term tests are thus carried out at various temperatures and different conditions of light. Also effects of short-term exposures to, e.g., high temperatures (simulating a transport situation) or moist air (simulating normal laboratory use) are studied. In some cases a stability

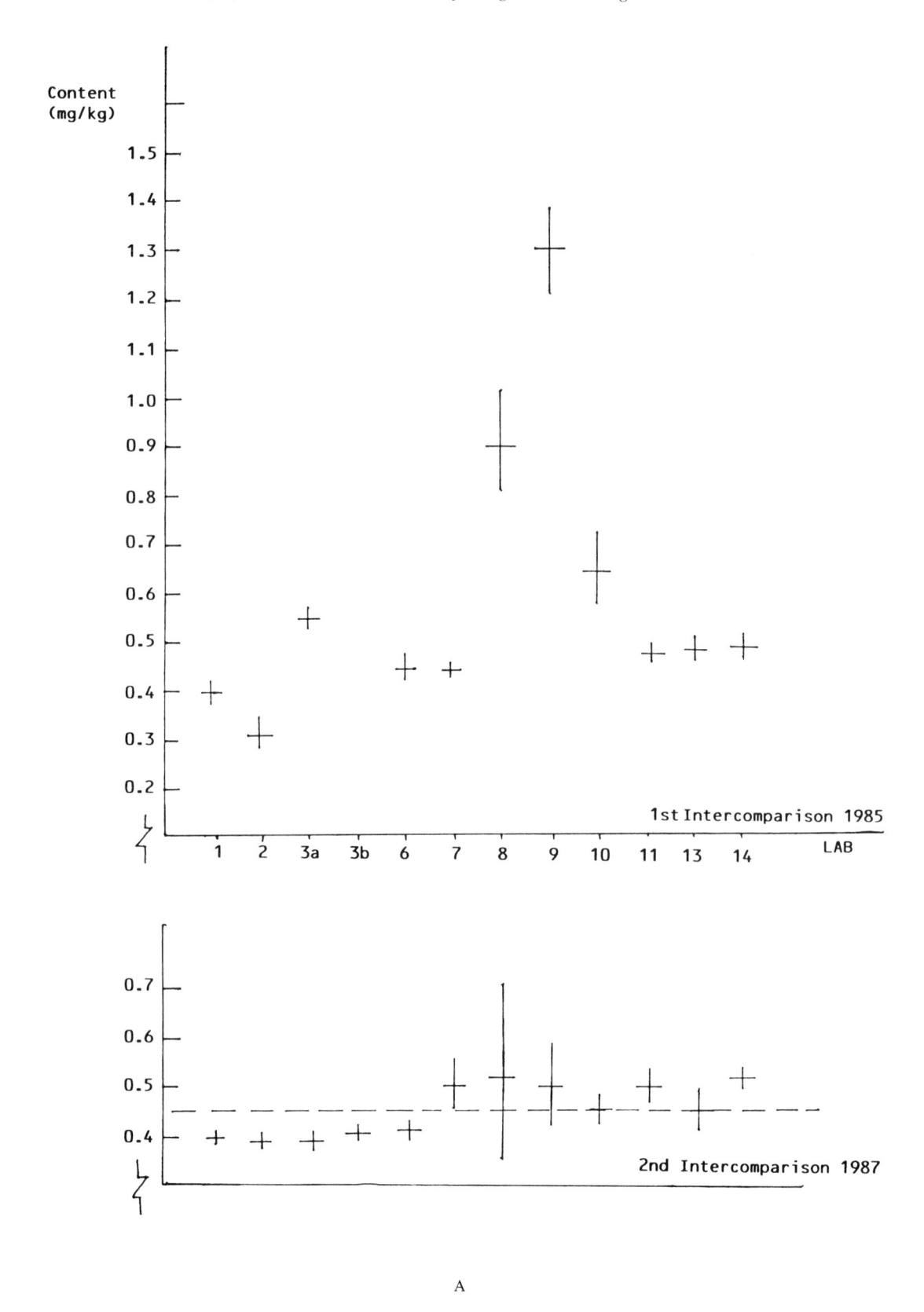

FIGURE 4. (A) Results of two intercomparisons on the determination of chlorinated biphenyl IUPAC no. 18 in fish oils. (B) Youden plot, MeHg in spiked extract vs. MeHg in raw extract. Horizontal and vertical continuous lines are the means of the laboratory means, dotted lines being the standard deviation of these means. The length of the bars are equal to the standard deviation (five replicates) of the laboratories.

Youden plot
spiked/raw extracts

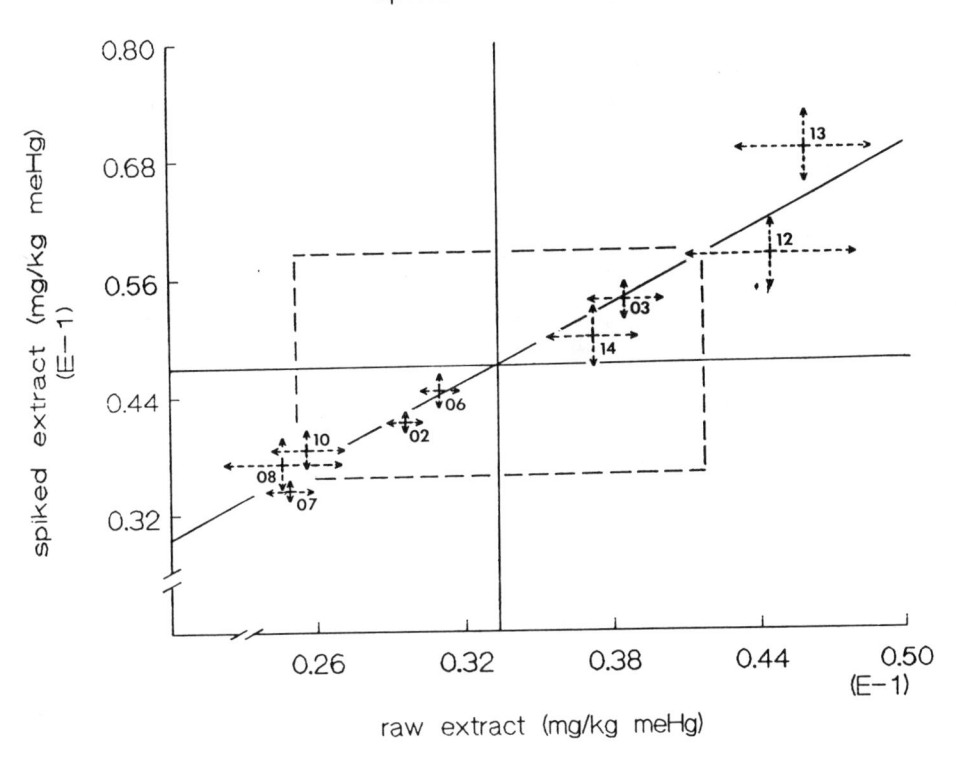

FIGURE 4B.

check is performed at regular intervals even when the materials are available.

3. Similarity with the Real Sample

When CRMs are used to verify the result of analysis of a certain matrix, the sources of error encountered in the analysis of the CRM should be of the same or of a more difficult nature (e.g., same matrix, comparable contents of analyte and interfering elements), as in the real matrix. In such a case, a good accuracy for the CRM may indicate a good accuracy for the unknown. This is often ignored.

4. Accuracy, Uncertainty, and Traceability

The certified values should be the best approximation of the truth. Different methods of the best accuracy should be applied by different outstanding laboratories. This is the only possibility to reduce systematic errors to such a level that they cannot be detected.

The uncertainty in the certified value should be sufficiently small to make use of the CRM for calibration or to be able to distinguish between a good and a bad result of the laboratory which uses the CRM for certification.

Traceability to the primary units is achieved by high standards in the certifying laboratories with regards to calibration of balances, volumetric glassware, and other tools of relevance to the value to be certified. Also, the calibration of the technique of final determination should be done with traceable compounds, which means that the laboratories verify stoichiometry or composition (e.g., for calibration of trace elements, the contents in the stock solution can be verified by gravimetry or titrimetry).

VI. SOME EXAMPLES OF CURRENT BCR PROJECTS

The main priority areas are

1. Biomedical analysis
2. Analyses related to food and agriculture
3. Environmental analysis
4. Analysis of industrial products
5. Applied metrology

A. BIOMEDICAL ANALYSIS

For the screening, diagnosis, monitoring, and prognostication of diseases a large number of substances are determined in human body fluids (e.g., blood, urine) and organ tissues. Those determinations that are performed *in vitro* constitute the field of biomedical analysis.

The priorities for undertaking activities under the BCR program were to a large extent established with the help of organizers of External Quality Assessment Schemes. The substances for the determination of which significant differences are observed between laboratories and/or between methods were selected as first priorities. Differences between results were appreciated according to clinical requirements.

It must be emphasized that accurate results are necessary especially when the substance concentration is close to the threshold of clinical decision.

The following projects are in progress under the current BCR program:

Electrolytes in human serum	Magnesium
	Lithium
Hormones in human serum	17β-Oestradiol
	Aldosterone
	Thyroxine
	Luteinizing hormone
	Follicle stimulating hormone
	Prolactin
	Chorionic gonadotrophin
Proteins (as highly purified preparations)	Apolipoproteins Apo AI, Apo AII
	Thyroglobulin
	Osteocalcin
Proteins in human serum	IgG, IgA, IgM
	Albumin, prealbumin
	Haptoglobin, α_1-antitrypsin
	Caeruloplasmin
	Transferrin
	Complement components C3, C4
	α_1-acid glycoprotein
	α_2-macroglobulin
	C-reactive protein
Proteins in human blood	Glycated hemoglobins
Enzymes (as partially or highly purified preparations)	Alanine aminotransferase
	Lactate dehydrogenase
	Creatine kinase
	Acid phosphatase
	Pancreatic α-amylase and lipase
Tumor markers (as highly purified preparations)	α-Foetoprotein
	Carcinoembryonic antigen

Possible work in discussion now includes creatinine, uric acid, urea, cholesterol, triglycerides, vitamins (e.g., B^{12}, A, D, and hydroxylated metabolites), trace elements (e.g., Se, Al, Zn, Cu, As, Pb, Mn, Ni, I), and drugs (e.g., theophylline, cyclosporin, and metabolites) in human serum; microbiology (Legionella) is also in discussion. Some 25 CRMs for hematology, clinical chemistry, and industrial toxicology are currently available.

B. EXAMPLES OF PROJECTS RELATED TO FOOD AND AGRICULTURAL PRODUCTS

With the items listed in Chapter 1, for various reasons the work devoted to growth promoting substances a veterinary drugs in farm animals is of great interest.

The use of drugs to increase the weight of farm animals is banned in the community, but some of these compounds can be used under strict conditions in veterinary treatment. Under a community directive, a monitoring program to check on possible illegal use of these compounds has been started. This work is being carried out by national laboratories approved for this purpose; they apply reference methods for which criteria have been listed, and which require certified reference materials for their validation. The BCR work involves the development of CRMs and blanks for the more commonly found compounds.

The CRMs in development are presented in Table 2; further activities are the drafting of a reference manual and the organization of intercomparisons between the national laboratories involved in the monitoring. (All drug residues in these CRMs are naturally incurred; spiking is not permitted.)

C. ENVIRONMENTAL ANALYSIS

The part of the BCR program devoted to environmental analysis focuses on the following:

1. Trace elements for which more attention will be paid to elements of newly arisen interest (e.g., Al) or to elements where difficulties were shown in the past (e.g., Cr, Mo)
2. Traces of organic toxic compounds, such as dioxins, chlorinated biphenyls, pesticides

TABLE 2
**Initial Projects for Illegal Growth Promoting Compounds
and Regulated Veterinary Drugs**

Compound	Material
Diethyl stilbesterol	Urine and muscle
Dienestrol, Hexeostrol	
Nor-testosterone	Urine and muscle
Thyreostatics	Urine and muscle
Trenbolone	Urine and muscle
Chloramphenicol	Muscle, meat and eggs
Sulphadimidine	Pork meat, liver, and kidney
β-Agonists (clenbuterol, cimmatrol)	Urine and muscle

Other projects of interest for human health (nutrition) are
- Vitamins (oil and water soluble) in several foods
- Dietary fiber in, e.g., cereals
- Cholesterol in oils, fats, milk, and meat
- Carbohydrates, sugar, protein, and fat in food
- Fatty acids in edible soil and fat

3. Trace element speciation (e.g., Sn, Hg, Cr, Al, Pb)
4. Workplace air monitoring
5. Analysis of wastes of different origin

The matrices of interest are normally chosen in such a way that an ecocompartment (e.g., water/sediment/aquatic plant) is covered. Table 3 summarizes some projects from all areas.

For occupational health measurements it is envisaged to study sampling from occupational air in addition to a study of the final measurement. To do so, participating laboratories will meet and sample from a specially designed atmosphere where vapors in known amounts homogeneously can be added.

D. EXAMPLE OF A PROJECT IN METROLOGY

Work will start soon on new methods and instrumentation for chemical and biological analysis and the measurement of physical quantities. The aims of this work are

1. Improvement of the accuracy where necessary by the development of improved measurement methods and instrumentation
2. Study of phenomena which could form the basis of new methods leading to novel instrumentation
3. Promotion of appropriate methods of calibration which should ensure traceability to the international units
4. Improvement of methods to collect analytical and metrological data and their utilization particularly in relation to quality control

Other projects cover the areas given in the introduction.

VII. POSSIBILITIES TO PARTICIPATE IN BCR WORK

A. PROPOSALS

For collaborative projects there is no need (unlike other Community R & D programs) to submit detailed proposals with detailed costings in the first instance. Any person, laboratory, or firm may submit suggestions to the commission, drawing attention to those measurements where improvements are necessary, especially for industrial products and industrial applications. This can be done simply by letter.

However, the proposers are requested to give the following details: explanation of the measurement or analysis concerned, the difficulties involved and discrepancies observed, the economic importance of the product concerned (size of the market), the economic consequences at the community level of the discrepancies in the measurement results (technical barriers, difficulties in trade with examples), and the situation of national and international standardization in the field of the possibilities for collaboration. Such suggestions are welcome at any time.

Laboratories with particular expertise could make themselves known even without proposing a specific project. They could be invited later to participate in projects corresponding to their capability. Therefore they should describe their field of activity and their specialization.

TABLE 3
Some Projects Illustrating the Work Done on Environmental Analysis

Material	Compounds studied	Stage of project
Rainwater	Na,K,Ca,Mg,Cl,NO3-,SO42-, NH_4^+,H+	Certification foreseen in 1991
Seawater	Cu,Zn,Ni,Cd,Pb,Cr	Certification foreseen in 1990
Plankton	As,Cd,Cr,Cu,Mn,Ni,Pb,Zn,Se	Certification foreseen in 1990
Fly ash extract	PCDDs and PCDFs ("dioxins")	Certification foreseen in 1991
Fly ash	PCDDs and PCDFs	Intercomparison in 1990
Waste oils	PCB	Certification foreseen in 1991
Milk powder	Incurred PCB	Certification foreseen in 1991
Pork fat	Incurred chlorinated pesticides	Certification foreseen in 1991
Soils/sediments	Industrial contaminants (e.g., phenols, sulphur, oil, PCB, pesticides, etc.)	Intercomparison in 1990
Water/sediment	Instable pesticides (atrazine, carbamates, phosphates, pytrethroids)	Stabilization studies to be concluded by 1991
Fish extracts	Methyl-mercury	Third intercomparison in 1990
Sediments/soils	Trace element speciation/binding	Intercomparison in 1990
Sediments	Tributyl tin	Intercomparison in 1990; certification probable in 1991
Solutions	Organo-Pb and -As	Intercomparison in 1990
Solutions (aq.)	Cr and Al species	Stability in 1990
Sorption tubes	Chlorinated alkanes esters/ketones and vinyl chloride	Intercomparison in 1990; stability in 1990

B. SELECTION CRITERIA

The commission will give priority to topics with higher economic importance for the community and where there is either

- A requirement for improvement through work of a technical and scientific nature
- A requirement for intercomparisons with a metrological approach
- A need for a transfer standard or a certified reference material

Preference will be given to collaborative work.

In addition, disputes concerning methods of testing which may differ from one country to another are matters requiring prior harmonization by the standards organizations and cannot be solved by this program.

For subjects which satisfy the criteria, the commission invites experts from all member states for further evaluation. If experts confirm the need for establishing a community project, they are invited to help defining the collaboration possible from each member state and the details of the work to be undertaken in the laboratories of the participants.

The draft project is then submitted to the advisory committee for management and coordination of the BCR program.

C. FINANCIAL SUPPORT TO PROJECTS

For projects involving a succession of intercomparisons, the community will cover the costs necessary for the collaboration (meetings, samples, evaluation of results, etc.), the costs of the measurements being borne by the participants. For projects which include a substantial amount of research and development, the financial contribution of the commission could be up to 50% of the cost of the work.

REFERENCES

1. **Tölg, G.**, private communication.
2. **Einerson, J. H. and Pei, P. C.**, *Environ. Sci. Technol.*, 22, 1121, 1988.
3. **Berman, S. S. and Boyko, V. J.**, ICES 6th Round Intercalibration for Trace Metal in Seawater, *JMG*, 6/TM/SW, 1987.
4. **Byrne, A. R., Camara Rica, C., Cornelis, R., de Goey, J. J. M., Iyengar, G. V., Kirkbright, G., Knapp, G., Parr, R. M., and Stoeppler, M.**, *Fres. Z. Anal. Chem.*, 326, 723, 1987.
5. **Subramanian, K. S. and Stoeppler, M.**, *Fres. Z. Anal. Chem.*, 328, 875, 1986.
6. **Leichnitz, K.**, *Sicherheitsing.*, 7, 24, 1986.
7. **Thier, H. P.**, *Mitt. Lebensm. Gerichtl. Chem.*, 30, 187, 1976.
8. **Boniforti, R., Ferraroli, R., Frigieiri, P., Heltai, D., and Queirazza, G.**, *Anal. Chim. Acta*, 162, 33, 1984.
9. **Herber, R. F. M., Stoeppler, M., and Tonks, D. B.**, *Fres. Z. Anal. Chem.*, 317, 246, 1984.
10. **Musial, C. J. and Uthe, J. F.**, *J. Assoc. Off. Anal. Chem.*, 66, 22, 1983.
11. **Knöchel, A. and Petersen, W.**, *Fres. Z. Anal. Chem.*, 314, 105, 1983.
12. **Tschöpel, P. and Tölg, G.**, *J. Trace Microprobe Tech.*, 1, 1, 1982.
13. **Heydorn, K. and Damsgaard, E.**, *Talanta*, 29, 1019, 1982.
14. **Tölg, G.**, Proc. *Anorganische Stoffe in der Toxikologie und Kriminalistik*, Verl. D. Helm, Heppenheim (D), 1983, 109.
15. **Griepink, B.**, *Fres. Z. Anal. Chem.*, 317, 210, 1984.
16. **Griepink, B.**, *Irish Chem. News*, 22, 1986.
17. General Requirements for the Technical Competence of Testing Laboratories, ISO-Guide, 25, 1982.
18. **Vijverberg, F. A. J. M. and Cofino, W. P.**, *Controll Procedures: GLP and QA*, Copenhagen, 1987.
19. **Kinsella, B. and Willix, R.**, *Analytical Quality Assurance in the Marine Quality Assessment Programme*, Western Australian Institute of Technology, 1985.
20. **Garfield, F. M.**, *TRAC*, 4, 162, 1985.
21. **Taylor, J. K.**, *TRAC*, 3, 11, 1984.
22. **OECD**, Principles of Good Laboratory Practice, 1981.
23. **Taylor, J. K.**, Handbook for SRM-Users, NIST, special publication, 1985, 260–100.
24. **Vogelgesang, J.**, *Fres. Z. Anal. Chem.*, 328, 213, 1987.
25. **Shewart**, *Economic Control of the Quality of the Manufactured Product*, D. Van Nostrand Reinhold, New York, 1931.
26. **Nordish Council of Ministers**, Handbook 1, Internal Quality Control, Project no. 180, 1984, 21–16.
27. **Dewey, D. J. and Hunt, D. T. E.**, Water Research Centre, Medmenham (UK) Technical report, 174, 1972.
28. **Kateman, G. and Pijpers, F. W.**, *Quality Control in Analytical Chemistry*, John Wiley & Sons, New York, 1981.
29. **Edwards, R. W. H.**, *Ann. Clin. Biochem.*, 17, 205, 1980.
30. **Westgard, J. O., Groth, T., Aronsson, T., and de Verdier, C. H.**, *Clin. Chem.*, 23, 1981, 1977.
31. **Siekmann, L. and Breuer, H.**, *J. Clin. Chem. Clin. Biochem.*, 20, 883, 1982.
32. **Siekmann, L.**, *J. Clin. Chem. Clin. Biochem.*, 22, 551, 1984.
33. **Lawson, A. M., Calam, D. H., and Colinet, E. S.**, The Certification of Cortisol in Two Lyophilised Serum Materials, Report EUR, 9661, 1985.
34. **Thienpont, L. M. R., de Leenheer, A. P., Siekmann, L., and Colinet, E. S.**, The Certification of Progesterone in Two Lyophilised Serum Materials, Report EUR, 12282, 1989.
35. ISO, 5727, 1981.
36. **Horwitz, W., Kamps, L. R., and Boyer, K. W.**, *J. Assoc. Off. Anal. Chem.*, 63, 1344, 1980.
37. **Borger, K. W., Horwitz, W., and Albert, R.**, *Anal. Chem.*, 57, 454, 1985.
38. **Wells, D. E., de Boer, J., Tuinstra, L. G. M. Th., Rekutergardh, L., and Griepink, B.**, Report on the Improvements in the Determination of Chlorobiphenyls, Report EUR, 12496, 1989.
39. **Griepink, B., Wells, D. E., and Frias Ferreira, M.**, The Certification of the Contents of Chlorobiphenyls, 28, 52, 101, 118, 138, 153 and 180 in Two Fish Oils, Report EUR, 11520, 1988.
40. **Gaskell, S. J., Collins, C. J., Throne, G. C., and Groom, G. V.**, *Clin. Chem.*, 29, 862, 1983.
41. **Marchandise, H., Ed.**, New Reference Materials; Improvement of Methods of Measurement, Report EUR, 9921, 1985.
42. **Youden, W. J.**, *Ind. Qual. Contr.*, 15 no. 11, 24–28, 1959.
43. **Youden, W. J.**, Statistical Techniques for Collaborative Tests, Statistical Manual of the Assoc. Off. Anal. Chem., 1, 1975.
44. **Aronsson, T. and Groth, T.**, *Scand. J. Clin. Lab. Invest.*, Suppl. 44, 172, 51, 1984.
45. **Griepink, B. and Marchandise, H.**, Referenzmaterialien, in *Analytiker Taschenbuch Band 6*, Springer Verlag, Berlin, 1986, 3.
46. **Marchandise, H. and Colinet, E.**, *Fres. Z. Anal. Chem.*, 316, 669, 1983.
47. **Griepink, B.**, *Fres. Z. Anal. Chem.*, 317, 210, 1984.

Chapter 36

REMARKS FROM THE SPANISH NATIONAL PLAN ON DRUGS

Santiago de Torres

I would first like to draw attention to the opportunity this symposium has afforded in discussing the latest issues involved in the analysis of metabolites of drugs of abuse in biological fluids.

In Spain, the reliability of these tests, given the consequences that may derive from false positive or negative results, has always been a matter of concern. For this reason, years ago, a quality control program was implemented in which 40 laboratories, the majority of whom are engaged in the urinalysis of drug addicts under treatment, acceded to take part.

The ultimate aim of this program was not only to control the quality of laboratory analyses, but also to make information available to and to improve the training of laboratory personnel involved in these tasks.

During the period in which Spain presided the European Council, the Ministers of Health passed a resolution inviting the European Commission to study the possibility of implementing a program of similar characteristics to that instituted in Spain to the European Community as a whole. It would seem logical, with the coming into force in 1993 of the Single Act, when people, goods, and capital will be able to circulate freely within the European Community, that the criteria established for carrying out these analyses as well as the consequences that positive results can have on individuals, should be unified, as far as possible.

Much has been done to improve the specificity and reliability of analytical techniques, but little progress has been made to define the cases, circumstances, aims, and above all, the consequences of carrying out these tests.

No decision has been taken to limit the use of these analyses and public opinion is therefore critical. It seems reasonable that certain jobs should be carried out by people we are sure do not consume any kind of psychotropic agent or drug of abuse. These would include bus drivers, armed personnel, members of the services, etc. This does not mean, however, that all job applicants should be subject to random urine testing independent of the kind of job he/she is applying for.

Analysts should be aware of this fact because if they are not, public opinion may be hostile and the objectives pursued by urine drug testing may be interpreted erroneously.

Every attempt should be made to improve the quality of the analytical techniques used, while at the same time carrying out more extensive research into the consequences, on therapeutic schedules or in the workplace, of the results of drug testing. Clinicians and analysts should work closely together to achieve a more realistic and more useful interpretation of analytical results.

Chapter 37

REMARKS FROM THE COMMISSION OF THE EUROPEAN COMMUNITIES

Alex Berlin

In 1989, the Spanish Presidency of the European Communities proposed to the Council of Ministers the adoption of a resolution aimed at improving the reliability of tests on body fluids to detect the use of illicit drugs. An essential component of this Resolution called for the setting up of a European Community-wide quality assurance program. However, the Council did not fully follow the proposal of the Spanish presidency, which was essentially a technical one.

A number of member states considered that adopting such a text would condone drug testing, especially on a random and routine basis. Instead, the Council adopted on May 16th, 1989, conclusions of a more political nature, and the following is quoted from them

The Council invites the Commission to firstly:

- examine the criteria currently used for reporting positive results, including the need to distinguish between screening and confirmation

- examine the existing quality assurance programmes,

- check on the availability of certified reference materials for illicit drugs and metabolites.

In parallel and at the end of 1989 within the framework of a Eurobarometer survey (a survey of European public opinion which the Commission carries out twice a year), questions were asked as to whether drug urine analysis is acceptable and, if so, under what circumstances. The survey was carried out in November and December of 1989 on 22,600 people in the European Community. Two thirds of the people interviewed were in agreement with the police being able to use this test when there is a problem. Two thirds were opposed to testing at the workplace, especially for hiring purposes. There was a greater acceptance of testing at the workplace in the case of problems and doubt regarding possible drug use. Finally, regarding testing for insurance purposes, opinion was equally divided. However, when people were asked if they would be willing to submit themselves to a test, about two thirds accepted the idea. On the basis of the above data, from the European Commission's point of view, we have to remain very cautious with respect to the rapidly spreading possibilities for routine screening and weigh very carefully the consequences of the growing availability of testing kits. In the industrial setting, we must ensure that presumptive positive results do not affect the workers in any way.

In conclusion, I hope that this symposium will have been the first step in establishing a network of high level collaborating analytical laboratories in the European Community and will foster international cooperation.

Chapter 38

DISCUSSION ON ASPECTS FOR HARMONIZATION

Szendrey: The overall field is very relevant for the U.N. Perhaps some of the attendants don't know that we have control programs. Last development was a special 2-day session during the Assembly devoted to that specific subject. Earlier, we were just dealing with the supply side (traffic, production of drugs), but in the last few years we were called on to extend our program in the demand reduction side, which means exactly this subject. The Division of Narcotics has a small laboratory with very limited resources and limited staff. This laboratory had to reshape its program for the last 3 days in the light of the Assembly, final resolutions, and what I heard today, is almost reflected word by word in my proposed program within this area. But I was extremely happy to listen for those speakers like Dr. San. As a medical doctor he gave me all the justification for my program. I have all the difficulties to try to sell proposals like why we will need drug testing in the development world. Today I heard a lot of strong arguments on the development world if we don't need that today we will need it tomorrow. I just came for a 2-week tour from India, and I repetitively heard the same request: "yes we have de-addiction centers, or we are developing them, but we don't have testing facilities".

In this area, the U.S. is a long way before us, as I can see now the E.E.C. countries are in a way of harmonizing their efforts and the internal procedures, and it is exactly the same what we'll have to do but in a totally different context, matrix. In the area of the developing world we must help to develop the very basic facilities, training, and also transfer whatever is transferable of these technologies already available. In this respect I believe it would be extremely useful for us to listen how the Twelve (European Community) will be successful in this undertaking, how far they can go, and what we can utilize in other parts of the world.

Fernandez (Barcelona, Spain): Creatinine is often used in order to investigate, in the laboratory, a possible masking or diluting action on the urines under analysis. The cutoffs however are always referred to mg/L or mg/ml. This means that even when a diluting effect is probable, the use of such cutoffs gives rise to negative results. The use of "normalized" cutoffs as mg/g of creatinine, as is being introduced in Industrial Toxicology or the refusal of a urine sample because of its creatinine or pH value, could be an alternative.

Berlin: A similar question regarding the creatinine level: can you use the creatinine concentration, or the density, or the pH as the criteria for eliminating a sample? We have had, in fact, the problem ourselves when we tried for the biological monitoring for lead in urine in the industrial setting to set lower and upper limits for creatinine levels for a sample to be considered acceptable from the dilution or concentration points of view. Here you have another assumption; you have the presumption that the sample might be tampered. In other words, how do you separate, let's say, an unsuitable sample from a tampered sample?

Widdop: There are some ways: creatinine concentrations, relative density. It is well known also that people add acid or alkalies to disturb some of the immunoassay tests, so you should test for the pH. People sometimes add bleach and you can smell it. Another problem is that liquid soap is available in some collecting washrooms, so you can shake the sample and you can see little bubbles in the top. I think, however, that if you have a proper chain of custody and you have samples that are collected under observation, properly sealed and documented, these other additional precautions which you can take are not probably necessary.

Sunshine: I think we have missed the intent of the question which I think was, "should you report results in terms not of milliliters of urine but of grams of creatinine to take care of the illustration of Dr. Wennig where the creatinine clearance makes the difference in the interpretation of the results". So, should creatinine be done on every specimen so that you can report that in all your work?

Wennig: If you have the doubt that there is something wrong in a particular case, i.e., when somebody in a rehabilitation program is going down at once and it goes up another way round, you have to check it. I just wanted to warn you that this is a possibility. I don't think you could do it in a routine base.

Unidentified Speaker: How long after absorption is useful the ratio between codeine/morphine concentration about 0.6?

Wennig: As far as I remember it is 24 to 30 hours, not more. You have also a gray line, which is called inconclusive results; you cannot say with certainty this comes from codeine or this comes from morphine.

Lopez Rivadulla (Santiago de Compostela, Spain): Have you experience about interpretation of results in other biological fluids or tissues, such as vitreous humor and kidney?

Moller: We have experience in coroner's cases where there is heroine overdose. The relation between the lungs, for example, and blood and liver is interesting.

Wennig: If you have a higher content in the lung than in the liver you have a quite short period after administration. If the ratio is the other way round; there is more in the liver than in the lung, it has been administered at least 8 to 10 hours before. So we have some idea when the administration has been done.

Sunshine: Prof. Donike you said you expect laboratories to perform quantitatively plus or minus 15% or two standard deviations of what? What constitutes the reference?

Donike: The reference is the mean of the results of all other laboratories. We do not rely on, lets say, the "gravimetric value".

Sutheimer: In order to stimulate some discussion on accreditation and quality control. Could we be accused of insuring our own existence prior to serving a common good?

Sunshine: Is something new on the "external blind control" being an essential part of the NIDA program?

Finkle: This was something that was discussed at the Consensus Conference. The principle of blind quality control is clearly the keystone of determining whether the laboratory is competent and achieving the right answers. It is probably the only method by which the complete process from sample collection to report submission can be quality checked in real time. Into that extent the groups that considered this, among other issues, at the Consensus Conference, believed that the achieving through blind quality assurance programs was the most important of all aspects.

Willette: Just a point of clarification: the Federal Guidelines of May 1989 required federal agencies to submit blind samples. Fifty percent of all samples submitted during the first 90 days with the new program and 10% thereafter. In December 1989, the Department of Transportation lowered its blind requirements to three blind samples per hundred specimens. The Nuclear Regulatory Commission still requires 10% because they are dealing in a more safety sensitive area with greater public visibility and a smaller workforce, perhaps 70,000 covered employees.

Finkle: A very important point is made here. Depending on how many samples the particular laboratory is handling, and depending on the size or requirements of the agency, the percentage of those quality control samples need to be adjusted.

Verebey: There is a consideration of lowering the cutoff on the THC to 50 ng/ml. Originally the cutoff was 20 ng/ml and was raised to 100 ng/ml in order to eliminate the possibility of passive inhalation, as studies have brought into focus that in this way nobody is going to be innocently accused. Nevertheless, I feel that going to 50 ng/ml might cause some problems. One hundred ng/ml is probably safer. What is your opinion?

Finkle: At the Consensus Conference (but remember that consensus does not means majority) the groups that reviewed these issues reached a consensus on that matter. That leaves a long, long way from being changed, and clearly before any change will be made there will be a great deal more discussion and opportunity of public announcement and so on. Do not panic.

Sunshine: What Dr. Vereby just said is for the presumptive test. There was no change made after the confirmation test which still is I think at 15 ng/ml, and, consequently, that is the controlling factor. No matter what the presumptive test is, you have to end up with the 15 ng/ml or greater for confirmation and that has not been changed.

Sunshine: It has been mentioned that the monoclonal amphetamine had an interference in the phenothiazines. I would not be too concerned about that because you can fairly easily check for phenothiazine interferences by spot tests. In fact any positive result you may have with the monoclonal test may be followed by a spot test which will indicate if you have a phenothiazine.

Widdop: I can agree with that, but in practice it is more easy to use the polyclonal antibody. And even sometimes the phenothiazine spot test is not so much reliable.

Segura: A question for Dr Myers. The BCR projects handle certified material and make intercomparison laboratories, but I understand you do not certify laboratories. I am afraid that because you are studying only the best laboratories in each country, the kind of work that other less experienced laboratories perform may be uncovered.

Myers: Our goal is to produce reference materials to spread the knowledge through these reference materials. To be efficient, a maximum of 20 laboratories is enough, especially with difficult determinations. We have groups of 20 laboratories and as long as we go on, for example, on PCB, we have had more and more candidates. Then we increased the number of laboratories and split the first group into more specialized groups. Now we have two groups of 20; one that is mainly analyzing food materials and the other one more environmental materials. And it is not impossible that we will create perhaps a third one of probably also 20 laboratories that would cover the surface water, soils, and so on. However there is a limit. We never can have a hundred. In microbiology, for example, Salmonella, we had 50 laboratories. Slowly some disappeared alone and for others the number needed to be reduced. A strong discipline is needed, and the manager of the project needs to be in close contact with the laboratories. If not, at the end you can just calculate the mean and only say you are out of range. If you want to go into the details of the methods, it is not possible with a lot of laboratories. What we ask here when we listen about national quality controls and accreditations in drug testing is that those good laboratories from one country may be confronted with others of the very best ones of the EEC, and this should be done with very good and very well prepared samples. This is specially important when we speak about accreditation, remarkably if EEC will act some day. It should be produced good, reliable, homogenous, stable reference materials to circulate through the laboratories. One possibility is to create BCR-like institutions in each country where BCR may help. Experience already exists in this regards.

Finkle: One comment that is pertinent to forensic toxicology and urine testing. NIDA was very severely criticized by many toxicologists because they believed that the standards were much too difficult, and therefore they believed that many laboratories would not be able to achieve a certification, but still would be good competent laboratories. My response to that is this: I believe that NIDA was very wise in making, initially, the guidelines and regulations very tight and very severe because as experience grows it will be relatively easy to relax some of these areas, and that was one part that was discussed at the Consensus Conference. After 2 years other areas can be relaxed without lost of quality in the program. Conversely, if NIDA had begun with relatively easy and loose guideline's regulations they would never had been able, after the fact, to make them tighter because they would have been a great rebellion and resistance among the laboratories. The second point is along the same lines and that could be of interest to our European colleagues. Many of us in forensic toxicologist laboratories believe then when we were inspected by a team of inspectors we were going to be inspected by our colleagues, our friends. And is a very small profession forensic toxicology in U.S. as it is relatively in Europe and so we knew that we would know these people that came to inspect our lab and we had work with them for years and years and so nobody feared these inspections. Let me tell you, who needs friends like these people? They are very tough on each other. I would never had believed how tough the inspectors are on their old friends and colleagues. Of course most of it is conditioned by the book of inspection regulations that they must follow. But if you think that you are going to have a friendly, easy experience the only consolation is that you will get your turn to go to their laboratory.

Berlin: Three questions (are) in common to Dr. Widdop. You are saying that *a priori* rendering the tests more economic is a benefit, and you have indicated that some countries are poorer and they should be able to do more testing if it does not cost so much. In fact, if you make the test more economical, the more you increase the possibility of testing and maybe of unnecessary testing. So, to what extent is that really an advantage?. Secondly, you were saying that by lowering the cutoff you are giving more positive results and are encouraging employers to test. What is the rational of this policy, *vis a vis* the impairment of the workers performance, because obviously the lower the cutoff the lesser will be the relationship between the results and the workers ability to perform. And finally something which worries me much more: you were saying that employers like a rapid turnover and that presumptive tests, specially if negative, should allow you to have an extremely rapid turnover. Does that mean that when you get samples, the negative ones that are presumptively negative are returned immediately and the ones are returned later? That would be, for the employer, a presumption that something went wrong.

Widdop: In regard to the first question on economics I can only speak on my situation. We are, at the present time, working for the National Health Services which is being rather cut financially. So we should go to this area funded by NHS and to perform proper toxicology. We are in this business to make a profit for the Health Services and also for the performing laboratory and therefore it pays to use test and reagents that are cheap. In regards to cutoff levels, what I really meant is that in the U.K. the industrial people are still not sure whether there is a problem or not to deal with here and must of them in fact are taking anonymous surveys just to see how big the problem is, and this is the main reason why we are picking the low cutoffs that we would not do in normal operation. The final question about the "rapid turnover" you have to delay the positive samples just because the amount of work involved in confirming those presumptive positive samples. And (at) the present time we handle this problem within a maximum of ten days, although most of our positive results are returned within four or five days. But it does create a problem because the employee is, for example, not allowed to go to special working tasks and this creates a suspicion. When there is more equipment and staff available we may increase the turnover of those samples and that will eliminate that particular problem.

Berlin: This last point is something that I thing should be considered much more carefully because in fact it creates, a presumption which is wrong most of the time and it may be totally counterproductive.

van Rossum: Do you do a quantitative test or only a cutoff level saying if the compound is there or not? I think the latter may be very wrong because you suppose everybody is equal and in fact it is not the case.

Widdop: In fact we quantitate in the confirmation by GC/MS. But if we are sending the results back to a clinician or a medical person with the levels there, they go to the phone and ask you to interpret, so you do some use of this. After that it is a medical decision, not an analytical one.

Szendrei: It is a really intriguing situation with the opiates. Just to add one word complication, whenever we are speaking of heroin addiction we assume that it is heroin, and pure heroin, but in most of the cases it is not. It contains sometimes substances: small amounts of codeine, acetyl codeine, etc. How to advise laboratories with limited expertise on how to interpret results. Sometimes in these countries they may have tremendous errors in advising the medical side.

Minty: Have you had any experience by using different immunoassays particularly with urines that are close to the cutoffs. You may have very different results with different immunoassays because of differences in the various antibodies.

Widdop: I have no experience at all because I always use the same EMIT assay. But really it is very difficult to compare, like comparing apples with pears. I do not have an answer for you.

Section V
Final Considerations

Chapter 39

EPILOGUE

Irving Sunshine

This epilogue will reflect on some of the preceding presentations in this book and present some supplementary comments.

A proper perspective of the nature and dimensions of the drug problem is essential before planning any program designed to combat that problem. The general conception is that society faces an unusual and overwhelming problem as a consequence of the misuse and abuse of chemical substances. An historical perspective may help frame this picture.

We have lived with drug use for centuries. One might say it started with the apple in Eden. Prehistoric societies used mood changing substances in their rituals. These practices have persisted into modern times. DTs from alcohol excesses and opiate usage have been described throughout recorded literature.[1] In the United States, in the mid-19th century, physicians prescribed cocaine and heroin. The very popular beverage Coca-Cola® contained cocaine. Dr. Widdop mentioned that one of the popes was partial to Mariani Elixir, a wine that contained cocaine. Just before the turn of the 20th century, recognition came that this indulgence was deleterious and remedial action was desirable. It took another 14 years to get the first national legislation passed — the Harrison Narcotics Act. At that time, 1 person in 400 was dependent on opiates, in 1930, 1 in 4000 was still dependent.[2] Reasonable containment of this drug problem was achieved when the Narcotic Farm Bill set up a rehabilitation program in Lexington, Kentucky, in 1935.

All this is cited to affirm that we are dealing with an age-old, cyclical problem. We have to develop a proper perspective on our current situation. A critical assessment is necessary. Are we on a bandwagon singing the tune "drugs of abuse are everywhere. We have a new, terrifying problem. We must do something about it." Remember the hippies in 1960? Woodstock? It took 15 to 20 years to overcome that problem.

So before we discuss analytical problems and control activities, we should determine the extent and nature of today's drug problems. How prevalent is drug abuse in each community? There are relatively few reliable epidemiological studies available, and some should be made. Only then can we realize the proper extent and nature of the problem. Denial is commonplace. "We have no drug problem here" is the usual statement, but when a demand for factual corroboration is made, no object reply is forthcoming. The fact remains that substances are abused all over the world, but how many people are involved and how damaging that usage is to the individual and to the society in which he lives needs objective evaluation.

This conference has not concerned itself with the need for concerted and extensive efforts to control a purported substance abuse problem. Epidemiological studies are essential to establish the extent and nature of this problem, and they should be implemented promptly so that proper judgments on programming can be developed.

If the decision is to be made to implement a drug testing program, who should be involved? Previous articles indicate that, in the United States, the following should be included: the armed forces, local police and fire departments, transportation personnel, federal employees, athletes, those involved in the criminal justice scene, and private employees. In the last category, pre-employment testing is prevalent and is growing. In addition to pre-employment testing, employee drug testing programs may include for-cause testing, meaning that someone suspects an employee to have a drug problem. Some of the different causes that make one suspect that a particular individual may not be functioning properly are that he comes to work late everyday, he is absent from work on Friday or Monday, or his productivity is not what it should be. One may want to test a person to see whether or not misusing drugs is the reason why his performance is less than optimal. For-cause testing is extensive, as is testing those involved in an accident.

An interesting aspect of this practice is deciding who of those involved in the accident should be tested. Following a railroad accident, the engineer, the fireman, and the brakeman may be tested. And that makes sense. But why do you test the porter, the conductor, or other people on the train crew who have nothing to do with the train's operation and possibly the accident? So even accident testing has some limitations. Another group of employees who are regularly subjected to urine drug tests are those in rehabilitation programs. An essential part of those programs is periodic urine testing to insure that the previous practice of abusing substances has ceased. Then of course, you have the big problem of compulsory random testing.

Should every employee be subject to a urine drug test on a random basis? This question has raised great furor, rightly so, within the United States. We have a very contentious society. The lawyers are everywhere. Their motivation may be to see to it that employees' legal rights are preserved, but thereby they are also preserving their own pocketbooks. So they are very eager to contest whether or not random testing should be the law of the land, applicable to all employees. Random testing is still unresolved and what will be accepted remains yet to be seen. Surely you have to consider which aspects of employee testing are desirable when you decide what you are going to do in your local programs.

To properly justify initiating a program, a cost/benefit ratio should be determined. The cost of an extensive program is high when reckoned not only in the high dollar cost of the testing program, but also in terms of the human problems that develop. What happens to the drug user, and whose responsibility is his/her future? Is rehabilitation possible and how can it be achieved? How does the potential harm one drug user can cause compare to the cost of a large testing program which uncovers a very small number of drug users? Dr. Berlin made an apt comment when he asked, "What happens if you withhold a positive finding until it's confirmed?". If you relieve the person of his responsibilities and then the presumptive positive is not confirmed, have you irreparably damaged his future success because of his alleged drug use? All these factors must be considered in calculating the cost of the program. The benefits of testing programs have been cited — decreased drug usage, improved job performance, decreased medical costs, etc. Most of these studies are uncontrolled subject reports that should be replaced by object controlled studies.[3] Then the real benefits of a drug prevention program could be assessed.

The United States Post Office tried to evaluate its drug testing program.[4] All applicants had to give a urine specimen for drug testing prior to being considered for employment. No applicant was refused employment regardless of the urine test result. This result was kept confidential. All those applicants who were hired were periodically evaluated. In this study, 5465 applicants were tested and 4375 were hired. Drug test results were not used to make employment decisions. The overall positive drug findings in these newly hired people was 8.83% (373 people). Of the positives, 67% used THC, 24% used cocaine, and 9% used other drugs. The absentee rate was 41% higher for the positives than the negatives. The positive group had a 50% higher number of involuntary separations (firings). The estimated cost in lost productivity associated with hiring those with positive findings totaled $17 million. Studies of this type are needed to assess the value of a drug testing program.

Little mention has been made of the extent of drug testing programs. In the United States, the Department of Defense has been testing all military personnel for over 15 years. That experience has been used to guide the recently mandated Federal Workplace Testing Program, which is directed by the Secretary of Health and Welfare through the National Institute for Drug Abuse (NIDA). All federal employees are covered by the program. The Department of Transportation has a similar program for employees in the transportation industry. A similar program is in force by the Nuclear Regulatory Agency. Legislation is pending in Congress to extent these programs to private industry. A 1988 survey of industries employing 50 or more people indicated that 91.7% did not then have a drug testing program. Of 950,000 employees tested, 9% were positive, but 12% of job applicants, in contrast, were positive. This study suggests that employees are less prone to use substances subject to abuse than are applicants. Were similar data from other studies available, the results would seem to justify pre-employment testing. No more recent studies are available on current practices, but current estimates suggest that more than 50% of the Fortune 500 companies have instituted drug testing.

Many, many of the multinational industries are extending this practice to their units in Europe. Drug testing laboratories in Europe probably will be belabored by the multinational companies, "We must have drug testing done here, just as it's done in the United States." That will be a real challenge to European drug testing laboratories because complying with the rigid accreditation requirements for a drug testing laboratory in the U.S. is challenging. Europe has a different legal system and should evolve a program that will satisfy *your* own needs as you decide them. If you have to set up two different laboratory procedures, one that will satisfy the multinational's desire to mimic their U.S. experience, and another that will satisfy your own needs, you will have a major problem.

The primary thrust of the presentations in this book is analytical. Many articles address various aspects of the analytical problems involved. There is a reasonable degree of similarity in the analytical techniques used in laboratories in the United States and in Europe. Dr. Blanke pointed out that evolving programs should critically evaluate existing programs in the United States and benefit from their mistakes. He points out that the NIDA program may be too rigid, as presently set up, and that its concepts rather than its specifics, should be its contribution to desirable practices. He, along with Drs. Gelpi and Barcelo, correctly points out that the technology necessary to keep up with the growing demands outstrips our ability to interpret the results.

Everyone agrees that the analytical results must be reliable and every effort has to be made to ensure this. Initially, you must address what Dr. Verebey and Dr. San mentioned several times, the problem of forensic vs. the clinical aspects of analytical toxicology. In forensic urine drug testing, you are asked to determine a specific number of analytes in a particular specimen. Whereas in the clinical situation, you are concerned with many different analytes and with different specimens (i.e., blood and urine). Patients may take any one of a host of different chemicals. If you want to determine whether or not any of these are present, surely the analytical techniques to be used are different than those used that were concerned with just forensic urine drug testing. The psychiatrist treating a patient wants to know whether or not his patient was using any substance, not, is it at the cutoff, above or below, but was he using any substance in the immediate past? That's part of the clinical problem. As Dr. San pointed out so well, clinical and forensic needs are different, they require a different approach and you have to decide which (or both) areas you want to encompass in your laboratory. In whichever area you choose to function, many presentations in this book have indicated how these analyses can be done accurately and reliably. There was no one who disagreed with the fact that if you use all the necessary attributes that are present in a good analytical toxicology program, you can produce reliable data. The required cornerstones on which an acceptable laboratory must rest to ensure this are a proper chain of custody, scientifically valid test procedures, competent staff, adequate equipment, and a quality assurance program. These requirements can be met with ease, provided that a lot of attention and a reasonable amount of financial support is forthcoming. The big problem I think is to decide what analytes should be included. You've heard of the NIDA 5; opiates, amphetamines, cocaine, THC, and PCP. This was a relatively arbitrary decision that was deemed sufficient by the people who set up that program initially. But when you get into the employee/employer relationship, the employers, in their wisdom or driven by the attorneys, suggest that they have to look for other substances beyond the NIDA 5. They want to include the barbiturates, benzodiazepines, alcohol, antihistamines, and, in some cases, diuretics. So you get close to the kind of a program that Dr. Donike was talking about in the Olympic doping control program. Such a broad program is unrealistic because you cannot do 4000 samples a day for that large number of analytes. That is the load one expects in a large forensic drug urine testing program. So you have to define the problem you are addressing and decide what it is you are required to do. The Hansen and Boone reference that is quoted time and again was written back in 1983 and indicated that drug testing was unreliable and inadequate. If you study that paper carefully, you will find that the authors were inadequate, that they made a lot of unfair comparisons that were not valid. Dr. Boone published another article in *JAMA* in 1987,[5] which reflects the current trend of the laboratory practice. In that article, he stated, "The science on which urine drug testing rests is solid. If these principles are followed, and if positive screening results are confirmed by GC/MS, no analytical false positives should occur." Everyone now subscribes to that statement. It represents the state-of-the-art in the laboratory today. It would have been nice if he had modified his statement to say GC/MS *or some other reliable confirmation technique*, because I think there are other confirmation techniques that ought to be considered.

Drs. Gelpi and Barcelo discussed how technological developments have advanced laboratory procedures so that a large number of specimens can be analyzed quickly, reliably, accurately, and inexpensively. The need to objectively demonstrate that the analytical procedure is under critical and careful objective control and that the laboratory can vouch safe its quality assurance program was emphasized by Drs. Willette, Cook, and Widdop. Everyone agrees that the laboratory must have internal security and document every step in the analytical procedure so that a reliable result is obtained.

What that result means provoked much discussion. Drs. Cami, Wennig, Bernet, and San indicated the limitations of both positive and negative findings. Their valid conclusion was that the test results indicate, with sufficient precision, that a person has or has not used a substance subject to abuse. It does not give any indication of impairment. The caution that a negative result does not indicate a person is not an abuser is well taken. As they point out, the test procedure encompasses a limited number of substances and does not exclude abuse of other substances that were not included in the test procedure. The laboratory report should clearly indicate its scope and limitations. Everyone involved should recognize that a limited analysis was performed. If the client requires information on other analytes than those in the original protocol, he should request that the laboratory satisfy his need by including the additional analyte. Several presentations suggested that in order to properly evaluate a laboratory report, a qualified physician's assessment of the test result, the patient, and the circumstances may be contributory.

Proficiency testing programs have been developed to ensure that laboratories produce reliable results. In the United States, the NIDA program has accredited approximately 70 laboratories. The rigid requirements of this program have been indirectly described by Drs. Sutheimer, Finkle, Willette, and Cook. There has been little mention of a comparable accreditation program under the auspices of the College of American Pathologists and the American Association for Clinical Chemistry that has accredited some 80 laboratories. There is an overlap of about 20 laboratories in these two programs. Various states have their own accreditation programs, independent of the two just mentioned. Whether these programs should be duplicated elsewhere is debatable. Drs. Christopherson, Lafarque, Moeller, and Segura have described the programs used in their respective countries. These seem to meet their needs. Whether, as time marches on, it will be necessary to develop one program that will satisfy the needs of the European Community was addressed by Drs. Berlin and Segura. As the latter pointed out, in 1993 there will be free passage of all citizens in the European Community. This mandates that they all should be accorded the same treatment. Problems will arise that need solutions — which substances should be included in the test profile, what methods will be acceptable, who will be tested, will physicians interpret the test results, and how will the entire process be controlled?

In all this planning, it would be desirable to benefit from the experiences acquired in the states. A meeting was held in November 1989 to get a concensus on the U.S. programming.[6] Dr. Finkle points out some of the revisions to the existing NIDA program that were suggested at that conference. These include permission to do on-site testing with confirmation in primary laboratories, use of other techniques than GC/MS for confirmation, elimination of the presumptive test cutoffs and using only the confirmation test cutoff to define a positive result, consideration of additional analytes beyond the NIDA 5, and evaluation of other noninvasive specimens, such as saliva and hair.

Another approach to accreditation of laboratory performance is external blind testing. In such a program, the laboratory would receive specimens containing known amounts of the analytes in question that would be submitted simultaneously with test specimens in an identical manner to those test specimens — the labels, the container, and the matrix would all be the same. Since the external blind specimen would be indistinguishable from others in the batch, it would be handled in the ordinary manner, not as a separate unit as is the case in proficiency studies. Evaluation of the laboratory's report on the external blind specimen would indicate its level of acceptable performance. By using external blind specimens in each batch of specimens submitted to the laboratory, routine, objective, and continuous monitoring can be achieved. This could eliminate the huge bureaucratic process in the present costly accreditation programs and insure reliable monitoring of the laboratories' routines. The major problem in the suggested external blind program is the ability to provide authentic specimens of known concentration in labeled containers identical to those of testees'. Were this achievable, there would be no need to inspect a laboratory or check on the details of its procedures. All that would be required to insure the laboratory's accreditation would be a correct report. The gospel supports this approach. "All I want to know is yea, yea, or nay, nay. And furthermore I need nothing."[7] Whether others will be converted remains to be seen.

Can present analytical procedures be modified to produce more reliable data more economically? Many innovations have been suggested. One has to do with the use of specimens other than urine and blood. Noninvasive specimens such as saliva and hair have been suggested by Dr. Moeller. Significantly more research is required before these specimens can be used for forensic practice. As this develops, it could confirm the valid use of these specimens. Hair has a potential value other specimens lack, not to detect the immediate past use of drug, it will not do that. But if you analyze segments of hair, it could indicate if an individual was using a drug. If the hair near the scalp is positive it suggests that the person has taken the drug within the last 7 to 10 days. Whereas if the analysis of the tip of that hair, which took a few weeks to grow, is also positive, you might infer a continuous use was involved, i.e., a chronic user. The technologies that Dr. Moeller described, using a pencil thick group of hairs, have been improved so you do not need quite as much hair to perform an analysis. In time, this approach may be very helpful. It might provide answers to questions, such as was a woman using cocaine when and just after she conceived, would that usage deleteriously affect her unborn child? An analysis of the mother's hair at her first trimester medical examination could determine whether or not she used cocaine in the recent past. Neither a urine or blood test, taken at that time, could answer the question of prior use, but hair analysis might. Surely, as more research efforts uncover its potential and limitations, analysis of hair specimens may become commonplace.

Many presentations were made on the value of chromatographic analysis for the confirmation of a presumptive positive preliminary drug test. No one addressed the potential for the older, reliable thin layer chromatography (TLC). It is an effective confirmation method and is far less expensive than GC/MS. TLC can detect 15 ng/ml of THC-COOH simply, easily, and inexpensively.[8] It is a very effective and reliable means for confirming other presumptive immunoassays, particularly the "amphetamines" result. It reliably separates the phenethylamines (methamphetamine, amphtamine, phenylephedrine, phenylpropanolamine) and is far less expensive than GC/MS. Its sensitivity satisfies the NIDA confirmation cutoffs for these drugs.

Another chromatographic technique which received little comment was dual column, dual detector capillary gas chromatography. It too is a splendid confirmation technique that can compete with GC/MS. As Dr. Fraisse indicates, the analytical prowess of GC/MS is exemplary. It can provide unique and specific quantitative data, but how many analysts have skills comparable to Dr. Fraisse's and the expensive equipment essential to GC/MS? GC/MS requires personnel who are experienced in the operation and maintenance of specialized instrumentation, but though few can now qualify, the number is growing.

Good forensic practice mandates that all results must be beyond a reasonable doubt, otherwise undesirable notoriety may result. Laboratory reports have to be like Caeser's wife, purer than pure. The good is buried with our bones, and the evil lives after. All we have to have is one mistake, and the media is on it. They impugn that everything you subsequently do is presumed to be incorrect. After one publicized mistake, everything you and your colleagues report is suspect. Everyone is then measured by the same yardstick.

However reliable the result, the following statement needs consideration. Clinical decisions cannot be made *only* on the basis of a laboratory analysis. Many may disagree with this. They must recognize that the laboratory can only provide an analytical result. It does not know the patient's background. The result is only a little part of the picture, and the whole picture must be visualized before one can interpret the result properly. That is not the role of the laboratory, that is the role of a consulting physician or some other person to whom that responsibility is relegated. Drs. Camí, San, and Wennig have presented excellent justifications of this philosophy.

However, whoever interprets the laboratory result must be aware of the concerns expressed by Drs. Barnett, van Rossum, and Baselt. The pharmacokinetics, pharmacodynamics, and pharmacogenetics of drug use must be known if any valid interpretations, beyond use, are to be made. Much more knowledge needs to be acquired in these areas.

No one questions that drug use caused the posting of many danger signs that suggest that we face a crisis situation. The Chinese symbol for crisis is made up of two characters, danger and opportunity. Today we are beset by the many dangers continued drug usage may bring to our communities. It is needless to report them here. However, few recognize the opportunity that minimizing or eliminating these dangers offers — an opportunity that should be seized by all concerned. We have an opportunity to provide the data that will demonstrate the extent of the problem. We have the opportunity to insure that reliable laboratory data can be used to identify drug abusers, and we have the opportunity to help monitor the rehabilitation of addicts so that they can return to productive activity. Replacing valued employees of long standing with naive, new personnel is expensive and time-consuming. Helping the addict to get rid of his "habit" and return to the workforce can be humanitarian and economical. Little has been presented in this volume on the value of good employee assistance programs. It is to the employers' advantage to encourage employee rehabilitation. If addicts are detected early on, the employee assistance programs can help employees return to gainful and productive activity. The need for early detection is apparent because recidivism is very high for those who revert back to drug use a second or third time. So seize the opportunity, avert the crisis, and insure a better world.

REFERENCES

1. **Westermeyer, J.,** The pursuit of intoxication, *Am. J. Drug. Alcohol Abuse,* 14, 175–187, 1988.
2. **Cowart, V.,** National Concern about drug abuse brings athletes under unusual scrutiny, *JAMA,* 256, 2465–2469, 1986.
3. NIDA Research Monograph #91, National Institute on Drug Abuse, Rockville, MD, 20857.
4. **Morgan, J.,** The relationship between drug test results and job performance indicators, *Am. Psychol. Assoc.,* abstract, 1989.
5. **Boone, J.,** Reliability of Drug Testing, *JAMA,* 258, 2487, 1987.
6. Technical, scientific and procedural issues of employee drug testing. Consensus report, Finke, B., Blanke, R., and Walsh, M., Eds., NIDA Publ. (ADM-1684), U.S. Government Printing Office, Washington, D.C., 1990.
7. *The Bible,* King James Version, Matthew, 5, 37.
8. **Fitzpatrick, D. L., Green, J., and Fowler, M. F.,** Comparison of 6 cannabinoid metabolite assays, *J. Anal. Toxicol.,* 9, 113–120, 1985.

Index

INDEX

A

AACC, see American Association for Clinical Chemistry
ABBOTT DATATRAC™ System, 118
Absentee rate, 268
6-Acetylmorphine, 156
Accreditation of laboratories, 31
Accuracy, improvement of by BCR program, 240
Adduct ion, 138
Adjustable threshold, 117
Administrative procedures, 214
Agriculture, analyses related to, 240
Alarm line, 243
Alleged drug use, 268
American Association of Bioanalysts, 100, 216
American Association for Clinical Chemistry (AACC), 87, 216, 270
7-Aminoflunitrazepam, 185
Amphetamines, 221
Analysts, 257
Analytical method, reliability of, 71
Analytical methodology, discussions on, 145–148
Analytical methods, 12
Analytical methods, overview on immunological and chromatographic, 73–82
  general considerations, 74–76
    extraction, separation, and detection, 74–75
    identification of analyte, 75–76
    standards and controls, 76
  methodologies, 76–81
    enzyme immunoassay, 79
    fluorescence immunoassay, 79–80
  methodologies, gas and liquid chromatography, 77
    immunoassays, 78
    interferences, 80–81
    mass spectrometry, 77–78
    paper chromatography, 77
    radioimmunoassay, 78–79
    thin layer chromatography, 77
Analytical noise, 85
Analytical reliability, 71
Analytical toxicology, forensic vs. clinical aspects of, 269
Antagonist maintenance programs, 201
Anti-inflammatory drugs, 87
Applied metrology, 240
Assay
  class drugs of, 147
  sensitivity of, 79

B

Banned substances, classes of, 227
Barbiturates, 221
Benzodiazepines, 221
Biomedical analyses, 240
Blind programs, 216
Blind samples, 228
Blood samples, collection of, 11
Budget, for running laboratory, 227
Buprenorphine, 200, 209, 223
Bureau Commuaitaire de Reference (BCR) program, possibilities and achievements of, 239–255
  certified reference materials, 249–252
  examples of current projects, 252–253

    biomedical analysis, 252
    environmental analysis, 253
    food and agricultural products, 252–253
    metrology, 253
  improvement of measurement quality, 247–249
  means to improve measurement quality, 241–247
    between laboratory measures, 246–247
    within laboratory measures, 242–246
  possibilities to participate in BCR work, 254–255
    financial support to projects, 254–255
    proposals, 253–254
    selection criteria, 254
  state of the art of chemical analysis, 241

C

Calibration curve, 146
Calibration table, 130
Calibrations, 240
Calibrators, 99, 107
Cannabinoids, 221
CAP, see College of American Pathologists
Centers for Disease Control, 216
Certified reference materials, 249
Chain of custody, 11, 19–25, 32, 214, 269
  handling in laboratory, 22–23
    access to specimens and aliquots during processing, 23
    separate specimen accessioning area, 22–23
    storage of positive specimens, 23
    transfer of aliquots, 23
    transfer of specimens, 23
  major steps in for drug testing, 21
  need for, 20–21
  records, 24–25
    complete, 25
    litigation presentation, 25
    retrievable for review, 24
    secure storage, 24
  reporting, 23–24
    control of data recording, 24
    evidence of review, 24
    transmission security, 24
    validation of accuracy of reports, 24
  sample collection and, 15–18
    cases of drug abuse testing, 16–17
    driving-while-intoxicated cases, 16
    methadone programs, 17
  specimen collection, 21–22
    collecting and shipping container, 22
    custody and control form, 21–22
    label, 22
    packing for shipment, 22
    seals for bottle and box, 22
  transport to laboratory, 22
    secured courier, 22
    shipping log and signed receipt, 22
  what is provided, 21
Chemical ionization (CI), 138
Choice, method of, 140
CI, see Chemical ionization
Clinical chemistry
  analyzer, 104
  use of RIA in, 122

Clinical practice, drug testing in, 199–207
  assessment of patient's compliance with therapeutic regimens, 201–203
    antagonistic maintenance programs, 201–202
    methadone maintenance programs, 202–203
  diagnostic confirmation of acute intoxication and/or dependence, 200
  follow-up of patients enrolled in therapeutic programs, 205
  health care repercussions, 205–207
    false negatives, 206–207
    false positives, 206
    voluntary fraud, 207
  monitoring changes in drug consumption patterns among patients seeking treatment, 201
  monitoring of drug consumption during detoxification treatment, 203–205
  promotion of contact between patients and health workers, 205
  test of reliability of information provided by patient, 200–201
Clinicians, 257
Cocaethylene (ethylcocaine), 185
Cocaine, 184, 221, 230
  base, 210
  interpretation of results, 155
Codeine, 156, 185, 231
  availability of, 125
  biotransformations of, 124
  dependence, 206
Collaborative projects, proposals submitted for, 253
Collection container, 22
College of American Pathologists (CAP), 87, 216, 270
Community directives, 240
Compulsory random testing, 267
Confirmation, standard for, 145
Confirmatory testing, 84
Consequences, of carrying out tests, 257
Control chart, 243
Control form, 21
Control limit, 243
Cost/benefit ratio, 268
Council of Ministers, 259
Cumulative sum charts, 243
Cutoffs, 98

D

Data validation, 71
Department of Defense, 268
Department of Health and Human Services (DHHS), 87, 99
Department of Transportation, 268
Derivative stability, 136, 137
Derivatization, 140
l-Desoxyephedrine (1-methamphetamine), 155
Deuterated internal standards, 78
Dextropropoxyphene, 184
DHHS, see Department of Health and Human Services
Diazepam, 184, 209
Diisopropyl alkylamines, 134
D.O.A., see Drugs of abuse policy
Documentation, 242
Dope agents, 226
Doping control, qualitative analysis in, 134
Drug abuse, metabolism of, 153–157
  cocaine, 155
    case 4, 155
    case 5, 155
  methamphetamine, 154–155
    case 1, 154
    case 2, 155
    case 3, 155
  opiates, 156–157
    case 6, 156
    case 7, 156–157
Drug abuse, prevalence of, 267
Drug influence, 10
Drug testing, legal issues in development of, 62
Drug testing, pharmacokinetic approaches on, 171–181
  absorption process, 174
  concentration profile at observation site, 175
  drug input by inhalation, 174
  drug input profiles, 173
  observing specific drug metabolites, 177–179
  profile of body transport function, 172–173
  urine profile of drug, 175–177
Drug testing process, 147
Drug testing program, implementation of, 267
Drug use, 10
Drug-drug interactions, relevance of pharmacogenetics and, 183–191
  drug interactions, 185–187
  polymorphic metabolizing enzymes involved in metabolism of drugs of abuse, 184–185
    acetyltransferase, 184–185
    debrisoquine hydroxylase, 185
    pseudocholinesterase, 184
    S-mephenytoin hydroxylase, 184
  relevance of pharmacogenetics on drugs of abuse testing, 184
Drugs of abuse (D.O.A.) policy, 90
Drugs of abuse testing, current issues on, 151–152
Du Pont aca® discrete clinical analyzer, drugs of abuse methods for, 103–111
  advantages of automated drug screening on the aca®, 110–111
  background, 104–105
    screening assays, 104
    toxicology testing, 104–105
  drug screening technology on the aca®, 105–106
    EMIT® assay methodology, 105
    principles of instrument operation, 105–106
    results reporting and cutoff values, 106
  limitations of urine drug screening procedures, 110
  performance characteristics of urine cocaine metabolite screening assay, 108–110
    comparison of methods, 109
    interferences, 109–110
    recovery, 108–109
    reproducibility, 108
  quality assurance considerations, 106–108
    calibration, 107
    quality control, 107–108
    specimen collection and storage, 107

E

EEC, 99
EI, see Electron impact
EIA, see Enzyme immunoassay
Electron capture, 138
Electron impact (EI), 138
Emergency drug screening, 110
EMIT® enzyme immunoassays, 97–101
  accuracy and reliability, 100–101
    legal credibility, 101
    NIDA certified laboratories, 100–101
    scientific, 100

applications on chemistry analyzers, 99–100
assay principle, 98–99
assays today, 98
history, 98
menu and cutoff, 98
Employee testing, 268
Endocrinology, use of RIA in, 122
Endogenous compounds, exogenous compounds compared to, 147
Environment, analyses related to, 240
Enzyme immunoassay (EIA), 12, 31, 79
Enzymes, determination of, 240
Epidemiological studies, 267
Errors, appearance of, 214
Eurobarometer survey, 259
Europe, urine drug testing in, 216–217
European drug testing laboratories, 268
European Economic Community, 217, 259
External blind testing, 270
External Quality Assessment, 122, 252
External quality control, 215

F

False negative analyses, 226
False negative results, 74, 206–207, 220
False positive results, 74, 147, 205, 217, 220, 226
Federal guidelines, 132
Federal Workplace Testing Program, 268
Field evaluations, 108
Flexibility, in choice of analyzer, 99
Flexible assay systems, 118
Flunitrazepam, 220
Fluorescein, 114
Fluorescence polarization immunoassay (FPIA), 31
Fluorescence polarization immunoassay (FPIA) systems, overview of systems in abused drug testing, 113–119
  diversity in testing systems, 117–118
    ADx® system, 118
    HTDx® system, 118
    MTDx® system, 118
    TDx® system, 117
  flexibility of methodologies, 116–117
    adjustable threshold, 117
    cross-reactivity, 116–117
    numerical and qualitative results, 116
  methodology, 114–116
  principle, 114
    rotation and polarization, 114
    sensitivity and specificity, 114
Fluorescence polarization, 79
Fluorescent tracer, 114
Food, analyses related to, 240
Food and Drug Administration, 98
Forensic constraints, 55–57
Forensic drug testing, 30–31
Forensic drug testing, future trends in, 59–66
  additional drugs, 63
  analytical laboratory aspects, 61
  analytical methods, 64
  cutoff, 64
  epidemiology of drug abuse in workplace, 60–61
  general recommendations, 63
  HHS-NIDA regulatory program, 61–62
  laboratory inspections and certification, 64
  monitoring laboratory performance, 65–66
  on-site, initial, screening-only testing facilities, 63
  overview on legal issues in development of drug testing at workplace in United States, 62–63
  performance testing, 65
  role of medical review officer, 65
  socio-political overview in United States, 60
  specimen collection, 64–65
Forensic Urine Drug Testing (FUDT), 87, 269
FPIA, see Fluorescence polarization immunoassay
FRAT, 98
FUDT, see Forensic Urine Drug Testing
Full scan mass spectra, 134

G

Gas chromatography, 77
Gas chromatography, liquid chromatography and coupled to mass spectrometry, 129–132
  drug analysis using GC/FT-IRD/MSD, 132
  drug analysis using GC/MS, 130–131
  drug analysis using LC/MS, 131
Gas chromatography/mass spectrometry (GC/MS), 130, 131, 145
Gas chromatography/mass spectrometry (GC/MS), correlative information by in doping analysis, 133–144
  chemical ionization, 138
  derivatization, 136–138
  gas chromatography information, 134–135
  negative chemical ionization (NCI), 138–139
  objective of mass spectrometry, 134
GC/MS, see Gas chromatography/mass spectrometry
Genetic polymorphisms, 184
Germany, drug testing in, 16
GLP, see Good laboratory practices
Good Laboratory Practice (GLP), 16, 214, 242

H

Hair drug testing, 16
Handling of samples, 22
Harmonization, 254, 261–264
Harrison Narcotics Act, 267
Health and Human Services-National Institute in Drug Abuse (HHS-NIDA), 61
Heroin, 156
HHS-NIDA, see Health and Human Services-National Institute in Drug Abuse
High performance liquid chromatography, 77, 122
High-performance sport, 228
Homogeneity, 249
Hormones, determination of, 240
Hospitals, suitability of Du Pont system for, 146
Hydrolysis, 75, 140

I

IDMS, see Isotope dilution mass spectrometry
Illegal growth promoting compounds, 253
Illicit drugs, use of, 259
Immunoassays, cross-reactivity of, 87
Impairment, indication of, 269
Inadvertent exposure, 85
In situ abuse drug detection, 89–96
  applicability of in companies, 96
  critical aspects in drug detection, 95–96
  current state of abuse drug detection, 90–91
  technologies, 93–95
  role of, 91–93

Instrumentation, 252
Intercomparisons, 246
Interferences, 80–81
Internal quality assurance, 214
Internal security, 269
Internal standard (ISTD), 71, 130, 145
International Amateur Athletic Federation (IAAF), 226
IOC accredited laboratory, right to inspect, 228
IOC medical commission, accreditation and reaccreditation of
		laboratories by, 225–237
	accreditation, 227–228
	concept of accreditation of laboratories, 226–227
	development of dope analysis, 226
	implementation, 228
	International Olympic Committee list of doping classes and methods,
		230–232
	medical commission of International Olympic Committee, 229–230,
	reaccreditation and proficiency test, 228
	requirements for accreditation of laboratories, 227–228
		essential equipment, 227
		letter of support, 227
		repertoire, 227
Ion-molecule reaction, 138
ISO guidelines, 247
Isotope dilution, 71
Isotope dilution mass spectrometry (IDMS), 145, 245
ISTD, see Internal standard
IUPAC, 249

J

Job applicants, 257
Job description, 214

L

Laboratories, performance of, 65
Laboratory inspections, 64
Laboratory quality assurance, concepts for, 53–54
Legal aspects, 9–14
	drug influence, 10
	drug use, 10
	evaluation of analytical methods, 12
	forensic toxicology, 11–13
		analytical control program, 12–13
		drug analyses, 12
		information on drug use, 11
		information to individuals, 11
		interpretation of results and reports, 13
		legal background, 11
		procedures at Institute of Forensic Toxicology, 11–12
		selection of biological material, 11
		specimen collection procedure, 11
	quality control procedures, 12
	standards of drug analyses, 12
Legal credibility, 101

M

Mass selective detector (MSD), 132
Mass spectrometry, 77
Mass spectrometry/mass spectrometry coupling, 145
Mass spectrum, 134
Matrix reference material, 245
Measurement quality, 241
Medical review officer (MRO), 64, 65

Metals, analysis of, 240
Methadone, 221
Methadone maintenance programs, 84, 202
Methanol extracts, 145
Methodology, specificity of, 78
Military, organization of laboratory for drug abuse testing in, 37–45
	aircrew, 39–40
		civil aviation, 40
		military aviation, 39–40
	centers participating in testing program, 38
	discussion, 42–45
		concept of passive smoker, 43
		mono-acetylmorphine in urines, 42
		positive reactions in urine tests, 42–43
		transformation of codeine into morphine, 43–45
	drug addiction testing procedure, 41–42
		treatment program, 42
		urine conditioning, 41–42
	drugs tested for, 38–39
	materials and methods, 38
	results on French armed forces, 40–41
		confirmatory results of control examination, 41
		screening test results, 40
	tested population, 39
Monoclonal antibodies, 87, 98, 145
Morphine-6-glucuronide, 122
MRO, see Medical review officer
MSD, see Mass selective detector

N

National Institute of Drug Abuse (NIDA), 87, 106
National Institute of Drug Abuse Guidelines, 216
Natural fluorescence, decay rate of, 80
Negative ions, 138
N-FID, see Nitrogen specific detector
National Institute of Drug Abuse Guidelines, 216
NIDA, see National Institute of Drug Abuse
Nitrogen specific detector (N-FID), 226
Nonspecific binding, 76
Nordiazepam, 184
Norway, drug testing in, 10, 11
Numerical quality control, 116
Numerical results, 116

O

Olympic doping control program, 269
Olympic Games, 228
Open programs, 216
Opiates, 88, 156, 221
Organizational aspects, discussion on for reliable drug testing, 67–68

P

Packing of samples, 22
Particle Beam (PB) LC/MS interface, 131
Passive inhalation, of cannabis smoke, 86
PB, see Particle Beam LC/MS interface
Performance, of laboratory, 246
Pharmacodynamics, 160
Δ-9 Pharmacodynamics, 163
Pharmacokinetics, 160
Δ-9 Pharmacokinetics, 163
Pharmacokinetics, relationship between pharmacodynamics and,
		159–170

nature of relationship, 163–168
  diphenhydramine, 166–168
  marijuana, 163–166
  pharmacodynamics, 162–163
  pharmacokinetics, 160–162
Phencyclidine, 209
Phenylpropanolamine, 220, 231
Polyclonal antibody, 145
Polycyclic aromatic hydrocarbons, 241
Poppy seed foods, 156
Pre-accreditation procedure, 227
Pre-employment testing, 267
Pre-employment urine specimen, 78
Precision, 84
Precolumn concentration, 131
Preliminary assays, 214
Presumptive analysis, 83–88
  comparison of assays, 86
  criteria for selection of cutoff level, 85–86
  essential characteristics of, 84
  precision, 84–85
  sensitivity and threshold, 84
  specificity of preliminary tests, 87–88
  threshold concentrations in common use, 87
Presumptive positive test, 147
Presumptive tests, 84
Proficiency testing (PT), 65
Proficiency Testing Programs (PTPs), 215, 220, 270
Propoxyphene, 221
Protonated molecular ion, 138
PT, see Proficiency testing
PTPs, see Proficiency Testing Programs

Q

QUAL, see Qualitative units
Qualitative analysis, 146
Qualitative (QUAL) units, 106
Qualitative urine screening assays, 105
Quality assessment, 242
Quality assurance, 242
Quality assurance program, 259, 269
Quality control material, 146
Quality control procedures, 12
Quality control programs, 213–218
Quality control programs
  for analysis of drugs of abuse, 1
  development of proficiency testing programs, 216–217
    Europe, 216–217
    United States, 216
  external programs, 215
  future developments, 217
  internal programs, 214–215
Quantitative results, 228
Quinine, 201

R

Radioimmunoassay, 78
Radioimmunoassay, drug measurements and, 121–128
  aspects of method, 122
  differentiating codeine from heroin or morphine use, 124–126
    analysis, 125
    results, 125–126
    samples, 125
  morphine and glucuronide metabolites, 122–124

  pharmacogenetics of codeine demethylation,
Random errors, 241
Random screening, 74
Random urine testing, 257
Ratio C/M, 125
Reaccreditation, 228
Recent abuse, 85
Reference materials, 240
Reference method, 244
Reference standards, 217
Rehabilitation program, 267
Relative retention times, 134
Reliability
  need for, 214
  of tests, 257
Reliable result, 269
Results
  archiving of, 242
  discussion on interpretation of, 209–210
  interpretation and reporting of, 193–197, 242
    analytical interpretation, 194
    future developments, 196
    international standardization, 196–197
    medical interpretation, 196
    negative result, 195
    positive result, 195
    sources of error in testing urine specimens, 195–196
    toxicological interpretation, 194–195
Retention indices, 134
Review committee, 228
Routine screening, 259

S

Sample reception, 214
Samples and results, general considerations of, 5–8
  contamination and interferences, 7
  identification, packaging, conservation, and transport, 7
  type of obtaining sample, 7
  type of sample, 6–7
Samples
  confirmation of, 130
  packing of, 22
Sampling, 242
Screening cutoff values, 61
Selected ion monitoring, 134
Selected ions, recording of, 134
Semiquantitative results, 116, 146
Sensitivity of measurement, 75
Sensitivity, lack of, 217
Shelf-life, of chemistry packs, 146
Single assay, 105
Six point calibration curve, 114
Soft ionization technique, 138
SOPs, see Standard Operating Procedures
Spanish national plan, remarks from, 257
Spanish National Plan on Drugs, 1
Spanish Presidency of the European Communities, 259
Spanish proficiency testing program, 219–224
  definitions, 220
  menu of substance and preparation of samples, 220
  results and discussion, 220–224
Specificity of measurement, 75
Specimen, blood as, 61
Specimen collection, 64
Split sample, 67

Spot tests, 76
Stability, 249
Stability studies, 108
Standard Operating Procedures (SOPs), 214
Storage of samples, 23
Suitable areas, considerations about, 47–51
Systematic errors, 241

T

Testing, sources of error in, 195–196
Δ-9-Tetrahydrocannabinol (THC), 163
TFA, see Trifluoroacetyl derivative
Thin layer chromatography, 77
Threshold, 84
Traceability, 251
Training periods, 217
Transport of samples, 22
Trifluoroacetyl (TFA) derivative, 136
Trimethylsilyl derivative, 136

U

U.S. Federal Guidelines, 106
Unconfirmed positives, 76
United States Post Office, 268
Urinary profile, 175–177
Urine samples
   problems of interpretation in screening, 124
   tampering with, 11

V

Variation, coefficients of, 249

Vicks inhaler, interpretation of results, 155
Vitamin B_2, 201
Voluntary fraud, 207

W

Work, quality of, 248
Work environment, 95–96
Workplace, drug testing at, 1
Workplace, testing at, 259
Workplace, organization of laboratories for drug abuse testing at, 27–35
   abused drugs tested, 32
   clinical drug testing, 28–30
      diagnostic drugs of abuse testing, 30
      emergency toxicology, 28–30
      rehabilitation toxicology, 30
   forensic drug testing, 30–31
      medical-legal testing, 31
      parole testing, 31
      workplace testing, 30–31
   history of drug testing, 28
   history of methodology, 28
   licensing agency policies, 31–32
      clinical testing, 32
      forensic testing, 31
   personnel, 34

X

X SYSTEMS™, 117